D0076471

Barry Stimmel, MD

Pain and Its Relief
Without Addiction
Clinical Issues in the Use
of Opioids and Other Analgesics

Pre-publication
REVIEWS,
COMMENTARIES,
EVALUATIONS . . .

"**B**arry Stimmel makes an important contribution to the crucial medical issue of pain relief. This book is chock full of pharmacological data and information about pain management and addictions."

David C. Lewis, MD
Professor of Medicine
and Community Health
and Director, Center
for Alcohol and Addiction Studies,
Brown University

"**I**f one is in need of a textbook for teaching a survey course about pain and its treatment, *Pain and Its Relief Without Addiction* fulfills this need. In addition, it addresses specific issues about pain treatment neglected in most books about pain, such as myths about addiction and drugs used for pain treatment; the need to aggressively treat pain in children; the elderly; sickle cell disease; and AIDS. This book also provides physicians with a rationale for shedding customary, outmoded practices of inadequate pain relief for modern practices of adequate treatment of pain."

C. Stratton Hill, Jr., MD
Department of Neurooncology,
Pain Management Section,
University of Texas
M.D. Anderson Cancer Center

Pain and Its Relief Without Addiction

Clinical Issues in the Use of Opioids and Other Analgesics

HAWORTH Therapy for the Addictive Disorders
Barry Stimmel, MD
Senior Editor

Pain and Its Relief Without Addiction
Clinical Issues in the Use of Opioids and Other Analgesics

Barry Stimmel, MD

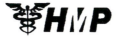

The Haworth Medical Press
An Imprint of The Haworth Press, Inc.
New York • London

Published by

The Haworth Medical Press, Inc., an imprint of The Haworth Press, Inc., 10 Alice Street, Binghamton, NY 13904-1580

DISCLAIMER

Medicine is an ever-changing science. As new research and clinical experience broaden our knowledge, changes in treatment and drug therapy are required. While many suggestions for drug usages are made herein, the book is intended for educational purposes only, and the author, editor, and publisher do not accept liability in the event of negative consequences incurred as a result of information presented in this book. We do not claim that this information is necessarily accurate by the rigid, scientific standard applied for medical proof, and therefore make no warranty, expressed or implied, with respect to the material herein contained. Therefore the patient is urged to consult his or her own physician prior to following a course of treatment. The physician is urged to check the product information sheet included in the package of each drug he or she plans to administer to be certain the protocol followed is not in conflict with the manufacturer's inserts. When a discrepancy arises between these inserts and information in this book, the physician is encouraged to use his or her best professional judgement.

Cover design by Marylouise E. Doyle.

Library of Congress Cataloging-in-Publication Data

Stimmel, Barry, 1939-
    Pain and its relief without addiction : clinical issues in the use of opioids and other analgesics / Barry Stimmel.–2nd ed.
        p.   cm.
    Rev. ed. of: Pain, analgesia, and addiction. © 1983.
    Includes bibliographical references and index.
    ISBN 0-7890-0126-8 (alk. paper)
    1. Analgesics. 2. Opioids. 3. Analgesia. 4. Analgesics–Side effects. 5. Opioids–Side effects. 6. Pain. 7. Medication abuse–Prevention. I. Stimmel, Barry, 1939-   Pain, analgesia, and addiction. II. Title.
    [DNLM: 1. Pain–drug therapy. 2. Analgesics–therapeutic use. 3. Substance Dependence. WL 704 S858p 1996]
RM319.S75 1996
616'.0472–dc20
DNLM/DLC
for Library of Congress   96-8993
                                                                                        CIP

To Matthew and Alexander
and to all those who have needlessly suffered pain

ABOUT THE AUTHOR

Barry Stimmel, MD, is currently Dean for Graduate Medical Education at the Mount Sinai School of Medicine of The City University of New York. He is Professor in the Department of Medicine and in the Department of Medical Education and has served as Dean of Academic Affairs, Admissions, and Student Affairs at the School of Medicine for over twenty years. A practicing internist and cardiologist, Dr. Stimmel is also Executive Director of the Narcotics Rehabilitation Center at the Mount Sinai Medical Center. He is editor of the *Journal of Addictive Diseases* and the author of over 100 articles and several books dealing with drug abuse, the effects of mood-altering drugs on the heart, and pain control. In addition, Dr. Stimmel lectures extensively on issues in medical education, substance abuse, and pain management.

CONTENTS

Preface

More than a decade ago, I observed that despite the persistent attention of scientists and physicians to the origins and treatment of pain, persons in pain still received less than satisfactory relief.[1] Since then I have remained impressed with the prevalence of unrelieved pain. This is not due solely to lack of knowledge or prescription patterns of physicians. Often many other health care providers and, at times, even those in pain, feel that the pain is not "real" but a manifestation of anxiety. Equally important is the concern that taking a narcotic to relieve pain is both morally wrong and medically indefensible. The fear of addiction is pervasive. As a result of these concerns, a person in pain is often overly sedated and unable to function well, or remains in continual discomfort.

These are not just my perceptions. A 1992 publication of the U.S. Department of Health Services noted that current medical practice fails to relieve pain in about half of all postoperative patients, contributing to unnecessary discomfort, longer recovery periods, and compromised patient outcomes.[2] Since prescribing analgesics for acute as compared to chronic pain is always more liberal, one would assume the percentage of those people in chronic pain receiving inadequate care is probably much higher. Indeed a recent poll by Louis Harris and Associates found 60 percent of persons in pain reluctant to take analgesics despite more than one-third of those in moderate pain being unable to work or perform routine activities for one of every three days of the year.

Over the years I have become increasingly convinced that the education of physicians who prescribe these drugs is a minimum, but not a sufficient requirement for relieving pain. Indeed, not infrequently, when orders are appropriately written, they are not effectively carried out. As the public becomes more informed and concerned about participating in their medical care, the ability to understand the causes of pain, as well as the best way to provide effective relief, become increasingly important.

This second edition is therefore directed not only toward physicians and other health care personnel, but toward an informed public as well. Although it belabors the obvious to observe that addressing a book to three distinct populations is far from an easy task, I have attempted to provide all with sufficient information to allow an individualized approach to pharmacologic care of a person in pain.

Each chapter is able to "stand alone" and need not be read in sequence. The first section reviews the anatomical, physiological, and psychological aspects of pain, as well as the basic concepts of drug dependence, tolerance, and withdrawal. The second section discusses the pharmacological actions and side effects of individual drugs used to provide or to enhance analgesia. The final section, which has been considerably expanded, discusses the general principles to be followed in pain management, as well as ways of treating pain in different populations.

Exceptionally detailed information is omitted, as ample references are supplied at the end of each chapter. These references have been updated and many of the older references have been deleted. A number of the older references have been retained, as it is felt they provide the best resource for those interested in obtaining more detailed information. Nonetheless, for some, the information provided may appear excessive. However, the text is liberally divided by subheadings to allow for rapid information retrieval regardless of one's background. All should be able to understand the introductory sections of each chapter, the basic concepts concerning dependence, and those chapters addressing pain management.

I should emphasize that only the treatment of pain with drugs is addressed. This is not to imply that nonpharmacologic methods of pain relief are ineffective. Indeed, depending on the setting, these techniques may provide more effective pain control. In addition, using some of these methods combined with analgesics may lessen the dose of an analgesic required to provide relief. The focus of this book, however, is to provide those who care for persons in pain, as well as those experiencing pain, with a working knowledge of what can be done to obtain relief if pharmacological intervention is warranted. At times pain may be impossible to avoid. However, it need never be tolerated unquestioningly.

NOTES

1. Stimmel B. *Pain, analgesia, and addiction: The pharmacologic treatment of pain.* New York: Raven Press, 1983.

2. U.S. Agency for Health Care Policy and Research. *Acute pain management: Operative of medical procedures and trauma.* Rockville, MD: U.S. Department of Health and Human Services, 1992.

Acknowledgments

A book such as this, of necessity, draws heavily on the experience of others, many of whom have devoted a major part of their professional lives to the field of pain. To some, such as Drs. Bonica, Sternbach, and Chapman, I continue to owe a particular unspoken word of thanks. To the many others equally committed, I have attempted to appropriately reference each chapter so that readers may return to both original and secondary sources if more information on a specific subject is desired. Equally important are the acknowledgments that must be given to those persons in pain whom I have been privileged to have under my care. Their feelings, concerns, and anxieties helped to form the last section of this book and provided me with a better understanding of the needs of those in pain.

On a more concrete level, I am grateful to Ms. Mary Kennedy, who has worked with me to produce yet another text, and to my editor, Ms. Peg Marr, for being exceptionally patient in receiving this manuscript as well as persistent in the thankless task of attempting to decipher my handwritten comments.

SECTION I:
PHYSIOLOGICAL CONCEPTS
OF PAIN AND DEPENDENCE

Chapter 1

The Anatomy of Pain

INTRODUCTION

The enigma surrounding pain dates back to antiquity. The most ancient interpretation ascribes pain as a punishment for offending the gods. Indeed, the word derives from the latin *poena*, meaning penalty or punishment.[1] However, although pain has been a source of concern to humans, the objective systematic study of pain was first undertaken by Aristotle. Aristotelian theory attributed pain to excessive stimuli arising from the skin and conveyed by the blood to the heart where pain is experienced. Pain was considered a feeling rather than a sensation and classified as a "passion of the soul," originating within one's heart.

Descartes was one of the first to dissent from the Aristotelian concept, postulating that pain originated from vibrations in the skin due to a noxious stimulus, which in turn activated a "delicate thread . . . attached to the spot of the skin," ultimately traveling to the brain, with pathways to the pineal gland.[2] Although other contemporary scientists, such as Galen and Vesalius, also attributed the sensation of pain to the brain, Aristotle's concept prevailed for almost two millennia.

Perhaps the major impetus to the modern investigation of anatomical properties of pain began in the latter part of the nineteenth century with the work of Mueller and Von Frey.[3] In 1840, Mueller hypothesized that the quality of a sensation depends on the properties of the neuroreceptor that is stimulated as well as the area of the brain in which the nerve terminates. Sensory pathways were felt to be the only means by which the brain received information about external objects, with each of the senses carrying a particular form of energy specifically for each sensation. In 1890, Von Frey postulated reception of pain to be due to the presence of receptors in recently discovered free nerve endings. Several years later, in 1894, Goldscheider described the critical determinants of pain as the central summation of repetitive sensory inputs.

THEORIES OF PAIN PERCEPTION

Specificity Theory

For the first half of the twentieth century, there were three major hypotheses advanced for explaining pain perception. The specificity theory proposed that free nerve endings, termed *nociceptors*, activated by mechanical deformation, chemical stimuli, or extremes in temperature, generated pain impulses carried by A-delta and C-fibers in peripheral nerves to the spinal cord. These fibers synapse and ascend in the ipsilateral Lissauer's tract for several levels before crossing to the lateral spinothalamic tract, and ascending to the thalamus. Within the thalamus, another synapse would occur with the fibers finally terminating in the cerebral cortex and the sensation of pain.[4]

Pattern Theory

The pattern theory described pain as a sensation resulting from spatiotemporal patterns of nerve impulses originating from nonspecific receptors rather than an individual stimulus-response phenomenon. The stimulus entering the cord through the dorsal root ganglia effects an activation of the "T cell" in the dorsal horn, which, in turn, transmits an impulse to the brainstem and the cerebral cortex. The T cell can be modulated by the brainstem. A variation of this theory proposed by Livingston[5] attributed the presence of noxious stimuli to initiation of reverberating circuits of differing velocities that affected synaptic transmission. The actual transmission of pain was processed through the more slowly conducting system. The existence of a fast and a slow system corresponded to a later description of myelinated and unmyelinated nerve fibers. The rapidly conducting system would have the ability to modify the input pattern transmitted in more slowly conducting multisynaptic fibers.

The pattern theory of pain, with input control and central summation, enabled the development of the duality concept of pain consisting of perception and reaction.[6] Perception, similar to other sensations, was considered a neurophysiological process affected by specific neuroreceptive and conductive mechanisms. Reaction was described as a complex physiological process influenced by multiple psychological factors, such as past experience and culture.

Both the specificity and the pattern theories, however, contained serious deficiencies. Specificity, allowing only for a 1:1 relationship between stimulus and pathway, was unable to explain pain in the absence of a specific input, such as causalgia or phantom limb pain. Furthermore, in both of these painful conditions, sectioning of appropriate peripheral nerves is often ineffective in relief of pain, whereas injection of local anesthetics in peripheral nerves may produce analgesia long after the effect of the drug has worn off. Although the pattern theory attributes initiation and perpetuation of pain patterns to the activity of brainstem or spinal cord nuclei, neuroanatomical evidence of these centers, however, is lacking.

Gate Control Theory

In an attempt to combine what was perceived as valid observations of both the specificity and the pattern theories that were concordant with existing neuroanatomical pathways, Melzack and Wall,[4] in 1965, described the gate control concept of pain. In brief, pain due to noxious stimuli transmitted through peripheral fibers was subject to the interplay between three spinal cord systems, which in turn could be modified centrally.

Peripheral fibers consisted of two parallel networks composed of either small fibers (facilitators) or large fibers (inhibitors). Certain small diameter fibers responded only to injury, whereas others would increase their discharge frequency with the intensity of the noxious stimulus. Cells of the substantia gelatinosa in the dorsal horn of the spinal cord, or cells in the nucleus of cranial nerve V, act as a gate to incoming stimuli, appropriately modifying these impulses prior to transmission to T cells in the dorsal horn. T-cell activation of neural mechanisms comprises the action system responsible for perception of and response to pain. This process is further influenced by fibers projecting through dorsal columns to the brain and descending control systems.

Firing of large fibers ultimately results in an inhibitory effect on substantia gelatinosa cells and a prevention of T-cell firing. Small fiber input can overcome this inhibition resulting in prolonged firing of T cells, which may become of increasing duration with each succeeding small fiber volley. The net result between the interplay of those two fiber systems, centrally modulated by descending control systems and peripherally modulated through ascending systems, comprises the physiologic basis for pain transmission.

Since Melzack's and Wall's initial description, an impressive volume of research has accumulated, making it clear that pain is a much more complex phenomenon that cannot be explained by any single system hypothesis. It is now believed that pain is carried through the central nervous system by several parallel pathways.

Discrete lesions of any single tract may not completely abolish the sensation. Interacting with these pathways are other central nervous system structures, which can greatly modify the transmission and perception of noxious stimuli.

CURRENT TAXONOMY

Modern explanations of pain must incorporate known neuroanatomical, physiological, biochemical, and psychological mechanisms in order to provide an understanding of the process by which pain is received and acted on. In the following sections, current knowledge with respect to neuroanatomical pathways concerned with perception of and reactions to pain will be reviewed. Prior to reviewing the neuroanatomical pathways believed to be associated with pain, it is helpful for those unfamiliar with this terrain to briefly and simply discuss the terms used to describe pain, as well as the relationship of the basic anatomical units involved in the awareness of pain. Those who have no interest in a more detailed description of anatomical pathways will be best served by moving to the chapter summary.

A common taxonomy to describe pain and pain syndromes developed by the International Association for the Study of Pain,[7] allows for a more precise description of phenomena surrounding pain while recognizing the importance of modifying factors (Table 1.1). Although pain may be described in a single sentence, its subjectivity as well as the importance of emotional or environmental factors is acknowledged. Pain is thus separated from the initiating noxious event, being able to exist even in the absence of proximate physical cause. Pain in the absence of tissue damage or obvious pathophysiological derangement is considered psychogenic (Chapter 4). It is extremely difficult, however, to distinguish the subjective experience of organically based pain from psychogenic pain. Psychogenic pain must, therefore, be accepted as a real experience and managed accordingly.

It belabors the obvious to observe that the coordination of the central nervous system by the brain rivals the most complex computer networks. The basic unit of this system is the nerve cell or neuron that consists of a nucleus within the cell body, dendrites that receive information from other neurons, and an axon that transmits information to other dendrites of nerve cells. Axons communicate to dendrites through spaces termed synapses (Figure 1.1). In general, chemical messages are received by the dendrites for the axons through neurotransmitters (Chapter 2), which are then converted into electrical impulses by ions of sodium potassium, chloride, and calcium, which move through the cell and its membrane to the axon and are then transmitted to other axons or nerve fibers.

Neurons, both sensory and motor, exist in many organs, as well as the central nervous system. Sensory neurons transmit signals to neurons in the

TABLE 1.1. Pain Terminology

Term	Definition
Pain	An unpleasant sensory and emotional experience associated with actual or potential tissue damage, or described in terms of such damage.
Allodynia	Pain due to a nonnoxious stimulus to normal skin.
Analgesia	Absence of pain on noxious stimulation.
Anaesthesia dolorosa	Pain in an area or region that is anaesthetic.
Causalgia	A syndrome of sustained burning pain after a traumatic nerve lesion combined with vasomotor and sudomotor dysfunction and later trophic changes.
Central pain	Pain associated with a lesion of the central nervous system.
Deafferentation	Loss of sensory input seen frequently in pain of central origin.
Dysaesthesia	An unpleasant normal sensation comparable to pain.
Hyperalgesia	Increased sensitivity to noxious stimulation.
Hyperaesthesia	Increased sensitivity to stimulation, excluding special senses.
Hyperpathia	A painful syndrome characterized by delay, overreaction, and aftersensation to a stimulus, especially a repetitive stimulus.
Hypoalgesia	Diminished sensitivity to noxious stimulation.

TABLE 1.1 (continued)

Hypoesthesia	Decreased sensitivity to stimulation, excluding special senses.
Neuralgia	Pain in the distribution of a nerve or nerves.
Neuritis	Inflammation of a nerve or nerves.
Neuropathy	A disturbance of function or pathological change in a nerve; in one nerve, mononeuropathy; in several nerves, mononeuropathy multiplex; symmetrical and bilateral, polyneuropathy.
Nociceptor	Receptors that respond selectively to noxious or painful stimuli.
Pain threshold	The least stimulus intensity at which a subject perceives pain.
Pain tolerance level	The greatest stimulus intensity causing pain that a subject is prepared to tolerate.
Paraesthesias	Sensations of pins and needles; numbness, tingling.
Referred pain	Pain experienced at a site distal from where the actual stimuli has occurred.
Trigger point	A discrete area usually located in muscle tissue which, when stimulated, results in pain.

FIGURE 1.1. The Neuron

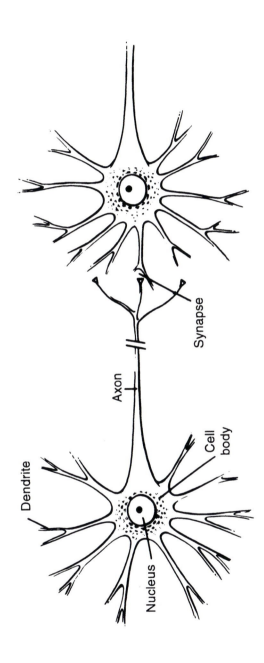

spinal cord which, in turn, can send messages out of the cord to muscles through motor neurons, or can travel through the cord to the brain to generate feelings or to modulate the impulses transmitted at the level of the spinal cord. Cells in the medulla, pons, thalamus, hypothalamus, and cortex (Figure 1.2) all have roles to play in the receiving and modifying of painful stimuli (Table 1.2).

It should be emphasized that the discussion below refers mainly to information obtained from animal models. Although it is certainly true that humans and other mammals do not share identical nervous systems, the information derived from these models has traditionally been found useful to the basic understanding of human neuroanatomical pathways. Subsequent chapters will address the role of neurotransmitters in the response to pain as well as the influence that emotions may have in modifying both the perception of and the reaction to this response.

PERIPHERAL NEURONAL SYSTEMS

Peripheral Nerve Fibers

The peripheral nervous system is composed of afferent neurons of both spinal and cranial nerves. Each neuronal cell body—located in spinal (dorsal root) or cranial ganglions—gives rise to a peripheral process that terminates distally in a receptor located in the body tissue, and to a central process that terminates in the central nervous system by synapsing with a second-order neuron.

Nerve fibers consist of A, B, or C fibers. The large myelinated A fibers are divided into α, β, $\aleph$, and δ fibers. The smaller thinly myelinated A-delta fibers carry noxious stimuli. B fibers are also myelinated but are not involved in transmission of painful stimuli. C fibers are nonmyelinated and slow conducting (Table 1.3). The fast conducting, large myelinated fibers innervate the sensitive mechanoreceptors and serve the functions of sensation (proprioception, touch, pressure) and reflex activity fibers; however, one-quarter of these fibers respond only to very strong mechanical stimuli that may damage tissues. These A-delta units supply the visceral muscle and other deep structures, as well as the skin and subcutaneous tissue.

Sensations induced by their firing are described as tapping or throbbing with stronger stimulation eliciting a "pricking" sensation. Approximately half of the unmyelinated C-fibers supply mechanoreceptors, with a few being sensitive to innocuous thermal stimulation. Approximately 25 percent of the remaining C-fibers are mechanical nociceptors and thermal

FIGURE 1.2. Components of the Human Brain
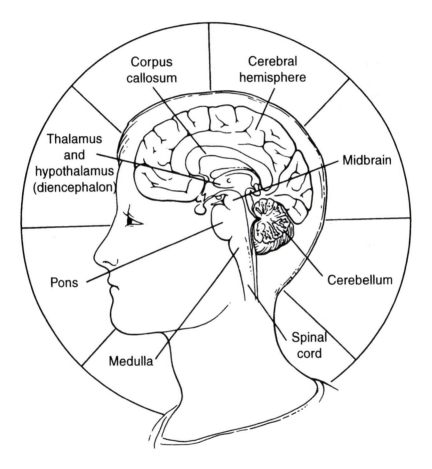

TABLE 1.2. Major Divisions of the Central Nervous System

	Basic functions
Spinal cord	• Motor and sympathetic reflexes • Afferent pathways
Brainstem	• Control of circulation and respiration • Activation by reticular system
Hypothalamus	• Homeostasis • Control of Neuroendocrine function
Basic ganglia, cerebellum	• Motor programming
Limbic system	• Affective-motivational components of behavior
Neocortex	• Cognitive components of behavior

TABLE 1.3. Classification of Nerve Fibers

	Size (micra)	Myelin-ation	Conduction (meters/sec)	Receptors
A- α (I) A- β(II)	Large (6-17)	Heavy	15-80	Mechanoreceptors
A-δ	Small (1-5)	Thin	10-25	Mechanoreceptors = 75% Thermoreceptors Nociceptors = 25%
C	Small (0.3-1)	None	0.4-1	Mechanoreceptors = 50% Nociceptors = 25%

nociceptors. Some may be polymodal, responding to both noxious heat and noxious mechanical distortion.[3] Both A-δ and C-fibers are essential for pain sensation.

Electrical stimulation of the two afferent fiber types transmitting pain reveals the A-δ fibers to evoke sharp pricking or fast pain, whereas the nonmyelinated C-fibers evoke a prolonged, dull, or burning sensation often termed slow pain. Repetitive C-fiber stimulation results in input summation and an increase in pain intensity. Deep or visceral pain is experienced with stimulation of visceral receptors and is transmitted through both A-δ and C-fibers.

Nociceptors

At present, considerable numbers of nociceptors have been identified. In addition, other receptors, such as mechanoreceptors and thermoreceptors, have also been isolated. Nociceptors have a high threshold to specific stimuli with relatively small receptor fields (Table 1.4). Their afferents are the small A-δ fibers and C-fibers. Nociceptors can be activated by strong mechanical stimulation (mechanical nociceptors), extremes in temperature (thermal nociceptors), chemical substances released in response to injury (chemonociceptors), and ischemia. Many nociceptors are polymodal, responding to several types of stimuli.

Nociceptors are found in visceral sites as well as in more superficial areas. The structure and functioning of visceral nociceptors are far less defined than those located superficially. It is not infrequently difficult to differentiate between visceral nociceptors and other visceral receptors. In addition, visceral neuronal pathways exist that evoke regulatory reflexes but elicit no sensory experience. It has been suggested that visceral receptors may be multimodal, serving either painful or other stimuli, depending on the frequency of discharge.[8]

Although most types of receptors become less responsive when subjected to repetitive stimulation, nociceptors do not exhibit this phenomenon. Following burns or other types of trauma, pain sensation persists. Indeed, repetitive noxious stimuli may sensitize the nociceptor, lowering its firing threshold such that subsequent innocuous stimuli cause activation and associated pain and hyperalgesia.[9] Although the reason for this is unknown,

TABLE 1.4. Characteristics of Nociceptors

High thresholds to mechanical or thermal stimuli
Small receptor fields
Repetitive noxious stimuli associated with a lowering of firing threshold
Persistent after discharges for suprathreshold stimuli

it is hypothesized that the tissue damage may simultaneously destroy a degrading enzyme, resulting in a prolonged depolarization of the transducer membrane with persistent firing in the pain fibers (Chapter 2).

The process by which painful stimuli are detected by nociceptors transmitted through afferent fibers and subsequently modified by the central nervous system is quite complex. Each pathway or region in the brain and spinal cord is influenced by interacting afferent impulses as well as descending control mechanisms. It is more than likely that no one structure is exclusively concerned with processing of painful stimuli from peripheral nerves on as 1:1 basis. Similarly, many of the divisions of the brain not usually concerned with pain perception may, under certain conditions, exert a modifying influence. The behavioral response to a painful stimulus will, therefore, be dependent on an interaction between parts of all of the major divisions of the central nervous system.

CENTRAL MECHANISMS

Although for decades the neuroanatomical pathways comprising the central nervous system transmission of nociception and pain have been described in considerable detail, controversy prevails over the role played by specific tracts. In contrast to the presence of a specific cortical sensory center for pain, current consensus holds that peripheral information concerning a noxious stimulus is transmitted through many central nervous system pathways to many parts of the brain. The complexity of the central nervous system, combined with the frequent disagreement as to the degree of participation of specific pathways in transmission of nociceptive information, make it quite difficult for the clinician to develop anatomical-clinical correlates of nociception and pain.

In the following discussion, an attempt is made to present a simplified concept of the central nervous system mechanisms involved in nociception and pain, fully recognizing that existing controversies will prevent this explanation in its totality from being completely acceptable to all investigators in this field.

Spinal Cord

The primary afferent spinal nerve fibers terminate within the dorsal horn of the spinal cord, with the subsequent transmission of impulses modified not only at the first synapse within the dorsal horn but also at multiple levels of the neuraxis. This sensory information transmitted through ascending systems to the thalamus and ultimately the cortex is affected by local, segmental, and supra-segmental factors. The information that finally reaches the cortex has thus been modified considerably since its entry into the dorsal horn cells.[10]

Structure

Rexed[11] has demonstrated that the dorsal horn of the spinal cord is a highly complex structure composed of a series of laminae that derive input from the periphery in accordance to fiber size. Six laminae are believed to receive nociceptive information (Figure 1.3). Immediately prior to entering the spinal cord, the large and small fibers in the dorsal roots become spatially organized so that the large myelinated fibers comprise the medial division and the small myelinated (A-δ) and unmyelinated (C) fibers form the lateral division. The A-δ fibers directly enter the Tract of Lissauer (fasciculus dorsolateralis) for one to two segments before penetrating the gray matter of the dorsal horn terminating in lamina I (marginal in the outer layer of lamina II and in lamina V.[12] The C-fibers end in lamina II. The Tract of Lissauer, however, extends the entire length of the spinal cord, merging with the trigeminal tract. Marginal neurons also receive input from fine primary afferents that end directly on dendrites, as well as from supraspinal sources that terminate on both dendrites and soma.

The cells in laminae II and III consist mainly of small inhibitory interneurons that send axons to the Tract of Lissauer, and a small number of large neurons that project to the ipsilateral and contralateral spinothalamic tracts. The termination of the large myelinated fibers in lamina II occurs through multiple small synapses. Laminae IV through VI (nucleus proprius or magnocellulars) contain the largest cells of the dorsal horn as well as a mixture of medium and small cells.

The large myelinated fibers (A-α and A-β) travel along the medial surface of the spinal cord, enter the gray matter deep in layers N and V, making synaptic contacts with laminae cells prior to terminating in the substantia gelatinosa. The axons of the large cells project into the substantia gelatinosa as well as to higher levels. Many of the cells in these three layers respond to nociceptive inputs. Those cells in lamina V that respond to such impulses in visceral fibers also receive nonnoxious input from other fibers. This may provide the basis for referred pain that can often be seen with visceral disorders. Cells in lamina V also may send ipsilateral and contralateral axons to the neurons comprising the spinothalamic tract. Cells in lamina VI receive contacts from other dorsal horn cells and dorsal root afferents that supply both superficial and deep structures.

FIGURE 1.3. Architecture of Dorsal Roots and Spinal Cord

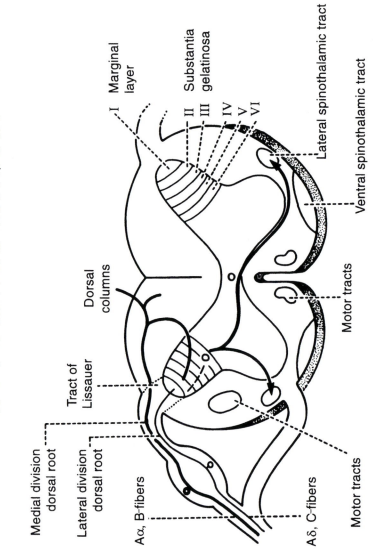

Transmission and Modulation of Pain

Functionally, it is felt that the A-δ and C-fibers terminating in the marginal zone as well as in lamina V through connections in the substantial gelatinosa are responsible for the excitatory synapse in the transmission of painful stimuli.[13] The substantia gelatinosa neurons interact in an inhibitory fashion with the marginal cells, forming a "feed forward" inhibitory circuit. The large myelinated fibers terminate in excitatory synapses of neurons in laminae II through VI. Since these fibers do not primarily carry nociceptive stimuli, it is felt that repetitive action in neurons in these laminae would result in increased inhibitory action on the marginal cells, allowing for a modulation in pain threshold.

Clinically, the inhibitory or modulating effect on pain of the high frequency, large myelinated fibers can be seen under a number of conditions. The ability of a counter-irritant to reduce pain is hypothesized to be secondary to the high frequency discharge initiated by thermal receptors reducing the transmission of small fiber impulses.[14] Similarly, pain following a cut on a finger can often be reduced by local pressure to nearby structures, increasing activity in large fibers serving to modulate the pain threshold.

The spinal cord, therefore, serves as far more than a relay station in transmission of nociceptive impulses. All sensory input is subjected to complex integrative and modulative processes with numerous synaptic events occurring prior to entry of the impulse into the ascending pathways.

Visceral nociceptive afferents may transmit stimuli through several pathways. Those of the thoracic and abdominal organs run through sympathetic pathways, cardiac nerves, and splanchnic nerves. Afferents from the genitourinary tract and reproductive system reach the central nervous system through the parasympathetic nerves of the pelvis. Branches of the thoracic and lumbar spinal nerves innervate the parietal pleura and the pericardium.[15,16] Due to the large number of superficial, as compared to deep afferent pathways, at times visceral pain may be "referred" to the slow or other superficial structures. Similarly, once an impulse from an organ is transmitted to the spinal cord, if proximate to other neurons, the pain may be perceived as originating from a different organ. An example would be esophageal or diaphragmatic pain being perceived by a person as coming from the heart.

Trigeminal System

Sensory input from the head is transmitted through sensory fibers in cranial nerves V, VII, IX, and X, which project to a brainstem trigeminal nuclear complex extending from the pons to the upper cervical segments of the spinal cord.[14] At this point of association with the sensory nucleus of the trigeminal nerve, a synapse occurs with second-order neurons. The central trigeminal nociceptor neurons comprise a complex structural organization, with their axons crossing both ipsilaterally and contralaterally to terminate in the medial and intralaminar thalamic nuclei.

Ascending Pain Pathways

There are four major ascending pathways involved in varying degrees in the transmission of nociceptive stimuli (Table 1.5). The Tract of Lissauer is believed to be concerned mainly with nociception.[16] As discussed above, this tract contains primary afferent fibers from the lateral division of the dorsal root (A-δ and C) as well as axons from the substantia gelatinosa neurons.

In humans, the lemniscal system, composed of dorsal columns consisting of large myelinated nerve fibers responsible for transmitting touch and proprioception, is felt to play an important modulating role. The rapid transmission of large fiber impulses to the brain allows an identification and subsequent modulation of response to noxious stimuli before impulses traveling

TABLE 1.5. Ascending Systems Transmitting Nociceptive (Painful) Stimuli

Tract of Lissauer	Relay nociceptive information A-delta and C-fibers
Lemniscal system	Inhibits dorsal horn transmission/triggers activity brain systems involved in analysis of input of other ascending pathways
Spinothalamic system Lateral spinothalamic	Spatial and temporal discriminative aspects of pain and touch
Ventral spinothalamic	Suprasegmental reflex responses of nondiscriminating aspects of pain
Spinoreticular multisynaptic system	Relays nociceptive information through reticular core and spinoreticulothalamic pathway
Dorsolateral fasciculus proprius	Supplementary route for nociception
Dorsal intracornu tract	Supplementary route for nociception
Spinocervical tract	Supplementary route for nociception

through A-δ and C-fibers reach dorsal horn. An increase in fiber activity inhibits dorsal horn transmission. The system may also function as a pathway that triggers the activity of brain systems involved in spatial and temporal analysis of input reaching the brain through other ascending pathways.[17]

The spinothalamic tracts (Figure 1.4), however, represent the main pathways for conveying pain impulses to the brain.[18] These neurons reside in laminae I and V of the dorsal horn. Although the majority of the neurons project to the contralateral side, ipsilateral connections also exist.

Lateral spinothalamic tract (neospinothalamic) fibers project to and synapse in the ventrolateral and posterolateral thalamic nuclei. These thalamic nuclei project fibers to the primary somatosensory cortex. Along its course, connections are also made with the reticular nuclei of the medulla and pons and cells of the periaqueductal gray area. The spinothalamic fibers, which run in close association with those of the medial lemniscus, have been considered responsible for spatial and temporal discriminative aspects of pain and touch sensation.[19]

The ventral spinothalamic tract (paleospinothalamic) is the older of the two divisions and is composed mainly of short fibers that project to the reticular formation of the medial spinal cord, the lateral pons, the midbrain, and ultimately, to the medial intralaminar thalamic nuclei. Rather than providing discrete or detailed somatotopic discrimination, the ventral spinothalamic tract is believed to participate in suprasegmental reflex responses concerned with aversive motivation and other nondiscriminative aspects of pain that are felt to be necessary to initiate a generalized response.[20]

The observation of persistent pain following mesencephalic tractotomies has led to the hypothesis of a spinoreticulothalamic pathway. This tract is believed to be responsible for transmission of diffuse slow pain as compared to the fast conducting system of the spinothalamic pathways. Other afferent systems that may participate in transmission of nociceptor signals have been summarized by Bonica.[3] The precise role played by these systems, however, remains to be clarified.

Reticular Formation

As discussed above, the reticular formation in the medulla and the pons is a major recipient of input from both of the ventral lateral tracts of the spinal cord as well as the trigeminal nucleus caudalis. Although nearly all bulboreticular neurons show a wide range of responsiveness, a number of cells respond only to noxious stimulation. The nucleus reticularis gigantocellularis is considered to be a relay nucleus for pain in the spinoreticulothalamic system, being activated by noxious somatic stimuli and A-δ fiber input. Conclusive documentation does not yet exist concerning the

FIGURE 1.4. Afferent and Efferent Systems Involved with Nociception and Pain

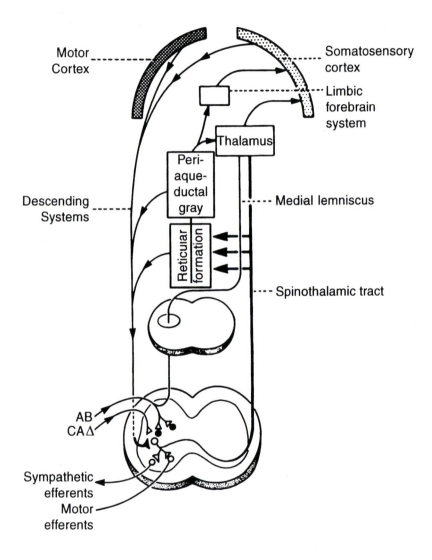

Key: A, alpha fibers; B, beta fibers; AΔ, delta fibers; C, C fibers. *Open triangles*, excitatory synapses; *black triangles*, inhibitory synapses.

importance of these pathways in the conscious awareness of reflex response to pain. The connection of the reticular system with the hyperthalamus and the limbic system, however, suggests that these connections may impact on motivational and affective states associated with human pain.[20]

The bulbar reticular neurons project to: the mesencephalic reticular formation; the medial and intralaminar nuclei of the thalamus and to the periaqueductal central gray matter. They run in the dorsal longitudinal fasciculus to the dorsal and posterior hypothalamus and the midline and intralaminar groups of the thalamus to reach the mesencephalic reticular formation. These pathways may be quite important with respect to function of descending control systems, which will be discussed in subsequent sections. The neurons of the mesencephalic reticular system are also believed to participate in pain mechanisms responding to noxious stimuli in laboratory animals, but their role in humans remains unclear.[21]

Thalamus

The thalamus may be considered to be divided into a ventral nuclear complex, a posterior nuclear complex, and medial and intralaminar thalamic nuclei (Figure 1.3). The fibers of the medial lemniscus also terminate in the posterior nuclear complex, as do fibers from the ventral lateral quadrant of the spinal cord and parts of the lateral spinothalamic tract. This region is considered to be part of a specific pain pathway involved in discriminative pain sensation, with cells responding to nonnoxious as well as noxious stimuli.

Sensory information from the ventral spinothalamic tract terminates either directly into the medial thalamic nuclei or indirectly through the bulbar reticular formation (Figure 1.4). The cells respond to both noxious and nonnoxious stimuli without any specific somatotopic organization. Lesions in the medial and intralaminar system are effective in relieving intractable pain while preserving somatosensory discrimination, suggesting that these areas are involved primarily in nondiscriminative aspects of pain.[20]

Cortex

Available evidence suggests that the primary area for receiving somatosensory information in the brain is not essential for recognition of pain.[10] This area, however, probably does play a role in modulating cognitive and noncognitive features of pain. It can be hypothesized that the receipt of this information allows the organism to evaluate the sensation through associations based on prior experiences.[3]

The thalamic neurons concerned with nociceptive information project to the retroinsular cortex as well as the striatum. Neocortical processes are felt to impact on sensory, affective, and motivational dimensions of pain through providing a capability of evaluating peripheral sensations.

Descending Control Systems

Although neuroanatomical correlates concerning transmission of painful stimuli to the brain have been well developed over the past two decades, more recent work has clearly established that the brain possesses a highly organized descending system for control of pain transmission. Tracts formerly considered to be exclusively motor pathways are now known to influence ascending transmission in all sensory systems. Subcortical structures with ascending fibers to the cortex receive descending cortical fibers (corticospinal, corticoreticular) that modulate transmission in subcortical areas, including the thalamus, reticular formation, and trigeminal system. Descending anatomical pathways have also been described in the (a) ventrolateral periaqueductal gray (PAG) matter through the nuclei of the raphe, the gigantocellularis, and the locus ceruleus, and (b) in the reticular formation in the medulla to the spinal cord through the dorsolateral funiculus, ultimately modulating neurotransmission in the substantia gelatinosa of the dorsal horn.[22]

The descending control system, therefore, influences synaptic transmission of sensory fibers at the dorsal horn level of the spinal cord as well as modulating ascending transmission at every level of the neuraxis. The functional integrity of the system is dependent on the release of biogenic amines as well as other neurotransmitters and neuromodulators. The interplay that these systems have with respect to neurophysiologic response to pain will be discussed in detail in Chapter 2.

Nociceptive Pain

Nociceptive pain is caused by stimulation of nociceptors, with transmission along the Alpha, delta (pricking or sticking pain), and the C- (burning or stringing pain) fibers, through spinothalamic tracts in the spinal cord. By alleviating the cause of this stimulation, by interrupting the anatomical pathways, or by the use of analgesics, the pain will be relieved. Permanent relief will only be obtained, however, through the first two methods.

Central Pain

Central pain is due to a loss of sensory input to or deafferentation in the central nervous system (Table 1.6). This may be due to diseases of the peripheral nerves or roots, the spinal cord, or the brain, most prominently the thalamus or cortex (Table 1.7). In central pain, it is often difficult to tangibly relate the immediate cause with the onset of discomfort. Indeed, characteristically there is a delay between the event and the onset of pain. This is best illustrated by phantom limb pain, pain occurring after the spinal cord has been sectioned or cell sensory input to the cord destroyed through injury, resulting in a loss of an extremity. Pain is perceived and localized to areas previously saved by the afferent nerve fibers.[23,24]

The feeling that is experienced may not be pain, as much as a drawing, burning, tingling, or numbing sensation. Central pain is most often chronic and may be accompanied by symptoms of depression, anxiety, or other psychiatric states. It is essential in addressing central pain that one not assume the discomfort is primarily related to the psychologic manifestations, rather than existing in its own right.

Despite our knowledge of the anatomy, physiology, and biochemistry of pain, most often it is the subjective complaints of a person that dominate. Our ability to define precise anatomic lesions is limited and our capability to relate the intensity of the pain experienced to the origin of the pain at times may be almost nonexistent. The interplay between emotion and pain remains complex. It is therefore essential to always remember that the experience of the pain must be addressed as actively as its cause. The reality of the discomfort cannot be dismissed if relief is to be provided. These concepts will be discussed in greater detail in subsequent chapters.

SUMMARY

In summary, despite the complexities that exist in clearly defining the neuroanatomical pathways conveying painful impulses, as well as the modulating influences exerted by the central nervous system, anatomically, pain can basically be classified as nociceptive or somatic pain and central or deafferentation. Noxious stimuli through activation of nerve endings in the skin send signals through the unmyelinated C fibers and small A fibers to the segmental dorsal root ganglia and then upward (proximally) to the dorsal horn of the spinal cord where they form synapses with second order neurons. These neurons in turn are subject to inhibitory signals from the brain, which are affected by neurotransmitters, including norepinephrine and serotonin and the endogenous opiates. The impulses then proceed upward through the contralateral spinothalamic tract, which in turn receives input from the brainstem and cortical areas, all of which results in the perception of the pain experience. [25]

TABLE 1.6. Potential Alterations in Neurons Deprived of Sensory Input

Activation of previously ineffective synapses
Development of new aberrant connections
Enhanced sensitivity to few remaining synapses
Enhanced sensitivity to neuroregulator substances

TABLE 1.7. Clinical States That May Be Associated with Pain of Central Origin or Deafferentation Pain

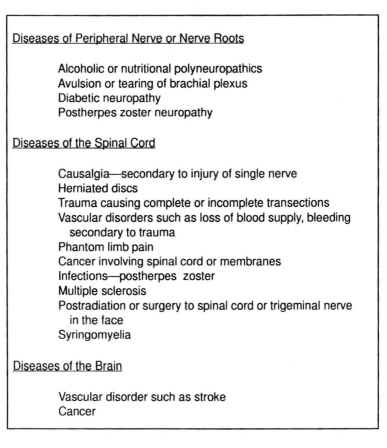

Diseases of Peripheral Nerve or Nerve Roots

      Alcoholic or nutritional polyneuropathics
      Avulsion or tearing of brachial plexus
      Diabetic neuropathy
      Postherpes zoster neuropathy

Diseases of the Spinal Cord

      Causalgia—secondary to injury of single nerve
      Herniated discs
      Trauma causing complete or incomplete transections
      Vascular disorders such as loss of blood supply, bleeding
        secondary to trauma
      Phantom limb pain
      Cancer involving spinal cord or membranes
      Infections—postherpes zoster
      Multiple sclerosis
      Postradiation or surgery to spinal cord or trigeminal nerve
        in the face
      Syringomyelia

Diseases of the Brain

      Vascular disorder such as stroke
      Cancer

Central pain, usually due to disease affecting the thalamus, can be modified by an injury to any sensory region of the central nervous system. However, it is not always to differentiate between the two (Table 1.8). In addition, the symptoms seen in each of these conditions may be modified by associated psychiatric disorders.

TABLE 1.8. Differences Between Somatic Pain and Central Pain

	Somatic Pain	Central Pain
Cause	• Firing of nociceptors	• Deafferentation with abnormal firing effected neurons
Description	• Occurs in direct response to stimulation of nociceptors	• Occurs sometime after initial injury
	• Pressing or cutting, clearly felt as painful	• Often described as burning tingling, "pins-and-needles" sensation
Examples	• Surgery, trauma, cancer infection, decreased blood flow to an organ	• Systemic disorders affecting peripheral nerves: diabetes, alcoholism, spinal cord lesions, disorders of the brain
Treatment	• Removal of source of stimulation, analgesics, interruption of neuronal pathways	• Response to opiates variable Only temporary relief by interruption of neural pathways
		• Often relieved by drugs in barbiturate-tranquilizer group, possible relief by sympathetic block

REFERENCES

1. Dallenbach KM. Pain: History and present status. *Am J Psychol,* 1930, 52:331–347.

2. Descartes R. L'Homme. In: Foster M. *Lectures on the history of physiology during the 16th, 17th, and 18th centuries.* Cambridge, England: Cambridge University Press, 1901:261–269.

3. Bonica JJ. Anatomic and physiologic basis of norciception and pain. In: Bonica JJ (ed). *Management of pain,* Vol 1. Philadelphia: Lea & Febiger, 1990:28–94.

4. Melzack R, Wall PD. Pain mechanisms: A new theory. *Science,* 1965, 150:971–979.

5. Livingston WK. *Pain mechanism. A physiologic interpretation of causalgia and its related states.* New York: Macmillan, 1901.

6. Hardy JD, Wolff HD, Goodell H. *Pain sensations and reactions.* Baltimore: Williams & Wilkins, 1952.

7. Merskey H. Pain terms: A list with definitions and notes on usage. IASP Subcommittee on Taxonomy. *Pain,* 1979, 6:249–252.

8. Zimmerman M. Peripheral and central nervous mechanisms of norciception, pain, and pain therapy: Facts and hypotheses. In: Bonica JJ, Liebeskind JG, Albe-Fessard DC (eds). *Advances in pain research and therapy,* Vol 3. New York: Raven Press, 1979:3–32.

9. Perl ER, Whitlock DG. Somatic stimuli exciting spinothalamic projections to thalamic neurons in cat and monkey. *Exp Neurol,* 1961, 3:256–296.

10. Melzack R, Casey KL. Sensory motivational and central control determinants of pain. In: Kenshalo DR (ed). *The skin senses.* Springfield IL: Charles C Thomas, 1968:423–443.

11. Rexed B. The cytoarchitectonic organization in the spinal cord of the cat. *J Comp Neurol,* 1952, 96:415–495.

12. LaMotte C. Distribution of the tract of Lissauer and the dorsal root fibers in the primate spinal cord. *J Comp Neurol,* 1977, 172:529–547.

13. Kolmodin GM, Skoglund CR. Analysis of spinal interneurons activated by tactile and nociceptive stimulation. *Acta Physiol Scand,* 1960, 50:337–355.

14. White JR. Effects of a counterirritant on perceived pain and hand movement in patients with arthritis. *Phys Ther,* 1973, 53:956–960.

15. Bowsher D. Pain pathways and mechanisms. *Anaesthesia,* 1978, 33:935–944.

16. Kerr FWL. Neuroanatomical substrates of nociception in the spinal cord. *Pain,* 1975, 1:325–356.

17. Dennis SG, Melzack R. Pain signalling systems in the dorsal and ventral spinal cord. *Pain,* 1977, 4:97–132.

18. Gilman S, Newman SW. *Manter and Gatz's: Essentials of clinical neuroanatomy and neurophysiology.* Philadelphia: F.A. Davis and Co., 1992.

19. Price DD, Dubner R. Neurons that subserve the sensory-discriminative aspects of pain. *Pain,* 1977, 3:307–339.

20. Casey KL, Jones EG. Suprasegmental mechanisms. An overview of ascending pathways: Brainstem and thalamus. *Neurosciences Research Program Bulletin,* 1978, 16:103–118.

21. Becker DP, Gluck H, Nulsen FE, Jane, JA. An inquiry into the neurophysiological basis for pain. *J Neurosurg,* 1969, 30:1–13.

22. Fields HL, Basbaum, AI. Anatomy and physiology of a descending pain control system. In: Bonica JJ, Liebeskind JC, Albe-Fessard DG (eds). *Advances in pain research and therapy.* Vol 3. New York: Raven Press, 1979:427–440.

23. Mekzack R, Loeser JD. Phantom body pain in paraplegics: Evidence for a central "pattern generating mechanism" for pain. *Pain,* 1978, 4:195–210.

24. Adams RD, Victor M. *Principles of neurology: Companion handbook,* 4th ed. New York: McGraw Hill, 1991.

25. Fields HL, Martin JB. Pain: Pathophysiology and management. In: Isselbacher KJ, Braunwald E, Martin JB, Fauci AS, Kasper DL (eds). *Harrison's principles of internal medicine. Thirteenth edition.* New York: McGraw Hill, 1994: 49–54.

Chapter 2

Neuroregulators and Pain

INTRODUCTION

The early hypotheses concerning the transmission of information in the central nervous system focused on electrical rather than chemical processes.[1,2] Information subsequently obtained from microelectrode recordings of single cells, however, was found to be irreconcilable with a purely electrical construct of neural transmission. Subsequent to von Euler's[2] discovery of epinephrine and Vogt's[3] demonstration of the relation between central nervous system norepinephrine and epinephrine to brain function, the field of behavioral neurochemistry expanded rapidly. At present, there are a number of possible central nervous system neuroregulators believed to modulate in some way response to pain (Table 2.1). These substances may be classified as neurotransmitters, neuromediators, or neuromodulators.

Neurotransmitters

A number of criteria must be met prior to considering a substance to be a true neurotransmitter[4] (Table 2.2). Basically, neurotransmitters convey information between adjacent nerve cells with the capacity for synthesizing the specific transmitter residing within the presynaptic elements or in the neuron itself. The noradrenergic receptor interaction can be used as a model of the function of a neurotransmitter (Figure 2.1).

Norepinephrine (NE) is synthesized within the granule of the nerve terminal through the conversion of tyrosine to dihydroxyphenlalinine (dopa) and then to dopamine (Figure 2.1). Synthesis of dopa and dopamine occurs within the cell cytoplasm. Dopamine subsequently enters storage vesicles and is converted to NE. Norepinephrine is discharged to the exterior by initiation of the nerve action potential, which may occur either spontaneously or after administration of sympathomimetic drugs. Following NE release and subsequent combination at the alpha or beta

TABLE 2.1. Neuroregulators Implicated in Mediating the Response to Pain

Acetylcholine	Histamine
Angiotensin	Indolamines
β Endorphins	Nerve growth factor
Bradykinin	Neurotensin
Catecholamines	Nitric oxide
Cydic AMP	Norepinephrine
Cholecystokinin	Prostaglandins
Cytokines	Protons
Dopamine	Serotonin (5 Hydroxytryptamine)
Epinephrine	Somatostatin
Glycine	Substance P
Glutamate	Thyrotropin releasing hormone
Gamma-aminobutyric acid or	Vasopressin
Gamma aminobutyrate (GABA)	

adrenoreceptor sites of the effector cells, excess NE either reenters the nerve terminal where it may be metabolized by monoamine oxidase (MAO), or is metabolized extracellularly by catechol-O-methyltransferase (COMT). Norepinephrine that is not metabolized is stored in vesicles until subsequently released. Compounds with similar structures are also taken up into the vesicle. Noncatechol sympathomimetic amines can exert a pharmacologic effect through a direct action on adrenergic receptors or through an indirect effect, resulting in a release of NE from the storage granules. Drugs exerting a predominantly indirect effect enter the adrenergic neuron by the same uptake mechanism.[5]

Neuromodulators

Neuromodulators, in contrast to neurotransmitters, are synthesized from nonsynaptic sites, yet they alter neuronal activity without the direct

TABLE 2.2. Characteristics of Neurotransmitters

Precursors, synthetic enzymes, and substance must be present in presynaptic elements of neuronal tissue or in neuron.

Stimulation of afferents cause physiologically significant release of substance.

Direct application of substance to synapse produces identical response to stimulation of afferents.

Specific receptors should be present in close proximity to presynaptic structures that interact with substance.

Interaction of substance and receptor induces changes in postsynaptic membrane excitability leading to appropriate potentials.

Specific inactivating mechanisms should exist to stop interactions of the substance with its receptor within a physiologically reasonable time frame.

Source: Modified from Snyder[4]

transfer of a nerve signal through the synapse.[1] Neuromodulators might affect synaptical activity through influencing the neurotransmitter by affecting synthesis, receptor binding, reuptake, or biotransformation. Alternatively, a neuromodulator might act directly on a large number of neurons at some distance from the release site. In addition to endogenous neuromodulators, a number of drugs have been shown to affect neurotransmitter function at all points in the transmitter-receptor interaction. Since many of these drugs are prescribed in the treatment of pain, a knowledge of their interactions with these systems is important.

Neuromodulators, therefore, act either to convey information between adjacent cells or to modify existing neuronal activity. As such, they are not involved primarily in either the metabolic activities of the cell or in mediating the response of a cell to the neurotransmitter. At times it may be difficult to precisely determine whether a substance is a neuromodulator or a neurotransmitter. Indeed, for a particular substance, this distinction may not be critical as long as its role in transmission of the neuronal impulse is understood.

FIGURE 2.1. The Adrenergic Neuron

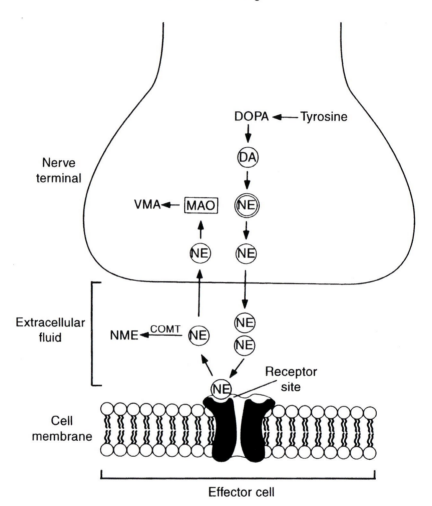

Synthesis, uptake, and metabolism of NE. Norepinephrine is synthesized within the nerve terminal from tyrosine through formation of dopa and dopamine. It is then stored in granules until released by incoming nerve impulses. The NE released in the extracellular fluid may attach to adrenergic receptors on effector cells or diffuse into the circulation. Norepinephrine stores in the nerve terminal are replenished by biosynthesis and the amine transport system of the axonal membrane. Degradation of NE occurs through catechol-O-methyl transferase (COMT) and monoamine oxidase (MAO).

Neuromediators

Neuromediators allow a cell to respond to the effects of the neurotransmitter at the post synaptic junction. One of the most common neuromediators involved in transmission of "painful stimuli" is cyclic AMP (adenosine monophosphate),[3,5] termed second messenger.

ENDORPHINS AND ENKEPHALINS

The endogenous opioids are among the most recently described neurotransmitters. In 1973, three independent laboratories almost simultaneously identified the presence of opioid receptors in the central nervous system that were no known to be responsive to any currently existing neurotransmitters.[6,7,8]

Distribution

The direct measurement of the opioid receptors on brain membranes became possible through radioimmunoassay techniques. All natural and synthetic opiates were found to bind to the opioid receptors; however, their binding capabilities varied greatly, depending on the specific opiates involved (Chapter 6). The distribution of the opiate receptors in the central nervous system has been extensively studied by dissection and autoradiographic visualization.[9] Almost all brain areas contain opiate receptors, with the exception of the cerebellum. Dense clusters of receptors have been identified at the synaptic areas of the ventral spinothalamic tract, the substantia gelatinosa of the spinal cord, the periaqueductal gray area (PAG), the intralaminar nuclei of the thalamus, and the extrapyramidal system, with the amygdala being one of the richest receptor regions.[10] Those receptors located in the limbic system have been associated with opiate-induced euphoria or dysphoria, as well as the affective components of pain perception.

Recently opiate receptors have been identified peripherally as well in the vicinity of peripheral nerve terminals.[11] Although not easily detectable in normal tissue, they can be identified in the presence of inflammation. Similarly, the local administration of morphine within joint spaces in doses that are ineffective when given systemically, has produced analgesia similar to that seen with local anesthetics and is able to be blocked by naloxone, further suggesting the presence of opiate receptors.

The interactions between opiates and the opiate receptors, as well as their role in dependence and withdrawal, are discussed more fully in Chapter 3 and 6. It is important to note, however, that recent evidence suggests that there are several types of receptors, with at least five distinct types being confirmed: mu (μ), delta (Δ), sigma (δ), kappa (ϰ), and epsilon (∈). Although each of these receptors display similar chemical properties, they clearly have different affinities and functions (Table 2.3). It is the μ receptor, however, that is felt to be the primary site of action of morphine and related analgesics. However, with respect to individual opioids, reactions may occur at several receptors that can vary from pure agonist to antagonist.

Not unexpectedly, the identification of these receptors gave rise to the hypothesis of an endogenous opiate system with a morphine-like substance acting as a neuroregulator. This hypothesis was also supported by the observation that electrical stimulation of the brain was associated with the activation of an endogenous pain-relieving system capable of providing prolonged analgesia. In 1975, Kosterlitz and Hughes,[12] and Hughes et al.,[13] isolated a morphine-like substance from pig brains. This substance, composed of the pentapeptides—Metenkephalin and Leuenkephalin—was felt to contain the neurotransmitters of an endogenous opiate system. Evidence suggesting that enkephalins functioned as neurotransmitters consisted of their (a) direct identification in regions of the brain paralleling sites of opiate receptors and (b) localization in nerve endings concerned with excitation. Additional circumstantial evidence was provided by the identification of exceedingly high concentrations of enkephalin in intestinal tissue. The high density of enkephalins in brain and intestine parallels the location of other peptides known to be neurotransmitters. However, the absence of proven reuptake mechanisms or evidence of rapid enzyme inactivation suggests that these substances may function more as neuromodulators than neurotransmitters.

Classification

Over the last several years, a large number of enkephalin analogues have been synthesized.[14,15] All of the endogenous opiates are felt to be related to β-lipotropin, a pituitary hormone consisting of 91 amino acids. At the present, three major types of neuropeptides have been identified: the enkephalins, the Beta endorphins and the dynorphins. Each group is derived from a separate precursor (Table 2.4) and each is located in different areas of the brain, although there is considerable overlap between the enkephalins and the dynorphins. The Beta endorphins are concentrated mainly in the pituitary and hypothalamus. The precursors of the enkephalins (proenkephalins) can be found in areas of the central nervous system, specifically involved with pain.

TABLE 2.3. Opiates, Receptors, and Their Functions

	Mu (μ)	Delta (Δ)	Sigma (δ)	Kappa (κ)	Epsilon (ε)
Site	Morphine and related opiates	Ketocyclozine	Enkephalins	Benzomorphan	B-Endorphins
Effects Analgesia	+	+ (spinal)	+		+
Pupils	Constriction	Constriction		Dilatation	
Heart Rate	Slow	-------	Rapid		
Affect	Indifference	Sedation	Delirium		
Opiate Activity Agonists[1]	++	+	Inhibits		
Antagonists[2]	Inhibits	Inhibits			
Mixed Agonist[3]-Antagonists	Inhibits	++			

1. Pure agonist activity
2. Naloxone
3. Pentazocine, Buprenorphine, Nalbuphine

TABLE 2.4. Endogenous Opioid Peptides

Precursor	Endogenous Opioid
Proenkephalin A	Enkephalin
Proopiomelanocortin	β-endorphin
Proenkephalin B (Prodynorphin)	Dynorphin

Mechanisms of Action

Enkephalins exert an inhibitory action on neuronal brain cells resulting from a reduction in the depolarizing flow of sodium across cell membranes. Enkephalin released at excitatory neuronal synapses also bind to the opiate receptors, increasing sodium conduction accompanied by a partial depolarization of the membrane terminal. The arrival of a second nerve impulse at the terminal would result in a net decrease in depolarization and a corresponding decrease in the amount of excitatory transmitter released.

The presence of enkephalins and opiate receptors in the regions of the central nervous system concerned with pain transmission supports the hypothesis of an endogenous pain suppression mechanism. Indeed, considerable circumstantial evidence has accumulated suggesting the involvement of an endogenous opiate system in pain relief (Table 2.5).[16,17,18,19] However, opposing evidence also exists (Table 2.6).

Release of other neuroregulators involved in the response to pain can also be effected by the endogenous opiate system. Simulation of enkephalin interneurons can inhibit release of Substance P, acetyl choline, dopamine, and norepinephrine.[33]

Summary

In summary, existing evidence supports the concept of an endogenous analgesic system modulated by endorphins. Teleologically, this system would be of great importance to survival, as it allows pain to be experienced as an early warning of tissue injury before the damage becomes severe.

Conclusive evidence of an endogenous analgesic role for the endorphins is dependent on demonstrating specific alterations of endorphin levels or turnover during painful states or during analgesia. This remains to be consistently confirmed. The numerous publications concerning the effect of naloxone (a pure opioid antagonist) on pain present contradictory findings. It is also

TABLE 2.5. Evidence for the Existence of an Endogenous Enkephalin-Mediated Analgesic System[a]

Interaction at opiate receptors known to be responsible for opiate analgesia
Opiate receptors located in central nervous system pathways known to be involved in pain transmission
Opiates selectively inhibit firing of nociceptive neurons in substantia gelatinosa
Direct injection of endorphins into cerebral ventricles results in analgesia
Analgesia produced by electrical stimulation of enkephalin-rich areas
Cross-tolerance exists between SPA and opiate analgesia
Endorphin levels significantly increased in organic pain as compared to psychogenic pain
Opiate activity decreased in spinal fluid of patients with trigeminal neuralgia
EA associated with increase in opioid activity in CSF in chronic pain
Naloxone demonstrated to lower pain threshold in mice and rats
Reverse SPA and EA in humans
Reverse placebo effect in postoperative pain
Lower pain threshold in persons with congenital hyposensitivity to pain
Enkephalin inhibition of potassium-stimulated release of Substance P from dorsal root ganglion

SPA, stimulation-produced analgesia; EA, electroacupuncture; CSF, cerebrospinal fluid.

[a]See references 25 and 28.

possible that an opiate analgesic system may coexist and interact with that of the endogenous opiates. Further information is still necessary to define clearly the role of endogenous opiate system in the manifestation of pain.

ACETYLCHOLINE

Acetylcholine (ACh) has been known to function as a neurotransmitter for decades. Cholinergic activity has been identified in the central nervous system as well as in autonomic ganglia, postganglionic parasympathetic nerve endings, and at the neuromuscular junction. Central nervous system sites of activity include the hippocampus, caudate nucleus, several thalamic nuclei, the lateral geniculate body, supraoptic nucleus, brainstem, and pyramidal cortical cells, as well as the cochlear nucleus. Evidence suggests that ACh may interact with the endogenous opiate system as well as exert hyperalgesic activity (Table 2.7).[20]

CATECHOLAMINES

The three major catecholamines that function as neurotransmitters in the brain are dopamine, epinephrine, and norepinephrine. Of these, dopamine and norepinephrine are prominent in transmission of painful stimuli and the response to path.

Dopamine

The central nervous system is a rich source of dopamine[21,22] whose major action is felt to be inhibitory. Dopamine is believed to be responsible for motor movements in the nigro-striatal pathway, as well as for thought disorders such as schizophrenia. Parkinsonism is felt to be due to damage to the dopamine neurons with a loss of their inhibitory effect on

TABLE 2.6. Evidence Against an Endogenous Endorphin-Mediated Analgesic System[a]

Beta-endorphin levels in CSF of pain patients low
Duration and severity of pain not correlated with CSF, β-endorphin levels
Direct intraventricular injection of enkephalins unassociated with analgesia
Intravenous injections of β-endorphin levels before and after electroacupuncture
Naloxone unable consistently to reverse electroacupuncture

[a] See references 17 and 19.

TABLE 2.7. Evidence Suggesting Role of Acetylcholine in Interaction with Opiates and Pain Pathways

---

Animal experiments

- ACh release inhibited by enkephalin and narcotic drugs can be reversed by naloxone

- ACh release increased by administration of naloxone

- Intraarterial injection of ACh associated with nociception

Clinical observations

- Pain produced by application of ACh to blisters or with intra-arterial injections

- Morphine analgesia enhanced by concurrent administration of physostigmine or neostigmine

---

the post synaptic neuron. Drugs blocking dopamine receptors, including the phenothiazines and butyrophenones, can produce Parkinsonism-like syndromes (Figure 2.2). Similarly, the ability of these drugs to bind to the dopamine receptors parallel their potency as antipsychotic agents. Agents that stimulate dopamine production, such as amphetamines and cocaine, may be associated with bizarre behavior. Dopaminergic mechanisms appear to play a role in modulation of pain as well as reinforcing addictive behavior. Intracerebral injections of dopamine have been demonstrated to enhance morphine analgesia. Similarly, administration of L-dopa has been associated with an increase in pain and contraction of areas previously rendered analgesic by rhizotomy.

Norepinephrine

Norepinephrine (NE) is released form discrete clusters of cells in the lateral reticular formation of the medulla, the locus ceruleus, and the PAG area, as well as the mesencephalon and diencephalon.[21,22] Many of these regions have also been identified as being rich in opiate receptors. Nociceptive activity can be considerably influenced by noradrenergic neurons.[23] Administration of norepinephrine can result in increase in causalgia and can be abolished by sectioning the sympathetic nerve fibers. Correspondingly, the use of an adrenergic agonists such as clonidine can relieve sympathetic mediated pain, as well as enhance narcotic analgesia.

FIGURE 2.2. Effects of Drugs on Dopaminergic Neurons

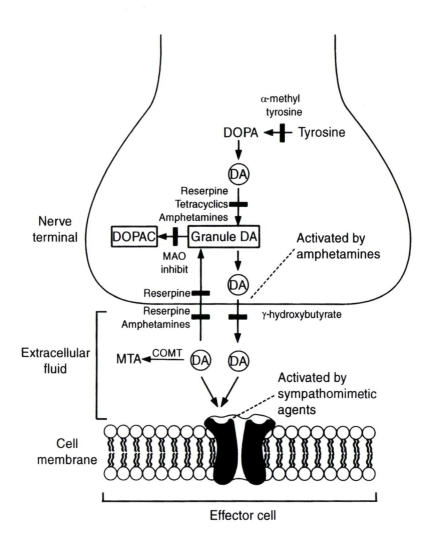

COMT, Catechol-O-methyltransferase; DA, dopamine; DOPAC, Dihydroxy-phenylacetic acid; MTA, 3-methoxytyramine.

In the PAG area of the brainstem, NE release may be associated with a potentiation in morphine analgesia. Similarly, NE release in the spinal cord may cause an inhibition of impulse transmission from pain afferents to motor neurons, dorsal roots, and several ascending spinal pathways.[24]

Many drugs affect the noradrenergic neuron (Figure 2.3). Those drugs that result in a central depletion of NE result in sedation, whereas drugs

FIGURE 2.3. Effects of Drugs on the Noradrenergic Neuron

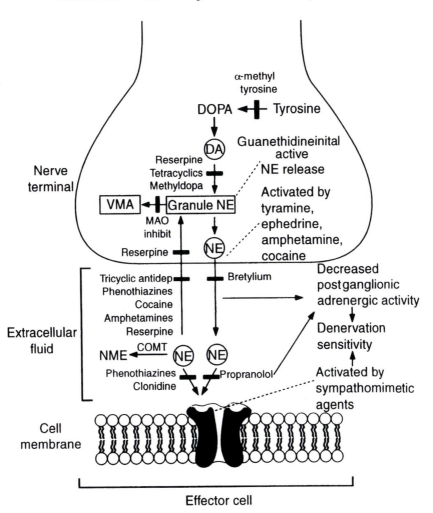

facilitating NE release or decreasing NE metabolism will result in increased wakefulness and motor activity, at times accompanied by an altered perception of pain. These observations may explain the effectiveness of amphetamines in enhancing morphine analgesia (Chapter 6).

HISTAMINE

Histamine can be identified throughout the brain, the highest levels located in the cerebellum, ventral hypothalamus, preoptic region, and hypophyseal stalk.[25] Histamine formed from histidine through the activity of histidine decarboxylase can be found in free-form or may be stored in synaptic vesicles. The precise role of histamine in neuroregulation of painful stimuli has yet to be defined. Intradermal injection of histamine can cause pain, whereas subdermal injection results in pain only when prostaglandin E is infused simultaneously. Turnover rates can be affected by stress and, on a peripheral level, histamine release from mast cells and other tissues has a prominent role in the inflammatory response.

SEROTONIN (5 HYDROXYTRYPTAMINE)

Serotonin (5-HT) is an indolamine that can be located in many regions of the body and plays an important role as a neurotransmitter in the central nervous system. Neurons containing serotonin (5-HT) extend through the medulla, pons, and mesencephalon, with fibers reaching into the spinal cord synapsing through the reticular formation.[21,22] As a result of its ubiquity, a number of 5-HT receptors have been identified and many psychoactive drugs have been shown to affect 5-HT secretions (Figure 2.4). The existence of painful stimuli is one of the many factors that can influence the activity of these cells.

The ability of 5-HT to cause a decrease in neuronal fiber discharge allows the possibility that its increased secretion may be associated with a diminished pain response (Table 2.8). As a result, serotonin or its precursor, the essential amino acid tryptophan, have been used to treat a variety of painful conditions. These include migraine, musculoskeletal pain, fibromyalgia, and postcordotomy pain. When successful, it has been hypothesized that serotonin can increase the pain threshold and diminish the tolerance to opioid analgesics without necessarily affecting pain perception. Similarly, depletion of serotonin can reduce the efficacy of morphine-induced analgesia. Ironically, intradermal injection of serotonin can actually produce pain by activating nociceptive neurons.

FIGURE 2.4. Effects of Drugs on the Serotonergic Neuron

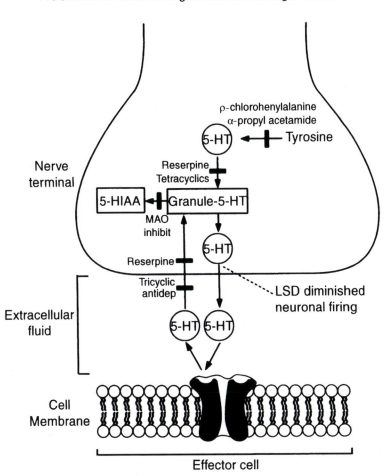

SUBSTANCE P

Substance P, one of the earliest described putative polypeptide neuro-transmitters, has a widespread distribution in nerve tissue, most prominent in the neurons of the dorsal horn.[26,27] Substance P meets several criteria for being a neurotransmitters: (1) it is present in appropriate neurons and their terminals; (2) it has been demonstrated to be transported to these terminals; (3) it is released on stimulation of dorsal root nerves; and (4) when applied

TABLE 2.8. Evidence Suggesting Analgesic Activity of Serotonin

Administration of drugs depleting serotonin accompanied by increase in nociceptive sensitivity

Opiate analgesia can be prevented by serotonin-depleting drugs and restored by intracerebral ventricular injection of serotonin

Destruction of nuclei-producing serotonin accompanied by increase in sensitivity to nociception

Electrical stimulation of serotonin turnover intensifies morphine analgesia

Morphine analgesia decreased with simultaneous administration of reserpine

to spinal neurons, it results in their excitation. Along with neurokinin A, it is felt to be responsible for a phenomenon termed "windup," the repetitive stimulation of C-fibers resulting in increased excitability manifested as pain. However, similar to the endorphins, there is no evidence that it is actually synthesized in sensory neurons or that a mechanism exists for its rapid metabolism or its neuronal reentry. It is possible that Substance P acts more as a neuroregulator than a neurotransmitter.

The importance of Substance P in modulation of painful stimuli is well recognized, although its precise role in this process remains to be determined. It has been hypothesized that Substance P is released in response to painful stimuli from dorsal root neuron cells, resulting in a slow depolarization of nerve cell preparation, exciting neurons similar to those activated by noxious stimuli in the peripheral nervous system. Drugs that deplete Substance P result in analgesia. Substance P is also present in other areas, such as spinal sensory ganglion neurons. It is also felt to play a role in the inflammatory response, potentiating other inflammatory mediators.

GLUTAMATE AND GABA

Glutamate is a neuroregulator present in highest concentrations in the branches of primary afferent sensory neurons.[21,22] Glutamate released from the brainstem and spinal cord nuclei acts on receptors of the postsynaptic neuronal membrane to cause rapid depolarization, exerting an excitatory effect. Inactivation subsequently occurs, followed by a sodium dependent reuptake into the presynaptic nerve terminal. Receptors for glutamate and aspartate, another "excitatory" amino acid, have been identified. One such receptor (NMDA) has also been identified as a possible site of action of PCP (Phencyclidine). NMDA receptors are felt to be responsible for the hyperexcitability seen in chronic pain states through increasing the discharge frequency of dorsal horn cells.

Glutamic acid is the precursor of gamma aminobutyric acid (GABA), a neurotransmitter that depresses cortical function (Figure 2.5). The precise role of glutamate in modulation of pain pathways remains to be clarified. However, GABA transmission has been associated with alleviation of anxi-

FIGURE 2.5. Gamma-Aminobutyric Acid (GABA) and the Benzodiazepine Receptor

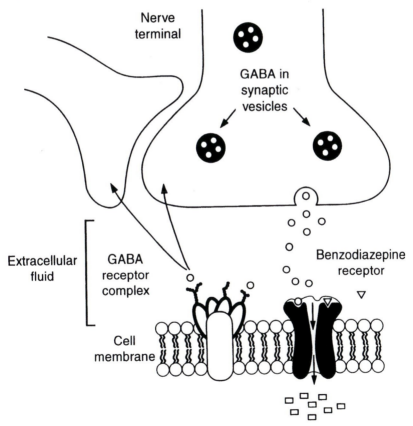

ety. Tranquilizing agents, much as barbiturates and benzodiazepines, facilitate GABA secretion (Chapter 9), and it is possible that interaction between these substances may exert a modulating effect on pain perception.

NEUROREGULATORS INVOLVED IN TISSUE DAMAGE

Damage to tissues secondary to inflammation, trauma, loss of blood supply, or other disorders is associated with release of a variety of neuroregulators and accompanied by pain. Several neuroregulators have been specifically identified with this response, although the precise role that each plays with respect to actual modulation of painful stimuli remains unclear. These substances include: bradykinins, histamines, prostaglandins, and substance P, all being able to stimulate nociceptors in varying degrees.

Bradykinins

Bradykinin neurons, identified in the hypothalamus, have fibers extending throughout the body.[28] Bradykinin receptors are found in areas involved with nociception and are potent stimulators of hyperalgesia. Their actions can be enhanced by prostaglandins and other substances produced during inflammation, such as interleukin and tumor necrosis factors. Correspondingly, bradykinin antagonists can inhibit superficial bradykinin induced pain in both animal and experimental models.

Prostaglandins

Prostaglandins (PG) are ubiquitous lipid-like molecules that may be synthesized in almost all tissues from phospholipids. Any noxious stimulus resulting in deformation of the cell membrane or activation of lipolysis will result in a hydrolysis-releasing arachidonic acid, which is subsequently transformed through prostaglandin synthetase to prostaglandin.

There are a number of prostaglandins and, as may be expected, there is considerable diversity with respect to their actions. Their major contribution to the inflammatory state is through either directly stimulating sensory nerve endings or by sensitizing these endings to other noxious stimuli. PGE and PGE_2 have been found to shift the dose response curves of bradykinin, Substance P, histamine, and acetylcholine to the left, indicating an enhancement of their algesic effects. This facilitative effect is cumulative and may persist for relatively long periods.

PG release can be inhibited by indomethacin, aspirin, and the nonsteroidal anti-inflammatory drugs (NSAIDs).[29] The peripheral hyperalgesic effect of prostaglandins can also be blocked by narcotic drugs, as well as by naloxone. In this instance, naloxone is felt to exhibit analgesic activity rather than function primarily as a narcotic antagonist. These preliminary observations of prostaglandin-opiate interactions, if confirmed, will lead to the development of effective analgesic narcotic agonists or antagonists with predominantly peripheral effects. Not all prostaglandins, however, have an algesic effect; PGF_{2a} can antagonize the algesic effects of PGE as well as decrease the algesic effects of bradykinin.[30]

Finally, inflammatory pain may also be intensified by the appearance of superoxide and its hydroxyl-free radical. These two agents are potent oxidizers that cause considerable tissue damage.

OTHER ENDOGENOUS SUBSTANCES IMPLICATED IN PAIN PERCEPTION

Gut and Brain Peptides

A number of other peptides identified in brain tissue have been indirectly implicated in pain perception through their localization in areas known to participate in modulation of painful stimuli (Table 2.9). Cholecystokinin cells originally isolated in the gastrointestinal tract have also been identified in the cerebral cortex, the hypothalamus, and the periaqueductal gray of the brainstem.[31] Cholecystokinin markedly enhances firing of cortical cells and may be involved in the integrative response to pain. Neurotensin is another peptide with a number of known peripheral actions. It has been suggested that neurotensin may play a modulating role in endorphin-independent pain pathways.

TABLE 2.9. Other Peptides Implicated in Pain

Cholecystokinin
Somatostatin
Thyrotropin-releasing factor
Vasopressin

Hypothalamic Releasing Factors

Several hypothalamic releasing factors may affect mood as well as pain perception. Thyrotropin releasing factor is believed to cause excitation in laboratory animals and mood changes in humans.[4] Somatostatin neurons have been identified in many brain areas, including primary sensory neurons and dorsal root ganglia cells.[4]

Nitric Oxide

Nitric oxide (NO) is produced in neurons in the dorsal horn or in sensory ganglia. NO is felt to play a role in the induction and maintenance of chronic pain. Experimentally, agents that inhibit NO receptor activity can diminish both inflammatory and neuropathic pain whereas Substance P and bradykinin cause a release of NO from the vascular endothelium.

Vasopressin

Vasopressin (antidiuretic hormone) cells are located in the supraoptic and paraventricular nuclei of the hypothalamus. Stimulation of brainstem reticular formation in animals results in increased vasopressin release. Clinically, vasopressin release in response to stress and pain has been well documented.[32] Most of the investigations, however, have been done in surgical patients who were also given anesthetic agents. Kendler, Weitzman, and Fisher [33] measured plasma arginine vasopressin concentrations pAVP in patients in pain seen in an emergency ward and in control subjects. pAVP was significantly higher ($p > 0.01$) in the patients in pain as compared to controls, although no difference in plasma osmolality was detected. These findings suggest that, in the absence of confounding factors, pain is associated with elevation of pAVP unassociated with changes in plasma osmolality.

SUMMARY

Neuroregulators have been shown to play a prominent role in the perception of and response to pain. Their location in the nervous system proximate to neuroanatomical pain pathways provides a rational explanation of nociception and existing modulating forces. The interaction between the neuroregulators, as well as the ability of drugs to modify their secretion, allow for the development of a pharmacologic approach to treatment of pain. Many agents that affect neuroregulator activity have the potential to be useful analgesics or, if devoid of analgesic activity, may potentiate analgesia induced by other drugs. The neuroregulators also affect the development of dependence on and tolerance to the narcotic analgesics. This subject will be reviewed in Chapter 3.

REFERENCES

1. Barchas JD, Akil H, Elliott GR, Holman RB, Watson SJ. Behavioral neurochemistry: Neuroregulators and behavioral states. *Science,* 1978, 200:964–973.

2. VonEuler US. *Noradrenaline: Chemistry, physiology, pharmacology, and clinical aspects.* Springfield: Charles C Thomas, 1956.

3. Vogt M. The concentration of sympathin in different parts of the central nervous system under normal conditions and after the administration of drugs. *J Physio,* (London) 1954, 123:451–481.

4. Snyder SH. Brain peptides as neurotransmitters. *Science,* 1980, 209:976–983.

5. Iversen LL. *The uptake and storage of noradrenaline in sympathetic nerves.* London: Cambridge University Press, 1967.

6. Pert CB, Pasternak G, Snyder SH. Opiate agonists and antagonists discriminated by receptor binding in brain. *Science,* 1973, 182:1359–1361.

7. Simon EJ, Hiller JM, Edelman I. Stereospecific binding of the potent narcotic analgesic (3H) Etorphine to rat-brain homogenate. *Proc Natl Acad Sci USA,* 1973, 70:1947–1949.

8. Terenius L. Characteristics of the "receptor" for narcotic analgesics in synaptic plasma membrane fraction from rat brain. *Acta Pharmacol Toxicol, (Copenhagen),* 33:377–384.

9. Kuhar MJ, Pert CB, Snyder SH. Regional distribution of opiate receptor binding in monkey and human brain. *Nature,* 1973, 245:447–450.

10. Bunney WE, Jr, Pert CB, Klee W, Costa E, Pert A, Davis CC. Basic and clinical studies of endorphins. *Ann Intern Med,* 1979, 91:239–250.

11. Stein C. The control of pain in peripheral tissues by opioids. *New Eng J Med,* 1995, 332:1685–1690.

12. Kosterlitz HW, Hughes J. Peptides with morphine-like action in the brain. *Br J Psychiatry,* 1977, 130:298–304.

13. Hughes J, Smith TW, Kosterlitz HW, Fathergill LA, Morgan BA, Morris, R. Identification of two related pentapeptides from the brain with potent opiate agonist activity. *Nature,* 1975, 258:577–579.

14. Collier HD, Hughes J, Rance MJ, Tyers MB. *Opioids: Past, present, and future.* London: Taylor & Francis, 1984.

15. Hollt V. Opioid peptide processing and receptor selectivity. *Ann Rev Pharmacol Toxicol,* 1986, 26:59–77.

16. Adams JE. Naloxone reversal of analgesia produced by brain stimulation in the human. *Pain,* 1976, 2:161–166.

17. Oyama T, Jin T, Yamaya R, Ling L, Guillemin R. Profound analgesic effects of beta-endorphin in man. *Lancet,* 1980, 1:122–124.

18. Almay BGL, Johansson F, Von Knorring L, Terenius L, Wahlstrom A. Endorphins in chronic pain. Differences in CSF endorphin levels between organic and psychogenic pain syndromes. *Pain,* 1978, 5:153–162.

19. Simon EJ. Opiate receptors and endorphins: Possible relevance to narcotic addiction. *Adv Alcohol Substance Abuse,* 1981, 1:13–31.

20. Keele CA, Armstrong D. *Substances producing pain and itch.* London: Edward Arnold, 1964.

21. Bjorklund A, Lindvall O. Catecholaminergic brain stem regulatory systems. In: Bloom FE, Mountcastle VB (eds). Section 1, *The nervous system, handbook of Physiology.* Vol. 1 V Sect. 3. Ed. Bloom FE, Mountcastle VB, Vol. IV:155–235. Bethesda, MD: American Physiological Society, 1986.

22. Gillman S, Newman SW. *Manter and Gatz's: Essentials of clinical neuroanatomy and neurophysiology.* Philadelphia: FA Davis and Co, 1992.

23. Kerr FWL, Wilson PR. Pain. *Annu Rev Neurosci,* 1978, 1:83–102.

24. Yaksh TL. Central nervous system sites mediating opiate analgesia. In: Bonica JJ, Liebeskind JL, Albe-Fessard DC (eds). *Advances in pain research and therapy. Vol 3.* New York: Raven Press, 1979:411–426.

25. Bonica JJ (ed). *Management of pain. Vol. 2.* Philadelphia: Lea & Febiger, 1990.

26. Skrabanek P, Powell D. *Substance P,* Vol. 2. Westmount, Quebec: Eden, 1980.

27. Hokfelt T, Johansson O, Ljungdahl A, Lundberg JM, Schultzberg M. Peptidergic neurones. *Nature,* 1980, 284:515–521.

28. Steranka LR, Manning DC, DeHass CJ, Ferkany JW, Borosky SA, Connor JR, Vavrek RJ, Stewart JM, Snyder SH. Bradykinin as a pain mediator: Receptors are localized to sensory neurons, and antagonists have analgesic actions. *Proc Natl Acad Sci USA,* 1988, 85:3245–3249.

29. Ferreira SH. Site of analgesic action of aspirin-like drugs and opioids. In: Beers RF, Bassett EG (eds). *Mechanisms of pain and analgesic compounds.* New York: Raven Press, 1979:309–322.

30. Juan H. Prostaglandins as modulators of pain. *Gen Pharmacol,* 1978, 9:403–409.

31. Dodd J, Kelly JS. Excitation of CA1 pyramidal neurones of the hippocampus by the tetra— and octapeptide C—terminal fragments of cholecystokinin (proceedings). *J Physiol* (London), 1979, 295:61P–62P.

32. Husain MK, Fernando N, Shapiro M, Kagan A, and Glick SM. Radioimmunoassay of arginine vasopressin in human plasma. *J Clin Endocrinol Metabol,* 1973, 37:616–625.

33. Kendler KS, Weitzman RE, Fisher DA. The effect of pain on plasma arginine vasopressin concentrations in man. *Clin Endocrinol,* 1978, 8:89–94.

Chapter 3

Basic Concepts of Dependence, Addiction, Tolerance, and Withdrawal

INTRODUCTION

The alleviation of pain with potent analgesic agents is often fraught with anxiety on the part of the patient and approached with excessive caution by physicians. In discussing these feelings, the words that most often surface are dependence, addiction, tolerance, and withdrawal. Patients in considerable pain are frequently afraid to ask for narcotics because of the fear of becoming dependent and subsequently "addicted" to the drug. Although this attitude may be understandable among the public, it is unfortunate that many physicians hold this fear and, as a result, may deny patients in severe pain the ability to obtain relief.

Physicians' concern in administering narcotics has been well demonstrated by the study of Marks and Sachar,[1] who recorded the presence of inadequate treatment with analgesic agents in 63 percent of patients in severe pain requiring narcotics for adequate analgesic. The prominent reason given for this hesitancy was the fear of producing addiction. Almost two decades after the appearance of Marks and Sachar's paper and, despite the importance of adequate pain control that has been emphasized by many professional groups, many people are still needlessly suffering with one recent review estimating that although 90 percent of persons in pain can obtain satisfactory relief, 80 percent fail to do so.[2,3,4]

The irrationality of the excessive fear of addiction to narcotics can be illustrated by the liberal manner in which other drugs capable of producing an equal degree of dependence are prescribed. This is most notable with respect to the barbiturates and benzodiazepines. Contrary to common belief, prolonged use of all the central nervous system depressants capable of altering mood can be misused and can produce dependence. It is therefore quite important for everyone, be they physicians or patients, to understand clearly the terms describing drug use (Table 3.1), as well as the behavioral,

TABLE 3.1. Common Terms Defining Drug Use

Term	Definition
Appropriate	Medication taken as prescribed by physician or manufacturer for specific indications.
Misuse	Unintentional inappropriate drug consumption.
Abuse	Intentional consumption of a drug to obtain a specific effect that usually differs from the primary indication for that particular drug.
Habituated	Continued drug taking after the initial reason for taking the drug has resolved. Intervals between drug taking are sufficiently long to prevent dependence, but drug use is unable to be discontinued due to emergence of anxiety.
Dependence	The need to continue taking a drug to experience its effects or to prevent the appearance of symptoms (psychological or physical or both).
Tolerance	The loss of a specific effect of a drug after a constant dose is taken at a fixed interval for a period of time.
Addiction	Compulsive drug-seeking behavior superimposed on the dependent state.

biochemical, and cellular concepts underlying dependence, tolerance, and withdrawal. The specific roles that physicians play in inadequately relieving pain, as well as in producing dependence, will be discussed in Chapter 15.

TERMS DEFINING DRUG USE

Drug Misuse

Inappropriate drug use is due either to misuse or abuse. Drug misuse is the unintentional consumption of a drug in other than the commonly accepted manner. This may result from inappropriate prescribing on the part of the physician or, more frequently, from a misunderstanding by the patient. Many drugs are misused daily, with over-the-counter analgesics and cold remedies probably being most common.

Drug Abuse

Drug abuse is a deliberate attempt on the part of the patient or the physician either to use a drug in other than the accepted manner or to use drugs not approved for any medical purpose, such as cocaine, marijuana, or heroin. Although the term abuse is not grammatically correct, as it is really not possible to "abuse" an inert substance, nonetheless, the term has become an integral part of common language. Since the two major scientific institutes for addressing drug dependency have incorporated this term into their names (National Institute on Drug Abuse, National Institute on Alcohol Abuse and Alcoholism), it is not likely that "abuse" will disappear from common terminology in the near future. In almost all instances of drug abuse, the primary effect desired is an alteration of mood. Continued drug abuse at sufficiently frequent intervals may lead to habituation, dependence, or addiction.

Habituation

Frequent use of mood-altering drugs, regardless of initiating cause, may result in a continuation of use after the primary problem has been resolved. Discontinuing the drug often is associated with the appearance of anxiety, necessitating continued drug taking. At this point, the taking of the drug (as much as the drug itself) becomes part of one's life pattern. Habituation is present if the intermittent use occurs at sufficiently separated intervals to prevent the development of dependence. Two most common examples of habituation are the need of many for a cup of coffee to start the day or, with smokers, the need to light a cigarette when having their first cup of coffee or their first alcoholic beverage at night.

Tolerance

Tolerance is present when there is a need to increase the dose of a drug that is taken at a regular interval in order to sustain its initial effects. Tolerance does not usually develop to all of a drug's effects nor may it develop at a uniform rate with a specific drug. The precise mechanisms by which tolerance develops have not been completely defined, but tolerance is felt to be related to the stimulation of enzymes that are responsible for breaking down the drug in the body or to a process called cellular adaptation. When one or more drugs act at identical receptors, cross tolerance to different drug groups may occur. This is most commonly seen with drugs in the alcohol-barbiturate benzodiazepine group.

Dependence

Habituation is usually followed by more frequent drug use and the development of dependence. Dependence is considered to be an adaptive state characterized by behavioral and other physiological responses, which include: (1) the need to continue to take a drug to experience its pleasurable effects, or to prevent withdrawal; (2) the appearance of disturbances, psychological or physiological, or both, when administration of the drug is abruptly suspended; and often (3) the need to increase the dose of the drug with continued administration to sustain the initial effects defined above. Tolerance need not be present in order for dependence to exist. However, not infrequently, depending on the specific drug, once dependence occurs tolerance develops.

Physical dependence occurs as a consequence of exposure to a drug, resulting in physiologic changes necessitating the continued presence of the drug to maintain normal function. Psychologic dependence may be associated with a similar requirement for a drug, but, on discontinuing the drug, objective physiologic changes cannot be identified. In such cases, the changes observed are subjective rather than objective. Psychological and physical dependence are not mutually exclusive; indeed, many drugs produce both. Further, as we learn more about the role of neurotransmitters in anxiety states and more clearly define the effects mood-altering drugs have on neuroreceptor function, it becomes even less meaningful to speak exclusively of psychological dependence.

A person may remain with a specific pattern of drug use or may progress through several patterns, finally becoming dependent. As an example, some people in moderate acute pain may appropriately begin to take a narcotic for analgesia. If the drug should be taken every four hours to provide effective relief from pain but, instead, is taken at much less frequent intervals, only when the pain becomes unbearable, this behavior constitutes drug misuse. A higher dose of narcotic will be needed to provide adequate analgesia, and the anxiety accompanying the increasing severity of pain will interfere with daily activities. If the narcotic is of short duration, the levels in the blood will fluctuate greatly and an increase in dose will most likely be accompanied by a degree of euphoria or sedation, which may be perceived as being quite pleasurable. If the misuse continues, the mood-altering effect may serve as reinforcement and the drug may be taken occasionally in the absence of pain, at the higher dose, specifically for its euphoric action. This now constitutes abuse rather than misuse. Continuation of the pleasurable reinforcement will result in taking the drug whenever the stresses of daily living become sufficiently anxiety provoking. This may occur at varying intervals; however, such behavior will usually lead to habituation and if frequent, will also result in a persistent level of the drug in the body and dependence. This scenario illustrates how inadequately prescribing a narcotic initially can produce exactly the effect that one wishes to avoid. Appropriate prescribing of analgesics for pain will be discussed in Chapter 13.

Addiction

Addiction is a sociologic term that has come to mean the presence of compulsive drug-seeking behavior, usually superimposed on dependence, and often tolerance. This drug taking is often accompanied by increasing the dose of the drug, even in the presence of adverse psychological or physical effects (frequent intoxication for example), due to the inability to terminate use. In general, the greater the ability of a drug to produce its psychopharmacologic effect the greater its addiction potential. Addiction, when applied in a medical setting, leaves much to be desired. This had been recognized by the Expert Committee on Addiction-Producing Drugs of the World Health Organization as early as 1967 when, in an attempt to provide a uniformity of terms, as well as nomenclature more consistent with medical practice, they recommended the term *dependence* be substituted for *addiction*.[5] However, despite their good intentions, by eliminating the term addiction, one often confuses appropriate dependency with inappropriate behavior.

The prescription of a dependency-producing drug to relieve pain and allow adequate function is not only appropriate but extremely beneficial. Such a person should not be considered to be addicted any more than a diabetic would be considered addicted to insulin, a cardiac patient addicted to Digoxin, an individual with psychosis addicted to phenothiazines, or a person with epilepsy addicted to phenobarbital or Dilantin.

Viewed in this light, most mood-altering drugs, whether taken to lessen anxiety, relieve pain, or produce a pleasurable effect, will to some extent result in dependence (Table 3.2). Different drugs, however, exhibit the features of dependence to varying degrees.

DEPENDENCE-PRODUCING DRUGS

Classification

Prior to discussing the role of dependency-producing drugs in relieving pain, it is appropriate to briefly consider the way in which drugs are classified, both in the mind of the public, as well as by law. Drugs with abuse potential may be grouped in a variety of ways: (1) public perception of their effectiveness; (2) their actual actions on various organ systems; (3) their mood-altering effects; (4) their sites of action on brain neurons; (5) what has been decided by legislation; or (6) their legitimate medical use. Legislation embodied in the Controlled Substances Act of 1970 regulates drugs with abuse potential into five schedules based on abuse potential and accepted medical use. These schedules must be adhered to by physicians when prescribing these drugs; the schedules have also been responsible for shaping public perception, and are often indirectly the cause for inadequate pain relief. A more detailed discussion of controlled substance schedules occurs in Chapter 15.

Drugs commonly associated with dependency are listed in Table 3.2. It should be emphasized that there are other agents effective in relieving pain or enhancing analgesia that are not known to be associated with dependency. These drugs include aspirin and the nonsteroidal anti-inflammatory agents, acetaminophen, the antidepressants, and certain of the phenothiazines. The role of these drugs in relieving pain is discussed in subsequent chapters.

In viewing the categories of dependency-producing drugs, it is helpful to remember several characteristics of these agents. First, all drugs within a group are interchangeable when given in an equivalent dosage. A person dependent on alcohol can maintain this dependency on a barbiturate or a benzodiazepine such as Valium, without discomfort or withdrawal. Effects obtained from a drug in one group, however, cannot be produced by administering a drug from another group. A person in pain on inadequate doses of meperidine (Demerol) cannot have pain relieved by administering diazepam

TABLE 3.2. Dependence-Producing Drugs

Group	Drugs included	Dependence	
		Psychic	Physical
Alcohol, Sedative-hypnotics, minor tranquilizers	Alcohol, barbiturates, and other drugs with sedative effects, e.g., chloral hydrate, chlordiazepoxide, diazepam, meprobamate, methaqualone	+2 to +4	+2 to +4
Amphetamines	Amphetamines and certain other stimulants	+2 to +4	+/−
Cannabis	All preparations of cannabis sativa	+2 to +3	+/−
Cocaine group	Cocaine and coco leaves	+2 to +4	−
Hallucinogens	Lysergic acid and hallucinogenic amphetamines	+2 to +3	−
Khat	All preparations of Cathaedulis forssk	+2 to +3	+/−
Opiates and opioids	Includes narcotics with morphine-like effects	+3 to +4	+4
Volatile solvents	Glue, some cleaning fluids	+2 to +3	+/−

− = None, + = little, +2 = mild, +3 = moderate, +4 = marked

(Valium). However, administering drugs from different groups simultaneously can have additive effects on organ tissues, especially the brain. Administering Valium and Demerol, while not enhancing analgesia, can enhance depression of the central nervous system and cause respiratory depression.

Second, the location within a specific group may not be completely accurate, as a single drug may have more than one action. As an example, initially alcohol serves as a stimulant and becomes a depressant as the concentration in the brain rises. The pharmacodynamic classification focuses on the molecular side of drug action in the brain.

Finally, tolerance to one drug within a group is usually associated with tolerance to another drug within the same group, when given in equivalent doses. This is important to remember when changing narcotic analgesics in order to obtain better control of pain, and will be discussed more fully in subsequent chapters. An important exception to this rule that must be remembered, however, concerns drugs in the alcohol-barbiturate group. Although chronic use of alcohol can be associated with a tolerance to benzodiazepine or barbiturate, acute use of large doses of these drugs can actually result in the opposite effect. For this reason, use of sleeping pills after excessive alcohol consumption can result in respiratory depression and, at times, fatal overdose.

Alcohol-Hypnotics, Sedatives, and Minor Tranquilizers

Alcohol, barbiturates, most nonbarbiturate hypnotics and sedatives, and the minor tranquilizers may be associated with physical and psychological dependence to such a marked degree as to impair considerably individual functioning with chronic use. The degree of psychic dependence produced is directly related to the route by which the drug is administered as well as the dose that is given. In general, there is a direct relationship among the development of dependence, the rapidity of onset of action, and the presence of a steep dose-response curve. Tolerance has also been demonstrated with all of these drugs. With respect to the barbiturates and nonbarbiturate, nonbenzodiazepine sedative hypnotics, although a considerable degree of tolerance may develop to their sedative effect, continued use results in only a slight tolerance to the lethal effects. It is, therefore, possible for an individual to escalate the dose rapidly to achieve a sedative effect with resulting toxicity.

Narcotics

Continued use of narcotic agents is also associated with both psychological and physiological dependence. However, narcotics, when used solely for pain relief, even when associated with a considerable degree of dependence, can, in fact, improve functioning through the removal of the incapacitating effects of severe pain. The use of narcotic agonist-antagonists (Chapter 7) for analgesia can also result in tolerance and physical dependence, which will vary considerably depending on the ability of the drug to produce an agonist as well as an antagonist effect.

Stimulants

Amphetamines can produce both psychological dependence and tolerance. Actual physical dependence is minimal, but withdrawal from these drugs is associated with minor physiologic syndromes. Chronic use of cocaine may be associated with hypersensitivity, a low degree of tolerance, and a mild physical dependence. A marked psychological dependence, however, may exist. Milder stimulants, such as nicotine and caffeine, can produce a mild physical dependence associated with a mild degree of tolerance and, not infrequently, a marked psychologic dependence. Considerable discomfort, as well as behavioral changes, can occur when these medications are withheld.

BEHAVIORAL ASPECTS OF DEPENDENCE

Cerebral Effects of Dependence-Producing Drugs

To develop the behavioral model of dependence further, it is helpful to review briefly the effects of opiate injection in both tolerant and nontolerant individuals. It should be emphasized that use of any dependence-producing drugs, such as those in the alcohol-barbiturate-tranquilizer group, will be accompanied by similar phenomena and, depending on the specific agent, may result in a greater degree of dependence than seen with many narcotics.

Administration of a narcotic to a drug-free, nontolerant (NT) individual will usually be accompanied by the experience of a mood-altering effect, even with a minimal, physiologically active dose. This person does not have a tolerance threshold (TT) for the drug.[6] As the brain level of narcotic increases, at some point the psychological effect is experienced, reaches a peak, and slowly diminishes with time at a rate consistent with the pharmacologic properties of the specific drug. A mood-altering effect will persist as long as the narcotic level in the brain exceeds a variable threshold. For a drug such as morphine, this may vary from three to six hours (Figure 3.1A). If administration of the drug is sufficiently spaced so as to occur when there is no narcotic level in the brain, the NT individual will remain NT, and a similar effect will probably be experienced with each dose.

If, however, the intervals between doses become sufficiently shortened so that there is always a minimal brain level of narcotic present, the person will develop a TT to the narcotic. This TT must be exceeded to experience the mood-altering effect. Correspondingly, repeated administration of the same dose of narcotic will be associated with a diminished intensity of the effect. The individual has now become tolerant to the drug. To experience fully the psychotropic effects, the TT must be exceeded by administering a greater dose (Figure 3.1B). In addition, since the homeostatic mechanism of the body has become reset at this new TT, the person has also become dependent on maintaining the TT. If the level of drug drops below the TT, discomfort will be felt and symptoms of withdrawal will appear. It is essential to remember, with respect to relief of pain with narcotic agents, that as long as the tolerance threshold is slowly increased, the amount of narcotics that can be administered is almost infinite. On the other side, if one exceeds the tolerance threshold too rapidly an overdose will occur, which may result in sedation, respiration, depression and, if severe, death.

The development of dependence commits a person to continue to take the narcotic to maintain his or her TT and, therefore, remain free of symptoms of withdrawal. However, at a fixed narcotic dose, the TT slowly increases until the mood-altering effects are no longer experienced (Figure 3.1C). This necessitates an escalation of narcotic dose (Figure 3.1D) and, in turn, is slowly accompanied by a further elevation of TT. This cycle can be broken in one of two ways. Drug taking can be discontinued abruptly. This result in withdrawal symptoms that may be of considerable severity (Chapter 6). More frequently, the amount of narcotic administered is slowly decreased. The TT is then able to be slowly lowered with minimal discomfort.

It must be emphasized that this description of dependence is simplistic and does not address the complex biochemical and physiological phenomena described below. There is also little evidence of a direct correlation between decreasing opiate levels and the appearance of specific withdrawal symptoms, suggesting the importance of interactions between psychological and physiological processes.

Animal-Human Correlates

The above model suggests that once dependence and tolerance develop, it is not a simple matter to stop drug-taking behavior. In fact, dependence, at times, may be perpetuated not only to obtain the positive reinforcement of euphoria but also to prevent the negative reinforcement of withdrawal. Although the problems associated with drug dependence in persons with chronic pain are well recognized, all too frequently this phenomenon is attributed more to psychological rather than to physiological causes. It is, therefore,

FIGURE 3.1. Development of Dependence and Tolerance with Repeated Drug Injection

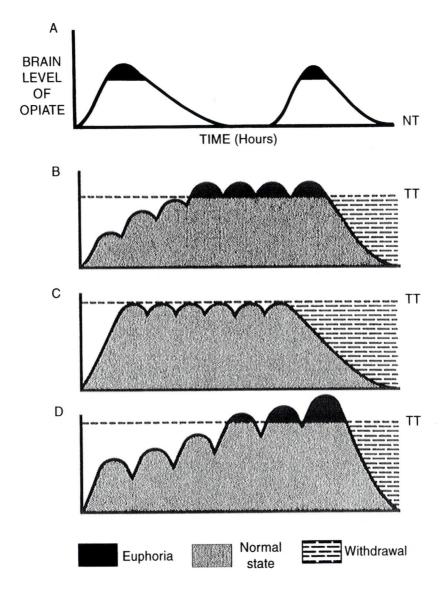

NT = Nontolerant; TT = Tolerant Threshold. Explanation in text.

quite instructive to review dependence, tolerance, and withdrawal in the animal model, moving from the laboratory to human behavior (Table 3.3).

Dependence

Narcotics readily produce dependence in laboratory animals and, once developed, will result in rats choosing morphine over water and self-administering the drug, even in the face of aversive stimuli.[7] Repeated administration of a narcotic for prolonged periods is not necessarily a prerequisite of dependence or withdrawal. Phenomena indicative of withdrawal can be precipitated by administering a narcotic antagonist one hour after a single dose of morphine in a laboratory animal.[8] Similarly, in humans, unequivocal physical abstinence phenomena can be precipitated by nalorphine injection after administration of analgesic doses of narcotics every six hours for as few as two to three days.[9] There is, however, an interval between injections of narcotics in which dependence and tolerance will not develop. In rats, this appears to be approximately 24 hours, whereas in human subjects perhaps two to three days.[9]

Once physical dependence develops, it need not persist for long periods to influence behavior. Rats previously made dependent, when narcotic free and offered a bitter tasting quinine solution, consume more solution than naive rats because of the prior association of bitterness with morphine reinforcement. Similarly, humans with a prior history of narcotic dependence, when expecting a narcotic effect, although receiving a placebo, will experience this effect.

The presence of anxiety or stress will facilitate the acquisition of drug dependence and, in the presence of a previously established dependence, necessitate an increasing dose of the narcotic to maintain homeostasis. In laboratory animals, the presence of anxiety facilitates self-injection. Clinically, the presence of anxiety will usually necessitate administration of large doses of narcotic agents to obtain relief from pain (Chapter 13).

Tolerance

The development of tolerance also will affect the self-administration of a drug, necessitating higher doses for a specific effect to be obtained. In laboratory animals, however, in the absence of adversive stimuli, self-administration of narcotics will increase for a period of time but then stabilize unless the animal is stressed.[10]

TABLE 3.3. Animal-Human Correlates of Narcotic Dependency

	Laboratory evidence	Clinical counterpart
Reinforcing qualities of narcotics	Selection of bitter tasting fluids in face of adverse stimuli	Precedence of narcotic-seeking behavior over all other forms of activity
	Choice of self-injection over food and water	
	Facilitating of self-injection by stress	Increased rate of narcotic and polydrug use with anxiety
		Acceptance into deviant subculture results in lessening of anxiety
Dependence and tolerance	Rapid development; some degree seen after 2-3 injections	Signs of dependence after maintenance of standard doses of analgesics for 2-3 days
	Self-injection stabilizes over 4-6 weeks once steady state tolerance develops	Object is euphoria rather than tolerance; dose constantly varies
	Persists in absence of narcotics for up to 12 months	Alteration of respiratory center to CO_2 for months postnarcotic state
Abstinence and withdrawal	Conditioned abstinence produced in narcotic-free state	Conditioned abstinence produced with saline injections
		Clinical signs of withdrawal develop in old environment even when narcotic free
	Persistence of physiologic signs associated with abstinence for 5 months postwithdrawal	Metabolic effects noted for up to 30 weeks postwithdrawal

Withdrawal (Abstinence Syndrome)

Physiological disturbances secondary to abstinence in the presence of narcotic dependence can be well demonstrated by the injection of a narcotic antagonist in both animals and humans. The intensity of the antagonist-induced withdrawal may not be related to either the degree of dependence or the dose of narcotic administered, but rather to the ability of the drug to bind to tissue sites and be slowly released back into the blood as blood levels fall. Methadone can produce considerable physical dependence as manifested by a rather prominent withdrawal reaction on injection of a narcotic antagonist. However, abrupt discontinuation of methadone is associated with a rather mild, although prolonged, abstinence syndrome. This is due to methadone being "a long-acting" analgesic agent, which is slowly released from the tissues. This property allows methadone to be an excellent drug for relieving chronic pain.

The appearance of withdrawal symptoms may be related not only to the actual physiologic effects of ceasing narcotic administration but can also be the result of conditioning. Narcotic-free rats will undergo withdrawal when placed in an environment previously associated with abstinence during physiologic withdrawal.[11] Monkeys that have been narcotic free for up to four months may experience withdrawal in response to a visual or auditory stimulus associated with the prior injection of a narcotic antagonist when dependent. Similar evidence of the conditioning effects of narcotics have been able to be demonstrated in humans by substituting saline injections for nalorphine in individuals with a prior history of narcotic dependence.[9,12] This phenomenon has been recognized by heroin addicts who, when narcotic free, experience withdrawal symptoms upon entering an environment where withdrawal had been previously experienced.

Withdrawal from narcotics, although most prominent in the first week to ten days subsequent to discontinuing the drug, may persist for a considerable time. Narcotic-dependent rats have exhibited signs of abstinence for as long as five months after withdrawal of morphine.[13] Rats will consume a significantly larger volume of morphine-containing solution as compared to control animals for up to one year after carbon dioxide have been shown to persist in up to 30 weeks postwithdrawal from a narcotic-dependent state.

BIOLOGY OF DEPENDENCE

Introduction

Numerous theories have been advanced to explain the phenomena of dependence, tolerance, and withdrawal (Table 3.4). Since the behavioral

TABLE 3.4. Pharmacologic Basis of Dependence and Tolerance

Activation of parallel biochemical systems

Disuse sensitization (denervation supersensitivity)

Alteration in neuroregulator function

Alteration in number of receptors

Opiate-specific neuronal kindling

Depression of cyclic AMP release

Alteration of neuronal membranes

aspects of opiate, sedative, and amphetamine dependence are quite similar, it is possible that common mechanisms may exist, although until quite recently, cross-tolerance had not been satisfactorily demonstrated among different classes of psychoactive agents. Evidence has now accumulated suggesting an interaction between narcotics and drugs in the alcohol-barbiturate group occur, most likely at the level of the opiate receptor.

In the laboratory setting, acute administration of alcohol will result in elevations of plasma endorphins similar to that seen with acute morphine administration. This rise can be prevented by administration of naloxone, a potent narcotic antagonist.[14] Naloxone has also been demonstrated to inhibit the development of alcohol dependence and diminish the central depressant effects not only of alcohol but also of toxic doses of benzodiazepines.[15,16]

These observations suggest the possibility of common receptor sites for dependency-producing drugs, allowing a hypothesis of a single model to explain the phenomena of dependence and tolerance. Some groups of drugs may share common receptor sites, whereas others might be associated with different sets of neuronal systems. It must be emphasized, however, that much more evidence is needed prior to an uncritical acceptance of these interactions. For those specifically interested in an explanation of the various theories of dependence and tolerance, a brief summary is provided below.

Cross-tolerance has been well established for the drugs within each group. As discussed earlier, each drug in each category in Table 3.2 is able to be interchanged with another drug in the same group after a suitable dose-adjustment is made. The following discussion of the biochemical models of dependence, however, will utilize the opiates as the prototype.

Alteration in Metabolic Pathways

One of the earliest theories to explain opiate dependence involved an alteration in biotransformation of narcotics with continued use. Metabolic tolerance could conceivably occur if administration of morphine was associated with stimulation of the hepatic enzyme systems responsible for its metabolism. The increased rate of biotransformation would require an increase in morphine dosage to obtain similar effects. Little or no evidence has been found, however, indicating significant differences in absorption, detoxification, or distribution between the dependent and naive animal.[17]

Cellular Adaptation

Cellular adaptation, secondary to changes in protein synthesis, has been postulated to be responsible for the development of tolerance. The administration of actinomycin D with morphine injections can prevent the development of dependence and tolerance in the laboratory animal.[18] If actinomycin D, however, is administered one hour subsequent to the morphine injection, tolerance is unaffected.

Redundancy

The redundance theory initially described by Martin[19] postulates the existence of functional systems with parallel pathways containing elements varying in sensitivity to morphine. Morphine-sensitive pathways may lie alongside resistant ones. Administration of morphine results in depression of the sensitive pathway with a compensatory hypertrophy of the second pathway associated with increased functioning. With time, this pathway may become tolerant to the drug effect. Removal of morphine results in the depressed pathway returning to its previous level of functioning, whereas the hypertrophied pathway continues to function at an increased level, resulting in the abstinence syndrome.

Disuse-Sensitization

The disuse-sensitization theory[20,21,22] is analogous to the phenomenon of denervation-supersensitivity observed in peripheral structures deprived of pharmacological input. Continuous morphine administration is accompanied by a depression of presynaptic release of excitatory neurotransmitters and a supersensitivity of postsynaptic receptors. Discontinuation of morphine is accompanied by restoration of presynaptic input and maintenance of postsynaptic hyperactivity, clinically manifested as withdrawal. This model may be able to explain the change in neurotransmitter and receptor activity as well as the specific biochemical alterations described below. However, evidence exists suggesting that hypersensitivity cannot solely account for dependence and abstinence. Certain drugs with considerable agonist actions do not uniformly result in dependence with chronic administration. In addition, the degree of hypersensitivity produced by pharmacologic denervation with potent neurotransmitter depleting agents is quite limited when compared to that seen with naloxone.

Opiate-Specific Neuronal Kindling

Villareal and Castro[23] have developed a model of dependence based on the known duality of morphine's ability to cause stimulation of certain brain areas and depression of others. Administration of morphine activates a pathway responsible for the observable acute opiate effects, such as analgesia, as well as a second pathway that results in a progressive development of sensitivity to specific "triggering" agents. This sensitivity through a "kindling" mechanism develops a progressive capacity to respond to certain agents that will result in an "explosive" release clinically manifested as withdrawal. The effects may be seen with (1) the use of a narcotic antagonist, (2) the administration of cholinesterase inhibitors, or (3) the termination of narcotic treatment. The ability of kindling mechanisms to remain intact may explain the precipitation of withdrawal phenomena by injection of a narcotic antagonist months after narcotic administration has been discontinued.

Neuroregulators

The role of neuroregulators in tolerance and dependence is being increasingly defined. Morphine may affect noradrenergic, dopaminergic, and cholinergic neurons (Chapter 2).

Noradrenergic Mechanisms

Norepinephrine neurons are found in greatest concentration in the locus coeruleus (LC). Opiate receptors have also been identified in high density in the LC and, when occupied by endogenous or exogenous opiates, are felt to be responsible for a selective decrease in firing of LC neurons with a subsequent decrease in noradrenergic activity. Chronic administration of morphine is associated with a diminished synthesis of endorphins. Abrupt morphine withdrawal is accompanied by a marked availability of receptor sites with an insufficient supply of endorphin, resulting in an increase in neuronal firing. This is followed by "rebound" secretion of norepinephrine, which is believed to be responsible for many of the symptoms seen during withdrawal. Naloxone can reverse the opiate-induced inhibition of LC firing but cannot by itself affect an increase in LC activity. It is of interest that clonidine, an alpha-2 noradrenergic antagonist used in hypertension, is also able to slow firing of LC cells, and is unaffected by the presence of morphine. This finding has led to the use of clonidine in alleviating the symptoms of withdrawal in humans being detoxified from narcotic drugs[24] (Chapter 6).

Dopaminergic Mechanisms

Measurements of serum prolactin, predominantly controlled by an inhibitory dopaminergic mechanism,[25,26] have been demonstrated to decrease during withdrawal, supporting the concept of underlying dopaminergic hyperactivity. Following alleviation of withdrawal symptoms, however, serum prolactin levels have not been found to return to base line, suggesting that although dopaminergic hyperactivity is present, it may not be related to withdrawal.[24,27]

Cholinergic Mechanisms

The surfeit theory advanced by Paton[28] relates the development of tolerance to morphine-induced depression of acetylcholine release at the terminal axons. This accumulation of acetylcholine increases until the actual fraction of transmitter released by subsequent nerve impulses is sufficient to overcome the morphine-induced blockage with resulting synaptic transmission. This may be manifested as tolerance. Increasing the morphine dose causes a further blockage necessitating another delay until sufficient acetylcholine accumulates. Discontinuing morphine results in the outpouring of accumulated acetylcholine manifested by the appearance of the withdrawal syndrome.

Serotonergic Mechanisms

The interactions of morphine with the serotonergic system are discussed in Chapters 2 and 6. Serotonin and its precursors have been specifically implicated in the development of the tolerance and dependence. Similarly, during naloxone-precipitated withdrawal, a marked sensitization to serotonin excitatory effects has been demonstrated.[29,30]

The Endogenous Opiate System

The isolation of enkephalins, dynorphines, and endorphins allows for the construction of additional models of dependence and tolerance (Chapter 2). In the basal state, binding to opiate receptors occurs, leaving a variable number of receptors unoccupied. Administration of morphine results in the binding of these remaining receptors with a potentiation of analgesic effect. With chronic morphine use, receptors are overloaded, resulting in free, extracellular morphine. This, in turn, activates a feedback loop to enkephalin and endorphin neurons, resulting in a diminished synthesis. At this point, since endogenous opiates are no longer available for binding, an increased binding of morphine occurs, clinically manifested as tolerance. When morphine is discontinued, the opiate receptors are exposed neither to morphine nor the endogenous opiates, resulting in the symptoms manifested as withdrawal.[31,32,33]

Alternatively, chronic morphine administration may induce an increase in activity of enzymes responsible for metabolizing the endogenous opiates. The decrease in available endogenous opiates might allow the receptors to become more available to morphine with subsequent dependence and tolerance. On withdrawal of the drug, the drop in endogenous opiate levels secondary to avid receptor binding might result in the abstinence syndrome. Although these hypotheses are quite attractive, it should be noted that alterations in enkephalin or endorphin levels have only been variably demonstrated in the brains of rats chronically exposed to morphine. However, improvement of withdrawal symptoms in humans has been reported following intravenous administration of 4 mg of endorphin.[34] Subjective symptoms due to endorphin injection subsided within minutes, whereas withdrawal symptoms were relieved for days. This observation further strengthens the possible role played by endorphins in dependence and tolerance.

Receptor Theory

Identification of opiate receptor sites (Chapter 2) has resulted in the hypotheses of several receptor theories of dependence. Chronic morphine administration associated with decrease release of neuroregulators has been proposed by Collier to be accompanied by the appearance of new receptors.[35] As the total receptor number is increased, function is maintained despite reduced levels of neuroregulators through morphine binding. Discontinuing morphine results in a loss of spare receptors, accompanied by a sudden release of accumulated neurotransmitters manifested as withdrawal. Although this hypothesis is attractive, other investigators have been unable to document changes in either receptor affinity or number of opiate-binding sites.

Alterations in Cyclic AMP

The administration of morphine has been shown to decrease cyclic AMP (cAMP) levels as well as to prevent the increase in cAMP usually seen with administration of prostaglandins. Morphine may also inhibit adenylate cyclase activity, the enzyme responsible for the synthesis of cAMP. With continued administration of morphine, the decreased level of cAMP slowly returns to normal, as does adenylate cyclase activity.[36] When these cells are placed in a drug-free medium, a marked overproduction of cAMP occurs. In laboratory animals accumulation of cAMP is associated with withdrawal. Administration of phosphodiesterase inhibitors to naive animals also results in an accumulation of cAMP. This, in turn, is associated with the appearance of symptoms closely resembling those seen during opiate withdrawal. The interaction between morphine and these neurotransmitters may also affect the development of tolerance and dependence. Just as the effects of morphine on cAMP can be blocked with the narcotic antagonist naloxone, the effects of norepinephrine and acetylcholine may be reversed by alpha blockers such as phentolamine or by atropine.[37]

Alterations in Neuronal Membranes

Alterations in neuronal membrane permeability have been associated with withdrawal syndromes. Changes in membrane permeability to Na^+, Ca^{2+} occur following opiate administration. Discontinuing opiate administration may result in an alteration of resting membrane potentials accompanied by a nonspecific hyperexcitability, clinically manifested as withdrawal.[38] Ionic change, however, although a concomitant of dependence and withdrawal, is probably in response to other existing biochemical alterations rather than being specifically responsible for development of dependence or abstinence.

SUMMARY

Recent advances in radioimmunoassay and neurochemical techniques have allowed for a clearer concept of the biochemical model of dependence. It should be emphasized, however, that no one model has been able to be conclusively shown to be solely responsible, and it is more than likely that these phenomena are explicable through an interaction of several models that have been presented.

More important than defining the precise mechanism by which dependence develops, however, is the realization that dependence in and of itself is

TABLE 3.5. Characteristics of Addictive Behavior Compared to Medical Dependence

	Addiction	Medical dependence
Primary Purpose	Euphoria (high)	Relief of pain
Dose and Frequency	Rapid dose escalates at increasingly frequent intervals as tolerance rapidly develops	Constant dose and frequency with slow incremental increases as tolerance develops
Ability to Discontinue Drug	Abstinence unlikely to be maintained despite frequent attempts	Can usually abruptly discontinue drug or if withdrawal occurs, successfully manage medically, with minimal discomfort
Functioning	Frequent periods of intoxification	Able to function productively; In acute pain states slight sedation effect may occur
Behavior	Focus on drug seeking to the exclusion of other socially productive activities	Able to engage in productive activity due to relief of pain
Side Effects	Common due to dose and way of administration; Continued administration despite complications	Mild. If present, can be adequately addressed
Polydrug Use	Frequent	Rare unless prescribed by physician

not to be avoided in the presence of either acute or chronic pain of defined origin. The characteristics of this dependence differ markedly from those observed in the presence of addictive behaviors (Table 3.5). The primary goal in the presence of pain is its relief and, with respect to chronic pain, to restore function. As will be described in subsequent chapters, when this is done appropriately, dependence is not an issue of importance.

REFERENCES

1. Marks RM, Sachar EJ. Undertreatment of medical inpatients with narcotic analgesics. *Ann Intern Med,* 1973, 78:173–181.

2. Odin RV. Acute postoperative pain: Incidence, severity, and the etiology of inadequate treatment. *Anesthesiol Clin of North Am,* 1984, 7:1–15.

3. American Pain Society, Committee on Quality Assurance Standards. *Quality assurance standards for relief of acute pain and cancer pain.* Amsterdam: Elsevier, 1990: 352–354.

4. Ferrell BR, Rhiner M. Hightech comfort. Ethical issues in cancer pain management for the 1990s. *J Clin Ethics,* 1991, 2:108–15.

5. WHO Expert Committee on Addition Producing Drugs. *WHO Tech Rep Ser,* 1967, 407:6.

6. Goldstein A. The pharmacologic basis of methadone therapy. In: *Proceedings of the Fourth National Conference on Methadone Treatment.* New York: National Association on Prevention of Addiction to Narcotics, 1972:27–32.

7. Stolerman IPL, Kumar R. Regulation of drug and water intake in rats dependent on morphine. *Psychopharmacologia,* 1972, 26:19–28.

8. Wikler A, Carter RL. Effects of single doses of N-allylnormorphine on hindlimb reflexes of chronic spinal dogs during cycles of morphine addiction. *J Pharmacol Exp Ther,* 1953, 109:92–101.

9. Wikler A, Fraser HF, Isbell H. N-allylnormorphine: Effects of single doses and precipitation of acute "abstinence syndrome" during addiction to morphine, methadone or heroin in man (post-addicts). *J Pharmacol Exp Ther,* 1953, 109:8–20.

10. Deneau G, Yangita T, Seevers MH. Self-administration of psychoactive substances in the monkey. *Psychopharmacologia,* 1969, 16:30–48.

11. Wikler A, Pescor FT. Classical conditioning of a morphine abstinence phenomenon, reinforcement of opioid-drinking behavior and "relapse" in morphine-addicted rats. *Psychopharmacologia,* 1967, 10:255–284.

12. Wikler A. Dynamics of drug dependence: Implications of a conditioning theory for research and treatment. In: Fisher S, Freedman AM (eds). *Opiate addictions: Origins and treatment.* New York: Winston & Sons, 1973:7–21.

13. Wikler A, Pescor FT. Persistence of "relapse-tendencies" of rats previously made physically dependent on morphine. *Psychopharmacologia,* 1970, 16:375–384.

14. Ho AKS, Allen JP. Alcohol and the opiate receptor: Interactions with the endogenous opiates. *Adv Alcohol Substance Abuse,* 1981, 1:53–75.

15. Litten RZ, Allen JP. Pharmacotherapies for alcoholism: Promising agents and clinical issues. *Alcoholism: Clin and Exp Res,* 1991, 15:620–633.

16. Bell EF. The use of naloxone in the treatment of diazepam poisoning. *J Pediatr,* 1975, 87:803–804.

17. Dole V. The biochemistry of addiction. *Ann Rev Biochem,* 1970, 39:821–840.

18. Cohen M, Keats AS, Krivoy M, Ungar, G. Effect of actinomycin D on morphine tolerance. *Proc Soc Exp Biol Med,* 1965, 119:381–384.

19. Martin, WR. Pharmacological redundancy as an adaptive mechanism in the central nervous system. *Fed Proc,* 1970, 29:13–18.

20. Collier HOJ. A general theory of the genesis of drug dependence by induction of receptors. *Nature,* 1965, 205:181–182.

21. Collier HOJ. Supersensitivity and dependence. *Nature,* 1968, 220:228–231.

22. Jaffe JH, Sharpless SK. XVII. Pharmacological denervation supersensitivity in the central nervous system: A theory of physical dependence. *Res Publ Assoc Res Nerv Ment Dis,* 1968, 46:226–246.

23. Villarreal JE, Castro A. A reformulation of the dual action model of opioid dependence: Opioid-specific neuronal kindling. In: Beers RF, Jr, Bassett EG (eds). *Mechanisms of pain and analgesic compounds.* New York: Raven Press, 1979: 407–428.

24. Gold MS. Opiate addiction and locus coeruleus. *Psychiat Clinics North Am,* 1993, 16:61–73.

25. Ary M, Cox B, Lomax, P. Dopaminergic mechanisms in precipitated withdrawal in morphine-dependent rats. *J Pharmacol Exp Ther,* 1977, 200:271–276.

26. Lal H, Hynes MD. Effectiveness of butyrophenones and related drugs in narcotic withdrawal. In: Denker P, Thomas CR, Villeneuve D, Barnet-LaCroix D, Aarcin F (eds). *Neuropsychopharmacology.* Elmsford, New York: 1978:289–295.

27. Clemens JA, Smalstig EB, Sawyer BD. Antipsychotic drugs stimulate prolactin release. *Psychopharmacologia,* 1974, 40:123–127.

28. Paton WDM. A pharmacological approach to drug dependence and drug tolerance. In: Steinberg A (ed). *Scientific basis of drug dependence.* London: Churchill, 1969: 31–47.

29. Ho IK, Loh HL, Way EL. Influence of 5,6-dihydroxy tryptamine on morphine tolerance and physical dependence. *Eur J Pharmacol,* 1973, 21:331–336.

30. Schulz R, Herz A. Naloxone precipitated withdrawal reveals sensitization to neurotransmitters in morphine tolerant/dependent rats. *Naunyn Schmiedebergs Arch Pharmacol,* 1977, 299:95–99.

31. Simon EJ. Opiate receptors and endorphins: Possible relevance to narcotic addiction. *Adv Alcohol Substance Abuse,* 1981, 1:13–31.

32. Gold M, Miller MS. Seeking drugs/alcohol and avoiding withdrawal. *Psychiat Annal,* 1992, 33:430–435.

33. Malfroy B, Swerts JP, Guyon A, Roques BP, Schwartz JC. High-affinity enkephalin-degrading peptidase in brain is increased after morphine. *Nature,* 1978, 276:523–526.

34. Su CY, Lin SH, Wang YT, Li CH, Hung LH, Lin CS, Lin BC. Effects of beta endorphin on narcotic abstinence syndrome in man. *J Formos Med Assoc,* 1978, 77: 133–141.

35. Collier HOJ. A general theory of the genesis of drug dependence by induction of receptors. *Nature,* 1965, 205:181–182.

36. Snyder SH. Receptors, neurotransmitters and drug responses. *N Engl J Med,* 1979, 300:465–472.

37. Nathanson NM, Klein WL, Nirenberg M. Regulation of adenylate cyclase activity mediated by muscarinic acetylcholine receptors. *Proc Natl Acad Sci USA*, 1978, 75:1788–1791.

38. Johnson SM, Westfall DP, Howard SA, Fleming WW. Sensitivities of the isolated ileal longitudinal smooth muscle-myenteric plexus and hypogastric nerve-vas deferens of the guinea pig after chronic morphine pellet implantation. *J Pharmacol Exp Ther,* 1978, 204:54–66.

Chapter 4

The Effects of Emotion on Pain

INTRODUCTION

In the preceding chapters, the neurophysiological correlates of pain have been reviewed. Pain initiated by noxious stimuli activates peripheral nociceptors, with subsequent transmission through afferent systems. Transmission often can be modulated by accompanying afferent sensations or by centrally initiated activation of descending pathways. In fact, however, our reaction to pain is much more complex. Noxious stimuli may be present without pain being experienced and, similarly, elimination of the stimulus may not be followed by alleviation of pain. Pain may also exist in situations where no apparent stimuli can be detected or may persist long after the tissue injury has resolved and the offending stimulus removed.

The definitions of pain that are found in the literature are almost as numerous as those investigating this phenomenon.[1,2] Unfortunately, most definitions are really less than adequate in providing either physician or patient with the ability to understand and analyze the series of events occurring within a person that result in the expression of pain. The need to critically analyze the painful experience is extremely important. In daily practice it is all too common to make a quick decision as to whether the pain is organic or "psychogenic," with the relegation of this latter group to benign neglect or psychiatric referral. A person in pain is often made to feel that his or her suffering is excessive and not to be taken too seriously. In fact, the physiological basis of pain cannot easily be separated from the psychological. This must be remembered if pain is to be effectively managed.

The psychologic dimensions of pain are quite complex and the literature addressing this subject voluminous. The model presented, therefore, is meant to be neither overly detailed nor comprehensive. The objective is to provide a better understanding of the psychological factors surrounding the pain experience so that a rational approach may be developed toward its management.

THE IMMEDIATE RESPONSE TO PAIN

Almost simultaneously with a noxious sensory input, energy is directed toward survival or to removal of the noxious stimuli as rapidly as possible.[3] This is most prominent in acute pain and can be of sufficient intensity to suppress its immediate perception. This phenomenon has been observed in both animals and humans. Initially, a wounded animal's main concern is flight. It will run long distances apparently unaware of a wound until the distance between itself and the hunter is sufficient so as to preclude the possibility of further injury.

Beecher,[4,5] in a classic study, demonstrated the importance of the circumstances of an injury in determining the response to painful events. Of 215 men suffering serious battle wounds, only 25 percent were in sufficient pain to request a narcotic. A comparative survey of civilians found 80 percent with similar wounds to promptly a request medication. Beecher attributed the difference in reaction to the emotional significance of the wound, assuming that the soldiers recognized this as their "ticket home" and were so relieved that the actual experience of pain was not paramount. Another more probable interpretation was the primary concern to be immediately removed from the battlefield so as not to suffer additional injuries. Their energies focused on this need for removal rather than the extent of the injuries. In contrast, mild injuries may often give rise to an expression of anger prior to the actual perception of a painful sensation. Once the noxious stimulus has been terminated, the immediate anger subsides, and attention is then directed toward alleviating the pain.

PSYCHODYNAMIC CONSTRUCTS OF PAIN

Freud readily recognized the role of the psyche in the perception of pain. He described pain as occurring when a stimulus breaks through the body's "protective shield" and continuously acts on the sensory system.[6] This is associated with a "narcissistic cathexis" or attachment of psychic energy to the site of the pain at the expense of withdrawing energy from other areas of ego function. Anticipating Beecher's findings by decades, Freud observed the psychic influence of pain to be of such magnitude that at times, even the "most intense pain failed to arouse." At the same time, the focusing of psychic energy can be so great that the pain may persist independent of the initial stimulus.

The continued response to pain is then modified by an interplay of psychic energies, which in turn effect behavior. A slow transition occurs from the actual physical pain to the "mental pain." In such settings, pain may become a conversion symptom perhaps initiated somatically but extended and maintained by an existing neurosis.[7] Within this psychodynamic construct, the experience of pain is modified by the basic drives of sexuality, aggression, and dependency. Physicians caring for patients in chronic pain are well aware of the emphasis placed on the description of the pain. On occasion, the pain itself may be sufficiently stimulating so that attempts to relieve it are delayed until the last moment. Alternatively, the abuse of narcotic analgesics can produce a degree of sedation or euphoria that may serve as an outlet for sexual energy, thereby relieving anxiety over disinterest or an inadequate sexual performance.

The behavioral manifestations of aggression and hostility in chronic pain patients are well known and serve to fulfill permanent feelings of dependency that frequently result in both aggressive and regressive behaviors. This gratification of unconscious dependent needs, as discussed below, serves as a powerful reinforcer and must be addressed when developing a therapeutic approach to an individual in chronic pain. The conversion of anger into pain occurs quite frequently, often facilitated by the physician implying the absence of an organic basis. A study of the relationship of pain to anger in persons attending a pain clinic and those with pain in an ambulatory care setting, found the former group to be more likely to show hypochondriasis and affective disorders.[8] This phenomena is also frequently observed in emergency rooms where a person's anger over waiting for long periods is often accompanied by an intensity in the pain experienced.

ANXIETY AND PAIN

Numerous studies have documented the interaction between anxiety and pain.[9-16] Their findings can be summed up by observation that the presence of anxiety not only increases the intensity of the pain but, in addition, will result in a larger dose of analgesic to provide relief. In contrast, relief of anxiety with nonpharmacologic means by reassurance, adequate explanations, and other support is associated with a decreased need for analgesia and, in hospitalized patients, a shortened stay. The importance of addressing anxiety in the management of both acute and chronic pain is obvious yet all to often neglected (Chapters 13 and 14).

CONDITIONING EFFECTS
AND THE PERPETUATION OF PAIN

Acute pain initiated by a nociceptive stimulus sets into motion a series of events ultimately culminating in a reaction to the stimulus. Usually, the initial responses are reflexive or involuntary, mediated by the autonomic nervous system. This type of reaction is termed respondent pain.[17] Persistence of a stimulus, however, initiates voluntary reactions termed operant behavior. This behavior is often followed by repetitive responses reactive to the environment. In terms of behavioral theory, repetitive operant behavior and subsequent reinforcement may lead to recurrence of the behavior even in the absence of the initial nociceptive stimulus.[18] This is called operant pain. Respondent pain, seen in acute injury, if not managed effectively and expeditiously, may be replaced by operant pain.

In chronic pain of undocumented etiology, operant behavior dominates. Although many react to chronic pain associated with a loss of autonomy and ability to function with a deepening depression, others, paradoxically, may find that this state stabilizes or even relieves anxiety. At this point, conditioned reinforcement has occurred. There are also number of other reinforcers that serve to maintain operant behavior. The use of analgesics on an as needed (PRN) basis with accompanying sedation and occasional euphoria can become a potent reinforcer and, in the presence of physical dependence, can provide physiologic reinforcement as well. The constant attention that family members direct toward relief of suffering by providing continuous care enhances secondary gain, and thus reinforces maintaining the disability. With chronic pain, especially of unclear etiology, frequently a regression occurs in which the adult assumes the role of the child, thus requiring constant attention and support. And, as with the child, when this is not forthcoming from either family or physician, anger erupts.

Economic incentives may also be important reinforcers. Continued payment of medical disability insurance provides a powerful incentive toward remaining unable to work. This is especially true when payment is commensurate with or greater than the expected income after the disability has subsided. The limitation of functioning also allows avoidance of behavior that may be anxiety producing or otherwise unpleasant. Expressed in the simplest terms, if one is unable to work one cannot be pressured into obtaining a job. Similarly, if one is constantly distracted by chronic pain or the sedative effects of drugs, attention is diverted from the need to be an active participant in family life. All these factors may play a role in modifying the response to chronic pain and in preventing success with any therapeutic endeavor.

SUGGESTION AND PAIN:
THE ROLE OF THE PLACEBO

Suggestion frequently determines a person's response to pain. This phenomenon is best illustrated by the placebo effect. A placebo is any therapy deliberately used for a nonspecific psychologic or psychophysiologic effect but that is devoid of any specific activity for the condition being treated.[19] The placebo effect is, therefore, unrelated to any specific properties of the therapy administered. The response is affected by (a) the specific personality, beliefs, and expectations of the patient; (b) the beliefs and expectations of the physician; and (c) the quality of the physician-patient interaction. Although the response to a placebo is usually subjective, at times it may be able to be quantified with documentation of actual physiologic changes. It should be emphasized that at one time or another many therapies thought to be medically efficacious are now known to have been, in reality, placebos.

Although many studies have attempted to define the personality of those who obtain relief from placebos, the findings have been quite variable and inconsistent.[20,21] Most persons have the ability to respond to a placebo at least once with little evidence that subsequent responses would be equally effective. There are, however, some factors consistently associated with a positive placebo response. Since anxiety frequently accompanies pain, it is not surprising that the placebo effect may be most prominent in painful conditions. Beecher demonstrated that as many as 35 percent of persons given a placebo for relief of organic pain were able to obtain relief, with a direct relationship noted between anxiety level and relief obtained.[22] For this reason, a placebo is frequently much more effective for the relief of clinical pain compared to pain induced in the laboratory setting.[22] Similarly, although morphine on the clinical setting is an extremely effective analgesic when given in the laboratory setting, it may often be indistinguishable from a saline placebo.

The severity and the type of pain has also been found to influence the placebo response. Placebos may be half as effective as morphine for quick relief of pain, with the effectiveness being directly proportional to the severity of pain experienced. Persons reporting a low level of postoperative pain prior to placebo administration have been found less likely to obtain relief than those patients who reported higher initial pain levels.[23,24] Impressive response rates to placebos or inactive drugs can be found in chronic as well as acute pain states, in both the presence or absence of organic disease. A study of 288 patients with cancer found half to receive pain relief from placebo medication.[21] Similarly, a study of relief of angina in over 1,000 patients, found 85 percent to have achieved subjective relief of symptoms from drugs proven to be ineffective.[25]

Suggestion is probably most important in effecting the placebo response, just as the efficacy of active analgesics can be diminished following physician suggestion of their ineffectiveness. A study of 500 dental patients found that those receiving placebo accompanied by the suggestion that pain relief would occur reported less discomfort than those persons given either a placebo without this suggestion or even the actual anesthetic without prior instructions as to the expected effect.[26]

When described by the physician as powerful drugs or when given by injection rather than by mouth, relief with placebos increases. When administered with an active analgesic, they are often found to enhance analgesia.[27]

At times, the placebo effect may be of sufficient intensity to allow subjects to exhibit not only relief from pain but also experience suggested side effects. A study of placebo responders with pain due to cancer found these patients to experience a greater incidence of central nervous system side effects than did nonresponders.[21] A most impressive illustration of the power of suggestion occurred when patients suffering from vomiting and nausea were actually able to obtain relief with the ingestion of ipecac, a potent emetic.[28]

Finally, it should be noted that the identification of the endogenous opiates has allowed yet another link to be drawn between psychologic and physiologic phenomena. Naloxone, a pure opiate antagonist, has been demonstrated to be an effective binder of opiate receptors, displacing synthetic narcotics from these sites (Chapters 2 and 7). Naloxone has been shown to be able to block placebo analgesia, suggesting that the response to placebos may be mediated by endogenous opioids.[29]

The use of placebos by physicians has always been controversial. Why would a physician prescribe a placebo instead of a pharmacologically active substance to provide relief? Spiro addresses this in a most thoughtful way, describing how a placebo may be prescribed as: (a) a "gift" to relieve a person with no observable cause of pain yet, is clearly dysfunctional due to discomfort and anxiety; (b) a challenge to prove to him or herself that, in fact, the patient has no discernable organic cause for pain and therefore, no need for further evaluation; or (c) a means of removing a demanding or angry patient from the office.[30]

The risks to a physician from prescribing a placebo, despite well-meaning intentions, are many. Most important is the image of the patient in the mind of the physician as not having organic based pain. Should the pain return or become of increased intensity, the physician may feel that only reassurance or additional placebos are necessary. If the person responds to the placebo, which can occur in the presence of organic based pain, the physician may well be deluded into thinking that the pain is purely psychogenic, allowing an undetected disease process to progress. The success of a placebo response may be the first step in a physician's feeling that subsequent complaints may also not be a cause for concern. Finally, even when a placebo is successful and the patient duly appreciative, if this deception is realized, there will most likely be a severe rupture in the physician/patient relationship accompanied by a loss of trust.

In summary, the placebo response may frequently be responsible for relief of pain. Since many patients will respond one time or another to a placebo, and since this response does not indicate the absence of organic pain, the use of placebos by physicians to separate organic from psychogenic pain is unwarranted. In addition, the deliberate deception on the part of the physician in knowingly prescribing placebos does not allow their use in the ethical practice of medicine. This subject is reviewed again in Chapter 13.

DEMOGRAPHIC CHARACTERISTICS OF PAIN

A large number of studies have been published attempting to correlate reaction to pain with age, sex, personality type, and social and cultural background.[27,31-39] It is difficult to generalize from these surveys due to the diverse experiences of both subjects and investigators. The findings summarized below must, therefore, be viewed cautiously.

In general, women have been found to be somewhat overrepresented in surveys relating to painful states[31-34] and to be more likely to be given potent analgesics. These findings, however, may be related to the stereotypical beliefs concerning men's stoicism by both physicians and patients.[35] The elderly's response to pain has been reported to be somewhat altered (Chapter 16). Whether this is due to an actual change in pain threshold, to altered receptor activity, or to greater reluctance to label a stimulus as pain, remains to be determined.[36] It remains unclear whether there is a decreased need for analgesics, a greater sensitivity to a drug's effect, or, more than likely, the reluctance on the part of physicians to provide potent analgesia for fear of undesired side effects.

Several studies have attempted to document cultural or racial differences in reaction to acute pain. In general, the findings are conflicting and probably have little clinical relevance for an individual patient. Cultural constructs, however, can be important in the response to chronic pain. This may be especially true with respect to cultural biases that may exist among those responsible for relieving pain, namely nurses and physicians. A study of 4,000 nurses from 13 different countries revealed many differences in their perceptions of suffering and the actual experience of pain, based on their own, as well as their patients' backgrounds.[36] This study found that nurses in general, feel that persons from lower socioeconomic groups suffer more than those from more affluent states, with Jewish and Hispanic patients suffering the most, and Asian and Anglo Saxon the least. Black and Puerto Rican nurses were found to infer psychologic distress, rather than actual pain, regardless of the patient's cultural origins. Israeli nurses were found to infer relatively low levels of psychological distress and physical pain. English, American, and Belgian nurses expressed the lowest inference of organic-based pain. All of these feelings, whether valid or not, diminish the chances of the pain returning.[38,39]

PSYCHOGENIC PAIN

Attribution of pain to the purely psychogenic realm is unfortunately all too frequent when a discernible organic etiology is not readily apparent. This is not without considerable risk, as the physician may often miss a critical sign of serious organic disease. Under certain conditions, however, psychologic factors may clearly predominate and in some instances be the only discernible etiology.

The American Psychiatric Association has recognized the existence of the Somatoform Pain Disorder.[40] This state is defined by a preoccupation with pain in the absence of adequate physical findings to account either for the pain or its intensity. This diagnosis is made in the presence of: (1) a preoccupation with the painful state for at least six months without either organic pathology or an explicable pathophysiologic mechanism; or (2) the presence of organic pathology accompanied by an intensity of pain, resulting in impairment in excess of what would be expected. Although these criteria are clearly stated pragmatically, a "gray zone" exists that makes it hazardous to assume that a person's pain is due to purely psychogenic pain.

It is a common occurrence that psychologic conditions may accentuate organic pain. Such pain must be completely explored and defined. In fact, the emotional changes observed may result from the debilitation caused by the pain. To try to qualitatively assess whether an individual's experience of pain, in the face of a known organic lesion, is capable of producing the intensity of pain experienced is exceptionally hazardous and often followed by a failure in the physician/patient relationship. In the presence of any observable disorder, the patient should always be given the benefit of the doubt.

Although predominant "psychogenically" determined pain does have considerably different characteristics compared to predominant organic pain (Table 4.1), it is unusual clinically to find a symptom complex that allows for a clear separation.[39,41] In addition, pain of purely psychogenic origin may, in fact, be responsible for the initiation of somatic mechanisms, such as tension headaches, skeletal muscle spasm, and visceral dysfunction. This results in the perpetuation of symptoms originating from both psychologic and somatic components.

Psychological Testing

A considerable body of literature has accumulated in an attempt to identify those individuals with predominantly psychologic pain. Studies have reviewed the presence of abnormal findings on psychological tests and psychiatric interviews in patients with pain.[27] Administration of the Minnesota Multiphasic Personality Inventory (MMPI) to patients with pain believed to be of psychogenic origin, as well as to individuals with organic lesions whose expression of pain was greater than could be expected, was able to define different profiles associated with "excessive" pain perception.[39] Similar attempts have been made to identify predisposition toward psychogenic pain in individuals who are field dependent ver-

TABLE 4.1. Characteristics Between Predominantly Physically Determined and Psychogenically Determined Pain

	Physical pain	Psychogenic pain
Onset	Usually but not always clear-cut	Can often be related to a life event rather than specific physical endeavor
Site	Usually localized to area of demonstrated pathology	Ill-defined—may crossover areas of anatomical neuronal distribution
Characteristics	Well-described	Ill-defined—subjective symtoms often considerably greater than objective findings
Aggravating factors	Able to be localized— movement pressure most common	Ill-defined—intensity may increase over wide range of stimuli. Anxiety most commonly associated with increased intensity
Relieving factors	Analgesics, physical therapy	Analgesics often ineffective. Psychotropic drugs, alcohol often pain refractory to all treatment
Psychologic factors	Often secondary, appearing after symptoms	Usually identifiable prior to onset of symptoms

sus field nondependent, extroverted versus introverted, augmenters versus reducers, sensitizers versus repressors, and copers versus avoiders.

There have been many attempts to quantitate personality attributes associated with chronic pain that have led to the development of canonical correlation analysis and somatic input.[41-43] In the opinion of this author, the clinical relevance of the information obtained from all of these studies remains less than clear. Although psychological testing may be of some use in predicting the degree of response to various invasive procedures,[44] it should not be used as the sole indication of psychogenic pain as, clinically, the dichotomy between psychogenic and organic pain is more apparent than real.

Preexisting Disorders

The preexistence of certain neurotic traits has been known to be associated with the ability of psychogenic pain to exert a considerable influence on the intensity of pain experienced. As discussed above, anxiety will heighten levels of experienced pain with techniques designed to decrease anxiety, resulting in a diminished pain perception and decreased need for analgesic drugs.[45-47]

Depression

An association between depression and purely psychogenic pain has not been consistently demonstrated, although depressed persons may feel pain more severely.[48] The presence of chronic pain is frequently associated with the appearance of depression or the deepening of depression in a previously depressed individual varying in duration and severity. The causal relationships between pain and depression, however, remain controversial. Although some feel that depression may be the etiologic antecedent of pain, others have found the pain may appear in the place of anxiety and depression, being present less frequently in depression.[41,49-51]

Clinically, it is important to identify those persons in whom depression may be a major component of a pain response. In such individuals, even in the presence of organic pain, antidepressants may be of considerable value. Similarly, if the course of pain is determined and adequately treated, the depression is frequently alleviated.

Hysteria and Hypochondriasis

Hypochondriacal neurosis may be a frequent companion to pain. These neuroses may take the form of irrational fears (phobias) or undue concerns over the presence of actual disease. Mild discomforts are often experienced as severe pain accompanied by a certainty on the part of the patient that a severe disabling disease is present. Alternatively, in a case of somatic hypochondriasis, the fixation on the pain may be unaccompanied by anxiety. In such instances, the patient can focus on the pain in great detail, allowing this symptom to become the center of his or her feelings while being relatively anxiety free with respect to other areas of function.

Hysteria is also frequently associated with pain. Hysterics tend to tolerate pain poorly and characteristically exaggerate their response in the desire to obtain attention. Conversion reactions are common with the person focusing all of his or her energy on the pain and its effects. Denial, either in the form of a lack of concern over the actual illness or an unawareness of any contributing personal problems, frequently occurs. The anxiety becomes totally focused on the existing symptom and its accompanying disability.

Engel has described a cohort of patients with chronic disabling pain in the absence of any detectable lesion who share the common characteristic of guilt.[50] Such persons are unable to tolerate success and frequently enter destructive interpersonal relationships. Surprisingly, at such times, their response to pain is minimal. When their life setting improves, painful symptoms recur, once again accompanied by feelings of guilt, which are relieved by the punishment of pain.

Psychosis

In the presence of a psychosis, pain may be experienced as part of the delusional state accompanied, at times, by the existence of a specific though imagined condition. However, in general, persons with psychosis, such as schizophrenia, often have a diminished pain sensitivity and an elevation of their pain threshold. Depression as part of a psychosis may also be seen in patients complaining of pain as a primary symptom. This may occur as a hypochondriacal delusion of a magnitude to obscure other psychotic symptoms or may be readily apparent if the symptoms are attributable to ill-defined external forces. At times, hypochondriacal pain may be an early psychotic symptom indicating a less severe psychosis as the patient is able to express a more socially acceptable symptom rather than a dissociative state.

Psychotherapeutic Approaches

There are a number of psychotherapeutic and psychosocial approaches to the management of pain (Table 4.2). The choice of one or more will depend on the etiology of the pain as well as the contribution of the

TABLE 4.2. Pychotherapeutic Approaches to Pain

Behavior modification
Biofeedback
Distraction and reframing
Family and couple therapies
Hypnosis
Psychodynamic-oriented therapy
Therapeutic communities

functional component.[52,53] More often than not a physician may use several techniques when caring for a patient. For all in pain, however, the physician must take the time to explain the pathophysiology of the pain in language clearly understandable. The reasons for prescribing specific medications and their side effects, the probable need to adjust the dose prior to obtaining satisfactory relief, and stating that complete relief cannot always be obtained with chronic pain, provide an understanding that in itself may be therapeutic. Regardless of the psychotherapeutic approach selected, concurrent analgesic therapy is often quite helpful.

SUMMARY

Considering the difficulties inherent in separating psychogenic from organic-based pain, it is important that each person who is in pain have a careful comprehensive needs assessment (Table 4.3). This should begin with a complete medical examination including appropriate laboratory procedures to aid in identification of organic disease. It is important to determine the degree to which the observed pathology is explained by the presenting symptoms. Pain is a multidimensional experience consisting of both sensory and affective components. If, however, the patient's response to the pain greatly exceeds that expected or if the abnormality found is inconsistent with the symptoms, psychological factors may be a predominate role.

In such instances, the events preceding or surrounding the initiation of symptoms should be carefully reviewed. The extent to which these symptoms have interfered with functioning and the patient's response to these limitations is also quite important in understanding the pain response and will be addressed in the section dealing with the practical management of pain.

However, regardless of an underlying neurosis, it is often exceedingly difficult to separate, with certainty, psychogenic from organic pain. It has

TABLE 4.3. Assessment of Influence of Psychogenic Factors in Pain Response

Comprehensive medical examination with appropriate laboratory determinations

Correlation between symptoms and documented pathology

Relevant life events surrounding onset of symptoms

Extent to which symptoms have interfered with function

been suggested that with any given complaint of pain the chances are approximately equal that the symptoms may be either physically or psychologically determined. Indeed, with the recent rapid advances in neurochemistry, perhaps the physiologic basis of psychogenic pain will be able to be demonstrated. It is, therefore, quite important to be aware of the effects of emotion on pain as well as the need to integrate both psychological and physical responses into a treatment plan to provide effective analgesia.

REFERENCES

1. Sternbach RA. *Pain: A psychophysiological analysis.* New York: Academic Press, 1968.

2. Melzack R, Loeser JD. Phantom body pain in paraplegics: Evidence for a central "pattern generating mechanism" for pain. *Pain,* 1978, 4:195–210.

3. Chapman CR. Psychological aspects of pain patient treatment. *Arch Surg,* 1977, 112:767–772.

4. Beecher HK. *Measurement of subjective responses: Quantitative effects of drugs.* New York: Oxford University Press, 1959.

5. Beecher HK. Relationship of significance of wound to pain experienced. *JAMA,* 1956, 161:1609–1613.

6. Strachy A, Tyson A. *The standard edition of the complete psychological works of Sigmund Freud.* London: Hogarth Press, 1973.

7. Freud S, Breuer J. *Studies on Hysteria.* New York: Basic Books, 1982.

8. Pilowsky I. Psychodynamic aspects of the pain experience. In: Sternbach RA (ed.). *The Psychology of Pain.* New York: Raven Press, 1978:203–217.

9. Mason JW, Sachar EJ, Fishman JR, Hamburg DA, Handlon JH. Corticosteroid responses to hospital admission. *Arch Gen Psychiatry,* 1965, 13:1–8.

10. Fleischman AI, Bierenbaum ML, Stier A. Effect of stress due to anticipated minor surgery upon in vivo platelet aggregation in humans. *J Human Stress,* 1976, 2:33–37.

11. Volicer BJ. Hospital stress and patient reports of pain and physical status. *J Human Stress,* 1978, 4:28–37.

12. Johnson JE. Effects of accurate expectations about sensations on the sensory and distress components of pain. *J Pers Soc Psychol,* 1973, 27:261–275.

13. Egbert LD, Battit GE, Welch CE, Bartlett MK. Reduction of postoperative pain by encouragement and instruction of patients. *N Engl J Med,* 1964, 270: 825–827.

14. Mount BM, Ajenian I, Scott JF. Use of the Brompton mixture in treating the chronic pain of malignant disease. *Can Med Assoc J,* 1976, 115:122–124.

15. Spear FG. Pain in psychiatric patients. *J Psychosom Res,* 1967, 11:187–93.

16. Merskey H. Psychiatric patients with persistent pain. *J Psychosom Res,* 1965, 9:299–309.

17. Fordyce WE. Learning processes in pain. In: Sternbach RA (ed.). *The psychology of pain.* New York: Raven Press, 1978:49–72.

18. Skinner BF. *Science and human behavior.* New York: Macmillan, 1953.

19. Shapiro AK. The placebo response. In: Howells JG (ed.). *Modern perspectives in world psychiatry.* Edinburgh: Oliver and Boyd, 1968:596–619.

20. Lasagna L, Mosteller F, Von Felsinger JM, Beecher HK. A study of the placebo response. *Am J Med,* 1954, 16:770–779.

21. Moertel CG, Raylor WF, Roth A, Tyce FA. Who responds to sugar pills? *Mayo Clin Proc,* 1976, 51:96–100.

22. Beecher HK. The placebo effect as a non-specific force surrounding disease and the treatment of disease. In: Janzen R, Keidel WD, Herz A, Steichele C (eds.). *Pain: Basic principles, pharmacology and therapy.* Stutgart, West Germany: George Thiene, 1969:175–180.

23. Evans FJ. The placebo response in pain reduction. *Adv Neurol,* 1974, 4:289–296.

24. Levine JD, Gordon NC, Fields HL. The mechanism of placebo analgesia. *Lancet,* 1978, 2:654–657.

25. Benson H, McCallie DP, Jr. Angina pectoris and the placebo effect. *N Engl J Med,* 1979, 300:1424 – 1429.

26. Pollack S. Pain control by suggestion. *J Oral Med,* 1966, 21:89–95.

27. Weisenberg MI. Pain and pain control. *Psychol Bull,* 1977, 84:1008–1044.

28. Wolf S. Effects of suggestion and conditioning on the action of chemical agents in human subjects: The pharmacology of placebos. *J Clin Invest,* 1950, 29:100–109.

29. Levine JD, Gordon NC, Jones RT, Fields HL. The narcotic antagonist naloxone enhances clinical pain. *Nature,* 1978, 272:826–827.

30. Spiro HM. Placebos, patients, and physicians. *The Pharos,* 1984, 47:2–6.

31. Robins AH. Functional abdominal pain. *S Afr Med J,* 1973, 47:832–834.

32. Merskey H, Spear FG. *Pain: Psychological and psychiatric aspects.* London: Bailliere, Tindall & Cassell, 1967.

33. Laskin DM. Etiology of the pain-dysfunction syndrome. *J Am Dent Assoc,* 1969, 79:147–153.

34. Bakal DA. Headache: A biopsychological perspective. *Psychol Bull,* 1975, 82:369–382.

35. Pilowsky I, Bond MR. Pain and its management in malignant disease: Elucidation of staff-patient transactions. *Psychosom Med,* 1969, 31:400–404.

36. Davitz JR, Davitz LL. *Inferences of patients' pain and psychological distress: Studies of nursing behaviors.* New York: Springer, 1981.

37. Clark WC, Mehl L. Thermal pain: A sensory decision theory analysis of the effect of age and sex on d^1, various response criteria, and 50 percent pain threshold. *J Abnorm Psychol,* 1971, 78:202–212.

38. Fordyce WE. *Behavioral methods for chronic pain and illness.* St. Louis: Mosby, 1976.

39. Sternbach RA. *Pain patients: Traits and treatment.* New York: Academic Press, 1974.

40. Somatoform pain disorder. In: American Psychiatric Association. *Diagnostic and Statistical Manual of Mental Disorders,* 3rd ed. Washington, DC: Author, 1987, 264–266.

41. Bond MR. Psychological and psychiatric aspects of pain. *Anaesthesia,* 1978, 33:355–361.

42. Lynn R, Eysenicky HJ. Tolerance for pain: Extraversion and neuroticism. *Percept Mot Skills,* 1961, 12:161–162.

43. Black RG, Chapman CR. SAD index for clinical assessment of pain. In: Bonica JJ, Albe-Fessard DG (eds.). *Advances in pain research and therapy,* Vol. 1. New York: Raven Press, 1976:301–305.

44. Large RG. Chronic pain and the psychiatrist. *Aust NZ J Surg,* 1978, 48: 113–115.

45. Eysenck HJ, Eysenck SBG. *Manual of the Eysenck Personality Inventory.* London: University of London Press, 1964.

46. Parbrook GD, Steel DF, Dalrymple DG. Factors predisposing to postoperative pain and pulmonary complications. A study of male patients undergoing elective gastric surgery. *Br J Anaesth,* 1973, 45:21–23.

47. Bond MR, Glynn JP, Thomas DC. The relation between pain and personality in patients receiving pentazocine (fortral) after surgery. *J Psychosom Res,* 1976, 20:369–381.

48. Merskey H. The characteristics of persistent pain in psychological illness. *J Psychosom Res,* 1965, 9:291–298.

49. Pilling LF, Brannick TL, Swenson WM. Psychologic characteristics of psychiatric patients having pain as a presenting symptom. *Can Med Assoc J,* 1967, 97:387–394.

50. Engel GL. "Psychogenic" pain and the pain-prone patient. *Am J Med,* 1959, 26:899–918.

51. Sternbach RA. Clinical aspects of pain. In: Sternbach RA (ed.). *The psychology of pain.* New York: Raven Press, 1978:241–264.

52. Pither CE, Nicholas MK. Psychological approaches in chronic pain management. *Br Med Bull,* 1991, 47:743–761.

53. Graffam S, Johnson A. A comparison of two relaxation strategies for the relief of pain and its distress. *J Pain Symptom Management,* 1987, 2:229–231.

SECTION II:
DRUGS USED TO RELIEVE PAIN

Chapter 5

Nonopioid Analgesics and Nonsteroidal Anti-Inflammatory Drugs

INTRODUCTION

The nonnarcotic analgesics are among the most widely used "pain killers" considered by both the public and by physicians to be effective and extremely safe, and, depending on the specific drug, may be purchased as over-the-counter (OTC) medications without prescriptions. The avidity of the American public for these drugs make them the most frequently purchased OTC medications responsible for approximately $650 million in purchases annually.[1] Unfortunately, these analgesics are also among the most common causes of inadvertent poisoning. In susceptible individuals, excessive use may also be associated with a number of complications.

These drugs are quite effective analgesics for mild and, at times, even moderate pain. Some of the newer nonsteroidal anti-inflammatory drugs are capable of providing pain relief equal to that seen with the more potent oral narcotic agents. Unlike the drugs in the opiate or narcotic group, a maximum analgesic effect is usually reached with increasing doses and tolerance does not appear to develop.

THE SALICYLATES

History

Aspirin (acetylsalicylic acid) is the most extensively used nonnarcotic analgesic antipyretic and anti-inflammatory agent. The effectiveness of salicylates in relieving pain can be traced over 2,000 years ago when Hippocrates used the bark of the willow tree (salax) for relief of pain and fever. Many years later, in 1763, the Reverend Edward Stone reported the value of the willow bark in reducing fevers. The active ingredient of willow bark remained unknown until Laroux, in the early 1830s, was able to isolate salicin from the bark. This was followed by the preparation of salicylic acid from salicin, a substance found to exhibit all of the activity of the willow bark in much smaller doses. Synthetic production of salicylic acid was soon accomplished. However, its insolubility in water and its irritating and corrosive effects on the skin allowed only external application. The development of the sodium salt, sodium salicylate, and its subsequent use as an antipyretic for rheumatic fever in 1875, initiated recognition of their effectiveness.[2] In 1853, Von Gerhardt at the Bayer Chemical Works in Elberfield, Germany, synthesized acetylsalicylic acid (aspirin). It was not until a number of years later, however, that advantages of aspirin over sodium salicylate became well recognized with its use being widespread by the start of the twentieth century.

Available Preparations

At the present time, aspirin is the most extensively utilized of all the nonnarcotic analgesics, available in numerous OTC preparations (Tables 5.1 and 5.2) alone or in combination with mild narcotics to potentiate analgesia. A number of other salicylate preparations are also available (Table 5.3). Although some of these preparations differ from aspirin, with respect to absorption and toxicity, with the exception of diflunisal (Dolobid), none provide greater analgesia.

Available aspirin preparations can best be grouped as plain, buffered, or enteric coated tablets, timed-release caplets, and buffered solutions. Most recently, intravenous preparations of salicylate have been used to treat mild, postoperative pain. The following discussion concerning the effects of salicylates and their use as analgesics, however, will focus on aspirin as the prototype, unless otherwise noted.

Pharmacology

Absorption

Following ingestion, salicylates are absorbed from the stomach as well as the upper parts of the small intestine. All aspirin preparations, however, are not alike with respect to solubility or their ability to neutralize gastric acids (buffering capacity) (Table 5.2). Although plasma concentrations may be detected in less than 30 minutes after a single dose with ordinary aspirin tablets, maximal plasma levels may not be reached until more than two hours after ingestion. The administration of aspirin as a solution, such as effervescent aspirin, results in a maximum level within less than 30 minutes.[3]

TABLE 5.1. Selected Nonprescription Analgesic Combinations

Brand	Acetaminophen (mg)	Aspirin (mg)	Other[a]
Alka-Seltzer[a]		324	1,3,12
Anacin[a]		400	2
Anacin-3	500		2
Arthritis Pain Formula		486	1
Arthritis Strength Bufferin		486	1
Ascriptin[a]		325	1
BC Cold Powder[a]		650	13,2
Bufferin		324	1
Coma Arthritis Pain Reliever		500	18
Coma Inlay Tabs		600	1
Comtrex	325		3,8,12
Coricidin		325	3,4,12
Coricidin Sinus Headache	500		4,11
Dristan		325	2,3,11
Dristan A-F	325		2,3,11
Duradyne	180	230	2
Excedrin	97.2	194	2,13
Excedrin PM	500		14
4-Way Cold Tab		324	3,12
Gelpirin	125	240	2
Gemnisyn	325	325	
Midola		454	2,6
Momentum		500	18
Novahistine Sinus Tabs	325		3,16
Ornex	325		12
Pamprin ES	400		17
Percogesic	325		15
Premsyn PMS	500		17,18
S-A-C	150		2,13
Sinarest	325		3,12
Sine-Off		325	3,12
Sine-Off MS	500		16
Sinutab	325		12,15

TABLE 5.1 (continued)

Brand	Acetaminophen (mg)	Aspirin (mg)	Other[a]
Supac	160	230	2,13
Ursinus Inlay Tabs		325	16,18
Vanquish	194	227	1,2

KEY: (a) Various combinations of brand may contain other ingredients, as well as primary ingredients in different doses.
(1) antacid; (2) caffeine; (3) chlorpheniramine; (4) chlortrimeton; (5) citrate; (6) cinnamedrine; (7) calcium; (8) dextromethorphan; (9) guaifenesin; (10) ergocalciferol; (11) phenylephrine; (12) phenylpropanolamine; (13) salicylamide/salicylsalicylic acid; (14) pyrilamine; (15) phenyltoloxamine; (16) pseudoephedrine; (17) pamabrom; (18) other substitutes.

TABLE 5.2. Aspirin Preparations

	Average daily dose (g)
Aspirin	3.6
Buffered Aspirin	3.6
Effervescent Aspirin	3.6
Enteric-Coated Aspirin	3.6
Timed-Release Aspirin	1.8

The precise plasma level at which analgesic effect may be obtained has been unable to be quantified. Controversy also exists as to the clinical significance of rapidity of absorption of different preparations. However, it has been suggested that with ordinary aspirin tablets, contrary to popular opinion, at least one hour may pass before analgesia can be objectively detected.[4] This may be contrasted to the analgesic effect of aspirin given in solution, which may appear within 30 minutes.[3]

Absorption is rapid and mainly in the upper part of the small intestine, although absorption in the stomach can also occur. Increasing the pH results in a greater degree of ionization and a shortened time of dissolution. The first effect would tend to decrease the rate of absorption; the second would facili-

TABLE 5.3. Available Salicylate Preparations

	Trade Name	Unit dose (mg)	Analgesic effect
Acetylsalicylic acid (aspirin)	Many	Variable[a]	++++
Calcium carbaspirin[b]		300	++
Choline Magnesium Trisalicylate	Trilisate, Tricosal	500-1000	+
Choline salicylate	Arthropan	870/5 ml	++
Diflunisal	Dolobid	500 mg	++++
Magnesium salicylate	Doan's, Magan, Mobidin	325,500,545,600	+++
Methyl salicylate[c]	Aurum, Ben Gay, Listerine, Theragold, Cool Mint, Therapeutic Gold		0 +
Salicylic acid[d]	Many	500 mg	++
Salicylamide	BC Powder	325/650	+
Salsalate	Amigesic, Disalcid, Argesic, Mono-Gesic, Salflex, Salsitab	500/750	+
Sodium salicylate		325,650	+
Sodium thiosalicylate[e]	Asproject, Rexolate Tusal	50/ml	+

[a]Usual analgesic dose: 300 to 650 mg.
[b]Contains calcium, aspirin, urea.
[c]In liquid form, used as counterirritant.
[d]Absorbed in small intestine.
[e]Injectable, used mainly as anti-inflammatory agent.

tate it. The quantity of buffer actually present in buffered preparations, however, may not produce either a significant decrease in gastric acidity or a diminished incidence of gastrointestinal side effects.[5] The use of buffers to shorten the time to relieve pain therefore is marginally effective. Buffered aspirin solutions contain more buffer than tablets and may cause less gastric irritation and bleeding. However, their high sodium content and their ability to rapidly increase urine pH can be associated with increasing urinary salicylate excretion, preventing effective long-term administration.[4,6] In addition, some preparations contain insufficient quantities of buffers to effectively change the pH. Enteric-coated aspirin probably provides the best protection against intestinal mucosal injury.[5] Although a major drawback to the use of enteric-coated aspirin had been a variable dissolution and absorption, newer products are more dependable. These preparations are ideal for single dose administration. Time-delayed preparations, although able to be taken less frequently, are probably of limited value; with continued use of regular aspirin preparations, an extremely long half life in the plasma develops.

Absorption of aspirin may be delayed by the presence of food or other substances, the rate at which the stomach empties, the pH, and the concomitant use of antacids. Salicylic acid preparations that are nonacetated are associated with a lower incidence of gastrointestinal side effects. Both salicylic acid and methyl salicylate may be rapidly absorbed when applied cutaneously. Rectal absorption of salicylate is variable and slower than that seen with ingestion.

Distribution

Subsequent to absorption, aspirin is rapidly distributed to all body tissues, and rapidly hydrolyzed in the gastrointestinal mucosa and liver to salicylic acid so that plasma concentrations are usually difficult to detect. Plasma levels of aspirin are considerably higher when administered in solution. Approximately 80 percent to 90 percent of salicylate is bound to plasma proteins, predominantly albumin. The presence of hypoalbuminemia may be associated with a higher level of free salicylate, which may predispose to salicylate toxicity.

Biotransformation and Excretion

Metabolism occurs predominantly in the hepatic microsomal system. Excretion occurs mainly through the kidney as free salicylic acid (10 percent), acyl glucuronides (5 percent), and gentisic acid (less than 1 percent).[7,8] Renal excretion is so rapid that, under usual conditions, only salicylic acid can be detected in the body. Metabolism, however, is rate limited. Increasing aspirin doses above the body's metabolic capacity will result in an increase in the proportion of salicylic acid found in the urine.[8] Urinary pH greatly affects salicylate excretion. Alkalinization will be associated with over 30 percent excretion of free salicylate, whereas acidification of urine inhibits ionization and is accompanied by a back diffusion of salicylate, with the free salicylate excretion diminishing to as low as 5 percent.

Pharmacologic Effects

Analgesic Activity

Salicylates are effective analgesic agents best suited for relief of mild to moderate pain, especially when inflammation contributes to the painful experience. In such instances they are preferred to the more potent narcotic (opiate) analgesics. Tolerance does not develop and dependence is quite unusual. Aspirin and related drugs have long been considered peripheral analgesics; however, over the years, the evidence has accumulated suggesting that they may have an analgesic effect on the central nervous system as well.[8] The peripheral effects of aspirin are felt to be related to the blocking of impulse generation.[9] Pain, especially in the presence of inflammation, is felt to be initiated by prostaglandin release. Aspirin inhibits both synthesis and release of prostaglandins by blocking the activity of cyclooxygenase (COX), the enzyme that converts arachidonic acid into prostaglandin. Recently two isoenzymes of COX have been identified. COX-1 is felt to have a "protective" role on the mucosa of kidney and stomach, whereas COX-2 is involved in the inflammatory response and production of pain. Since aspirin is rapidly hydrolyzed to salicylic acid, which has minimal analgesic activity, other mechanisms may also be important. It is possible that aspirin may effect the release of an endogenous opioid, which in turn may contribute to analgesia.

Antipyretic and Anti-Inflammatory Effects

Salicylates also are extremely effective antipyretics and anti-inflammatory agents. In normal therapeutic doses, aspirin will reduce elevated body temperatures without affecting normal temperature. Antipyresis is believed to occur by a resetting of the homeostatic mechanism in the hypothalamus responsible for temperature regulation.[7] Salicylates also increase oxygen consumption and metabolic rate. With toxic doses, a pyretic effect may occur.

The anti-inflammatory effects of salicylates have been known for more than a century. The most likely mechanisms for the clinically observed anti-inflammatory effects of salicylates are inhibition of prostaglandin synthesis and release, as well as a direct interference with COX-2 and other enzymes or proteins involved in the inflammatory process.[10] It should be emphasized that, although the clinical symptoms of inflammation are suppressed by aspirin, subsequent tissue damage is often unaffected. In rheumatic diseases, this may result in a continued destruction despite symptomatic relief.

Cardiovascular System

In therapeutic doses, salicylates have little or no effect on the cardiovascular system. In increasing doses, salicylates have been associated with increases in plasma volume and in cardiac output, with dilation of the peripheral vasculature. The administration of 4 g of aspirin per day to patients with variant angina has been associated with an increased frequency of anginal episodes.[11] In this study, high-dose aspirin therapy was felt to reduce exercise capacity and provoke exercise-induced coronary artery spasm in susceptible patients. However, the clinical relevance of this remains to be determined. Low dose aspirin is known to be quite effective in diminishing the risk of recurrent myocardial infarction, as well as the chances of developing an acute coronary event, recurrent ischemia attacks, or stroke.

Gastrointestinal System

Gastrointestinal distress is the most frequent adverse reaction to aspirin. Some persons experience nausea and vomiting, others may develop gastric erosion as well as duodenal ulcer disease. Gastrointestinal bleeding can be documented with as little as three to eight aspirin tablets a day; however, the amount of blood lost is relatively small, being less than 20 mm a week. The use of larger doses, as seen in severe inflammatory states, may be clinically significant, increasing blood loss by fivefold.[12] Tolerance to the gastric irritant effect of salicylates does not appear to develop with continuous salicylate ingestion.[13]

The gastrointestinal effects of aspirin are related to its penetration of the lipid membrane of the gastric mucosal cell with subsequent cell damage. This allows a back diffusion of hydrochloric acid accompanied by tissue and capillary injury. Mucosal damage is also facilitated by aspirin inhibition of gastric mucous secretion through its effect on COX-1 resulting in a reduced synthesis of prostaglandin, which normally inhibits gastric secretion. A contributory factor promoting bleeding may be aspirin-induced inhibition of platelet aggregation.

In persons with chronic liver disease, salicylates, even at therapeutic doses, may cause liver damage with potential fatal outcomes. Similarly, the use of salicylates to treat fever in viral infections in children may promote the development of Reye's Syndrome, which may be fatal.

Hematologic Effects

Salicylates affect the hematologic system in a multitude of ways (Table 5.4), the most clinically relevant being prolongation of the bleeding time by inhibition of platelet aggregation. This effect may be seen after a single dose and may last up to seven days.

Metabolic Effects

Multiple metabolic effects may also accompany salicylate administration (Table 5.5). When used in analgesic doses, most of these effects are not of clinical importance. An increase in aspirin dose or the presence of aspirin overdose will be accompanied by marked metabolic abnormalities. This will be discussed further in the section dealing with salicylate toxicity.

Respiratory System

The ability of salicylates to uncouple oxidative phosphorylation results in an increase in oxygen consumption and carbon dioxide production accompanied by an increase in ventilation. Salicylates also act directly on the

TABLE 5.4. Organ System Effects of Aspirin

Cardiovascular[a]
    Peripheral vascular dilatation
    Increases in plasma volume and cardia output
    Exercise-induced angina in susceptible persons with coronary artery disease
Gastrointestinal
    Nausea and vomiting
    Epigastric distress
    Gastrointestinal bleeding
    Peptic ulcer disease
    Hepatic dysfunction
Hematologic
    Reduction erthrocyte survival time
    Lowering plasma iron concentration
    Hemolysis in presence of glucose-g-phosphate dehydrogenase deficiency
    Diminished platelet adhesion
    Reduction in plasma prothrombin
Renal
    Decrease in glomerular filtration and renal blood flow
    Analgesic nephropathy
Respiratory
    Increase in alveolar ventilation
    Stimulation of respiratory center or depression of respiratory center[a]

---

[a]In large doses.

TABLE 5.5. Metabolic Effects of Salicylates

Acid base balance
   Respiratory alkaloisis (compensated)
   Increased renal excretion by bicarbonate sodium, potassium
   Metabolic acidosis[a]
   Respiratory acidosis[a]
 	
Adrenergic activity
   Activation of sympathetic centers
   Epinephrine release from adrenals
 	
Aminoacidurea[b]
 	
Carbohydrate metabolism
   Hyperglycemia
   Depletion of liver and muscle glycogen
   Hypoglycemia in diabetics
	Fat metabolism
	   Inhibits incorporation of acetate into fatty acids
	   Inhibits epinephrine stimulated lipolysis
	   Displaces long chain fatty acids from plasmas protein
	
	Uncoupling of oxidative phosphorylation
	   Increases oxygen consumption
	   Depletion of hepatic glycogen
	   Hyperpyrexia[a]
	   Decreases aerobic metabolism
	
	Uric acid metabolism
	   Decreases urate excretion (low dose)
	   Uricosuria and hypouricemia (high dose)

[a]In toxic doses.
[b]Associated with negative nitrogen balance.

medulla and stimulate the respiratory center, resulting in hyperventilation. High doses of salicylates, however, exert a depressant effect with central respiratory paralysis, at times combined by circulatory collapse. This occurs in the presence of continued carbon dioxide production, causing a profound respiratory acidosis and, occasionally, pulmonary edema. Additional respiratory effects secondary to salicylates have appeared in a number of reviews and need not be discussed further.

Renal-Genitourinary System

Aspirin ingestion has been associated with clinically significant decreases in glomerular filtration and renal blood flow,[14,15] most pronounced in persons with underlying renal disease. This effect is due to salicylate inhibition of prostaglandin synthesis.[16] In normal subjects, however, administration of therapeutic doses of aspirin has been accompanied by either minimal or clinically insignificant changes in renal function.[15] In large doses, especially when combined with other analgesics, nephropathy may occur.

The effect of aspirin on urinary excretion of uric acid is dose dependent. Low doses may be accompanied by a decrease in uricosuria and a net uric acid retention.[17] Intermediate doses of 2 to 3 grams a day may not have any effect. Daily administration of aspirin at doses of greater than 4 grams will result in uricosuria accompanied by a fall in plasma urate concentration.[18] Aspirin can also prevent spironolactone-induced diuresis through inhibiting receptor binding on the tubular cell.[19]

Effects on Pregnancy

Aspirin crosses the placental membranes. Although under experimental conditions administration of aspirin in high doses has been found to be teratogenic, there is no evidence of an increase in birth defects in humans.[20] The use of aspirin in the late stages of pregnancy has been associated with a delay in onset of labor, increased bleeding in the newborn, stillbirths, pulmonary vascular disease, and low birth weights.[21,22]

Adverse Effects of Salicylates

The ubiquity of aspirin in a large number of OTC analgesics, antipyretics, and decongestants allows for a considerable potential for toxicity due to misuse or intentional overdose. Indeed, considering the widespread use of this drug, either alone or in combination with other analgesics and decongestants, and most recently to diminish the risk of heart attack, it is remarkable that so few serious reactions occur.

There is a considerable variability with respect to the dose of aspirin necessary to produce a fatal overdose. Toxic symptoms have been reported at dosages as little as 3 grams a day and have not appeared when up to 10 grams a day are given. The potential for fatality exists if anywhere from 10 to 30 grams of aspirin or sodium salicylate are ingested over a short period. Children may experience a fatal reaction after taking as little as four grams. The rapid absorption of methyl salicylate allows this drug to be associated with a fatal overdose at considerably lower dosages.

The correlation between symptoms and serum salicylate concentration is poor. In general, however, symptoms do not appear at serum levels under 150 mg/ml, whereas almost 50 percent of all individuals with serum salicylate concentrations in excess of 300 mg/ml will begin to experience gastrointestinal effects.[7] Salicylate intoxication can be either acute, as seen in overdose reactions or during the initial phases of acute aspirin therapy, or chronic, occurring with prolonged administration. Chronic intoxication may occur as a result of a cumulative effect of therapeutic doses.

Symptoms and Signs

The symptoms experienced with aspirin toxicity are listed in Table 5.6. In instances of acute severe toxicity, symptoms may progress rapidly, ending in respiratory depression and cardiovascular collapse unless treatment is quickly instituted. In the absence of suicide attempts, aspirin toxicity usually develops in people taking aspirin in increasing therapeutic doses over time. For this reason, symptoms may develop slowly and may not be readily recognized.

Acute Effects

Hypersensitivity reactions to aspirin can occur and may be associated with urticaria, angioedema, or an asthmatic diathesis. These reactions usually occur in patients with a prior history of asthma, nasal polyposis, or vasomotor rhinitis.[23,24] Although the mechanisms responsible for these acute reactions remain to be more clearly defined, it is possible that inhibition of prostaglandin synthesis may play a prominent role. Diminished levels of prostaglandin may be associated with a spontaneous degranulation of mast cells, accompanied by a release of histamine and subsequent allergic reactions.

Another early sign of aspirin toxicity is hyperventilation associated with symptoms consisting of excitement, restlessness, and conversational streams described as "the salicylate jag." If these symptoms are attributed to increased anxiety, the early warning signals of salicylate intoxication will not be detected.

Disturbances in Hearing

Symptoms due to chronic toxicity may develop quite slowly and, unless the physician or patient is aware of these, potential toxic effects may go

TABLE 5.6. Signs and Symptoms of Salicylate Toxicity

Mild	Moderate	Severe
Vertigo	Acneform eruption[a]	Hallucinations
Tinnitus	Diarrhea	Convulsions
Diminished hearing	Drowsiness	Coma
Nausea	Confusion	Cardiovascular collapse
Vomiting	Excitement	Petechial hemorrhages,
	Restlessness	pulmonary edema
	Hyperventilation	

[a]If salicylates administered more than one week.

unnoticed. Ototoxicity, manifested by tinnitus or deafness, can be an early sign. This is dose-related and usually reversible when the aspirin is discontinued. It is more frequent in the presence of diminished levels of serum protein (hypoalbuminemia) due to diminished aspirin binding to albumin with increased plasma levels of free aspirin.

Gastrointestinal Bleeding

The toxic effects of aspirin on the gastrointestinal tract have been described. The intensity of the erosive effect can vary with the type of salicylate ingested as well as the specific vehicle utilized. There is controversy whether adverse gastrointestinal effects can be minimized when aspirin is taken in solution rather than in tablet form.[25,26] Buffered aspirin has been associated with a greater blood loss than enteric-coated aspirin.[5,27]

As discussed earlier, the simultaneous administration of antacids may mitigate these adverse effects. However, the excretion of aspirin is also increased, and most buffered aspirin preparations do not contain enough antacid to be effective. Simultaneous administration of the Histamine H2 antagonists used to treat peptic ulcer (cimetidine [Tagamet], ranitidine [Zantac], or famotidine [Pepcid]) has been demonstrated to reduce the incidence of aspirin-induced gastric erosion. Nonacetylated salicylates, such as choline salicylate or choline magnesium salicylate for trisalicylate, are associated with a lesser degree of gastric irritation.[28]

Dermatologic Signs

Dermatologic signs of chronic salicylate intoxication may be quite frequent and include acneform eruptions, erythematous or scarlatiniform, or desquamative dermatitis. Occasionally, bullous eruptions may occur, as may hemorrhages within mucous membranes.

Hepatic Dysfunction

Aspirin-induced hepatic dysfunction has been reported, usually in persons with rheumatic or collagen diseases receiving high-dose aspirin therapy.[37] In children with rheumatoid arthritis, the incidence of abnormal liver function tests subsequent to aspirin administration may reach 40 percent, with reports of acute hepatic necrosis appearing in the literature.[29]

Metabolic Changes

The metabolic changes resulting from salicylate intoxication have been well described (Table 5.7) and will not be repeated in great detail.[30] The

TABLE 5.7. Metabolic Changes in Salicylate Intoxication

Respiratory alkalosis
Respiratory acidosis[a]
Metabolic acidosis[a]
Dehydration
Hyperthermia
Hypoglycemia

[a]In children or adults ingesting large doses.

prominent disorder is one of acid-base imbalance. Hyperpnea occurring early in the course of intoxication results in a fall in serum carbon dioxide and an increase in pH subsequently modulated by renal excretion of bicarbonate, sodium, and potassium ions. This results in a return of the pH toward normal, producing a compensated respiratory alkalosis.

Toxicity in Children and the Elderly

In children and the elderly, the signs and symptoms of salicylate toxicity may be different and more severe. High fevers are particularly prominent in children, often accompanied by dehydration intensified by associated vomiting and hyperventilation. Central nervous system excitation, especially with the ingestion of methylsalicylate, may also be seen.

In children, rather than a respiratory alkalosis, a respiratory acidosis and subsequent metabolic acidosis may be the prominent feature owing to (a) depression of the respiratory center, with carbon dioxide retention; (b) dehydration associated with impairment of renal function and hypotension, resulting in an accumulation of inorganic and metabolic acids; and (c) impairment of carbohydrate metabolism with accumulation of ketone bodies.

The symptoms of intoxication with the use of different salicylate preparations are rather similar, with the exception of marked central nervous system excitation noted with methylsalicylate, and an enhancement of adverse gastrointestinal symptoms because of the local irritative effect of salicylic acid.

Treatment

The principles of managing salicylate intoxication are based on (1) diminishing absorption of remaining salicylate; (2) correcting the hyperthermia, dehydration, and metabolic abnormalities; and (3) hastening excretion from the body (Table 5.8).

Elimination of salicylate from the gastrointestinal tract may be accomplished by inducing vomiting in the conscious patient who does not present with gastrointestinal bleeding, or by gastric lavage and absorption with activated charcoal. Although there is a considerable variation in appearance of symptoms based on serum salicylate levels, on an individual basis, determination of serum salicylates can be of great value in monitoring the subsequent course of overdose.

Dissociation of salicylate is dependent on body pH. Salicylic acid is highly ionized at the pH of blood, with relatively small changes in pH associated with a marked increase in proportion of non-ionizable salicylate acid molecules. A decrease in blood pH from 7.4 to 7.2 will essentially double the proportion of non-ionized salicylate. Acidosis, therefore, will facilitate the entry of salicylates into the tissues and may be the reason why acidemia is associated with an extremely poor prognosis.

The use of alkalizing agents through intravenous administration of sodium bicarbonate at a rate sufficient to produce an alkaline diuresis is, therefore, quite important. This maneuver is, however, associated with the potential hazard of pulmonary edema or too rapid a correction of the metabolic disturbance, so that careful monitoring is mandatory.

Diuretics that are carbonic anhydrase inhibitors (Acetazolamide, Diamox, AkZol, Dazamide, Neptazane) should be used with extreme caution in order to prevent acidosis. Acetazolamide results in a lowering in blood pH and a resultant increase in brain salicylate levels. It is important to emphasize that in laboratory animals, the lethality of sodium salicylate can be tripled if administered with a nonlethal dose of acetazolamide.[31]

TABLE 5.8. Principles of Therapy in Salicylate Intoxication

Decrease absorption of remaining drug
Diminish uptake by tissues—especially brain
Correction of pathological changes
Hyperthermia
Acid base abnormalities
Hypoglycemia
Dehydration
Hyperpyrexia
Hypotension
Increase renal excretion of salicylate

Hypoglycemia, if severe, may be associated with a marked diminution in cerebral functioning. Glucose administration will also correct the ketosis and help alleviate the metabolic acidosis, if present. Serum potassium should be carefully monitored, with replacement, if necessary, once renal output is adequate.

The presence of hyperthermia and dehydration, which may be of sufficient intensity to present an immediate problem, should also be quickly corrected. Hyperthermia may be managed with tepid water sponging. Hydration should be restored by the use of intravenous fluids containing appropriate electrolyte solutions.

The presence of central nervous system depression or excitation should not be treated with any specific mood-altering drug. Since salicylate intoxication may be associated with ingestion of a central nervous system depressant, addition of any other agent, such as barbiturates or narcotics, will result in a worsening of the depression, accompanied by increase in intensity in acidosis and coma. If necessary, artificial respiration to increase excretion of carbon dioxide and alleviate existing acidosis is preferred.

If the acidemia cannot be prevented and blood salicylate levels greater than 50 mg/ml persist, extra corporeal removal is often necessary. This can be accomplished through exchange transfusion, hemoperfusion, or peritoneal or hemodialysis. This technique should also be considered in persons with a serious underlying disease or when the symptoms are not resolved despite appropriate therapy.

Prompt recognition of salicylate toxicity and rapid institution of appropriate therapy should allow a favorable outcome in all but the most serious of salicylate overdoses. Recovery from salicylate overdose should occur almost routinely.

Aspirin-Drug Interactions

Although aspirin is used with impunity, its pharmacologic actions nonetheless place it in the group of drugs that have the potential for considerable drug interactions (Table 5.9). In general, aspirin-drug interactions occur through the actions of aspirin on the gastrointestinal tract, plasma protein binding, renal function, and coagulation pathways.

The irritant effects of alcohol and aspirin on the gastric mucosa, as well as the ability of both of these drugs to effect platelet adhesiveness, may result in an increased prevalence of gastrointestinal bleeding. As discussed earlier, gastric irritation can be decreased by the administration of antacids or with enteric-coated aspirin. Concurrent ingestion of aspirin and indomethacin will result in a decreased absorption of indomethacin associated with diminished plasma levels.

TABLE 5.9. Effects of Aspirin-Drug Interactions

Increase toxic effects of aspirin	Decrease in effectiveness of aspirin	Increase toxic effects of other drug	Decrease in effectiveness of other drug
Ascorbic acid ammonium chloride	Antacids	Chlorpropamide	Fenoprofen
Carbonic anhydrase inhibitors			Angiotension converting enzyme inhibitors
Nizatidine			Beta-adrenergic blockers
			Indomethacin
Phenylbutazone	Corticosteroids	Diphenylhydantoin	Spironolactone
Probenecid		Heparin	Nonsteroidal anti-inflammatory drugs (NSAIDs)
Para-Aminobenzoic acid		Methotrexate oral anticoagulants	Probenecid
Sulfinpyrazone		Para-Aminosalicylate Sulfonylureas	
		Valproic acid	

Competitive binding with plasma proteins may result in a hypoglycemic reaction in persons maintained on oral sulfonylureas. Similarly, the level of plasma diphenylhydantoin may be increased with a greater potential for toxicity. Plasma naproxen levels may also be increased; however, its clinical significance remains to be determined.

Displacement of coumarin derivatives from plasma proteins may potentiate hypoprothrombinemia, greatly enhancing the possibility for bleeding. This effect is intensified by the ability of aspirin to diminish platelet aggregation as well as to exert a direct effect in lowering plasma prothrombin levels when given in high dosages. Aspirin also has been associated with decreased plasma levels and half-life of many of the newer, nonsteroidal anti-inflammatory drugs.

A number of drugs may interact with aspirin at the level of the kidney. Acidification of the urine with ammonium chloride or ascorbic acid will result in increased absorption of aspirin with a greater potential for salicylate toxicity. Aspirin may interfere with renal excretion of chlorpropamide, which, when combined with competitive displacement of this drug from protein binding, can result in considerable hypoglycemia.[32]

The ability of corticosteroids to enhance glomerular filtration rate can result in a decreased plasma concentration of aspirin. This may become important in patients maintained on high doses of aspirin and steroids when the steroids are subsequently discontinued. The diminished excretion of aspirin may be associated with a potential for salicylate toxicity.

Drugs associated with increased excretion of uric acid, such as phenylbutazone, probenecid, and sulfinpyrazone, administered with aspirin, will result in inhibition of uricosuric activity accompanied by elevation of serum uric acid. The administration of aspirin and spironolactone is accompanied by an inhibition of the diuretic effect, possibly because of competition of aspirin at the spironolactone receptor site.

Diflunisal (Dolobid)

Diflunisal is a derivative of salicylic acid with analgesic and anti-inflammatory activity more potent than aspirin. Its absorption following oral administration is quite good, with an analgesic effect observable within one hour, reaching a maximum effect between two to three hours. Its plasma half-life is eight to twelve hours. Daily does of 500 mg to 1 gram are comparable to daily aspirin doses of 2 to 4 grams. It is effective for treatment of mild to moderate pain and is most frequently used to relieve the pain of arthritis. A loading dose of 500 mg-1000 mg is usually needed, followed by 250-500 mg every eight to twelve hours. The analgesia produced is believed to be comparable to that seen with aspirin or acetaminophen-codeine combinations. Since Diflunisal is a salicylate, its side effects are similar to those seen with aspirin, but not as severe.

PARA-AMINOPHENOL DERIVATIVES

Acetaminophen and phenacetin are the two para-aminophenol derivatives commonly used as analgesics. Since the analgesic activity of phenacetin is primarily due to its rapid biotransformation to acetaminophen, and since acetaminophen has far less toxicity, it is the drug most frequently used alone or in combination with other agents. It is an effective analgesic and antipyretic. However, it has no clinical significant anti-inflammatory activities.

The use of acetaminophen can be traced back to 1893; however, widespread use did not occur until after 1949, when acetaminophen was identified as the major active metabolite of the other analgesic para-aminophenols. At present, acetaminophen can be found under more than 150 different labels and is an active ingredient in more than 200 proprietary drug combinations.[33] It is actively promoted as being equal in effectiveness to aspirin without any of the commonly encountered gastrointestinal side effects. Due to its minor effects on coagulation, it can be used by patients taking oral anticoagulants or those with bleeding disorders. However, the increasing use of this drug has been accompanied by a respect for its potential toxicities, especially when taken intentionally in large doses.

Pharmacology

Absorption of acetaminophen from the gastrointestinal tract is rapid. Peak plasma concentrations occur within 30 to 60 minutes, with a plasma half-life up to three hours. Absorption is not only dependent on the rate of gastric emptying but, in addition, may vary greatly depending on its bioavailability in different preparations. Acetaminophen is widely distributed throughout the body. Binding to plasma proteins is variable, but in the presence of an overdose, may reach 50 percent. A good correlation does not exist between serum concentration and intensity of analgesic action.[34]

Metabolism occurs mainly in the liver, with approximately 80 percent conjugated with glucuronic acid. Hydroxylation and deacetylation result in the production of other metabolites. These pathways can be increased by activators of the hepatic microsomal system, such as phenobarbital. Excretion occurs in the urine, with approximately 3 percent of the drug excreted in free form. Renal impairment may be associated with a decrease in the excretion of conjugated acetaminophen without any notable increase in serum concentrations of the active drug.

Metabolism of phenacetin occurs predominantly through biotransformation to acetaminophen. Phenacetin, however, can be converted to a number of other metabolites which are responsible for the methemoglobinemia and hemolysis of blood cells sometimes observed during phenacetin therapy. The tendency toward methemoglobinemia and hemolysis is greater in individuals who genetically are limited in their ability to metabolize phenacetin to acetaminophen.

Pharmacologic Effects

The effects of acetaminophen on most organ systems are relatively minimal. Cerebral effects consisting of alteration of mood can occur. However, they are much more common with phenacetin.

Analgesic Activity

Acetaminophen has analgesic and antipyretic activities similar to aspirin. Its mechanism of action are not well defined. Acetaminophen directly acts on the hypothalamic heat regulating center, and has been shown to inhibit the action of endogenous pyrogens, which may explain its antipyretic effect. It is an active prostaglandin synthetase inhibitor; however, the intensity of this effect is much more prominent centrally rather than peripherally. This may explain its relative ineffectiveness in inflammatory states.

The analgesic efficacy of acetaminophen has been documented in several medically controlled studies. Approximately 600 mg of acetaminophen are felt to be equal in analgesic effect to 600 mg of aspirin, with the dose response curves of these drugs quite similar. Pain associated with inflammation, however, would be expected to respond much better to aspirin due to acetaminophen's relatively weaker anti-inflammatory effects.

Toxicity and Overdose

Analgesic Nephropathy

The use of analgesic combinations has resulted in the appearance of an entity termed analgesic nephropathy. Lesions in the kidney consist of papillary necrosis, chronic interstitial nephritis, and sclerosis of the capillaries in the lower urinary tract.[35,36] These conditions have been considered to be the result of a microangiopathy, accompanied by a compromised vascular supply with subsequent necrosis. Although initially controversial, it is now commonly agreed that analgesic nephropathy is a distinct form of interstitial nephritis specifically associated with long-term consumption of high dose non-narcotic analgesics. This has become of particular concern with use of over-the-counter combination analgesics, most often containing acetylsalicylic acid, paracetamol, and caffeine (APC). Specialists in renal disease both in the United States and in Europe have called for the withdrawal of these medications from the over-the-counter market.

It has been shown, however, that the risk of kidney disease is greatest in daily users of phenacetin, less but increased with daily acetaminophen use, and not increased with daily use of aspirin.[35] The use of one pill a day or 1,000 pills in a lifetime can double the risk of having end-stage renal disease. Since this entity occurs in the presence of ingestion of a number of other substances, including the aspirin nonsteroidal anti-inflammatory drugs, the exact etiologic role of these drugs remains to be clarified. However, recent evidence suggest that it is the users of acetaminophen or NSAIDs who have an increased risk of renal disease, rather than those who use aspirin.

Hepatic Disease

Although acetaminophen, when taken in recommended therapeutic doses, is a relatively safe analgesic agent, ingestion of increasing doses may be associated with severe hepatotoxicity.[37] The underlying mechanism of acetaminophen hepatotoxicity is an inability to excrete all of the ingested drug with the accumulation of toxic metabolites that subsequently bind to the hepatic macromolecules. This process may not solely be dose related, as liver disease may develop with long-term acetaminophen use of rather small doses. It is believed that alcohol use or fasting may predispose one to acetaminophen liver damage.

Initial symptoms, usually appearing after ingestion of a single dose of 10g, consist of nausea, vomiting, diarrhea, and abdominal pain. Laboratory evidence of hepatic dysfunction can appear within 24 to 48 hours; however, elevations of enzymes, indicative of hepatic dysfunction, may not reach their maximum for another two to four days. Severe intoxication may be associated with hepatic encephalopathy, coma, and death.

Mortality rates are variable, reported to be as high as 10 percent in patients treated only with supportive therapy. If recovery occurs, the hepatic lesions usually heal slowly, with subsequent development of cirrhosis being quite unusual.

Acetaminophen toxicity will occur after a single dose of 10 grams, although as little as 5.8 grams have been associated with severe hepatic dysfunction. Alcoholics seem to be particularly susceptible to this effect with serum liver damage occurring with as little as 3 to 4 grams.[32,38] It is important, however, to place this in perspective. If extended release acetaminophen is the form involved, then plasma acetaminophen levels should be measured four hours and then eight to ten hours after ingestion.[39,40] Despite billions of tablets of acetaminophen being consumed and millions of people believed to use alcohol excessively, the actual incidence of liver damage is quite small. Nonetheless, the use of acetaminophen in combination with frequent or chronic alcohol use does increase the potential for toxicity and should be avoided.

Treatment

Similar to therapy of all drug overdoses, initial treatment should be focused on eliminating the remaining drug from the gastrointestinal tract. This can be accomplished by use of gastric lavage to eliminate only unabsorbed pills. Since the principal antidote is the administration of oral n-acetylcysteine (Mucosal), activated charcoal should not be given. Treatment should be started within two hours but may be effective for up to 24 hours after ingestion. As noted above, measurement of acetaminophen levels can be helpful in determining whether acetylcysteine need be given. Elimination of absorbed acetaminophen by extracorporeal techniques has not been found to be effective even when attempted within 12 hours after ingestion.

Acetaminophen-Drug Interactions

Acetaminophen is associated with relatively few clinically relevant drug interactions. Although it can stimulate the hepatic microsomal enzyme system, at therapeutic doses interactions between other agents are infrequently observed. The administration of acetaminophen and oral anticoagulants may be accompanied by a slight increase in prothrombin time, usually not of clinical importance. Administration of metoclopramide and acetaminophen may result in increased acetaminophen absorption owing to stimulation of gastric emptying time.

As noted above, hepatic toxicity has been reported to be potentiated in the presence of enzyme inducers, most specifically barbiturates and alcohol.[38] Acetaminophen may also interact with chloramphenicol, resulting in a prolongation of chloramphenicol half-life when both drugs are used concurrently.[41]

Summary

In summary, acetaminophen is a useful analgesic for persons unable to take aspirin, and for febrile states associated with viral infections in children when aspirin is contraindicated. It is a useful nonnarcotic analgesic in individuals on oral anticoagulants or with hematologic disorders manifested by coagulation defects. The use of acetaminophen in therapeutic doses is rarely associated with any untoward effects other than allergic reactions. Toxic effects due to overdose, however, may be quite severe and, at times, fatal.

NONSTEROIDAL ANTI-INFLAMMATORY DRUGS

Commonly Prescribed Drugs

A large number of nonsteroidal anti-inflammatory agents (NSAID) have become available for use in this country over the past several years and are widely used, with up to 60 million prescriptions written annually (Table 5.10). Virtually all of these drugs are effective in relieving pain associated with inflammation. A few are equal to or more effective than aspirin or acetaminophen in relief of noninflammatory pain. Some are equal in analgesic effect to several of the narcotics (opiates). Extensive reviews concerning the actions of the NSAID agents have appeared elsewhere. The following discussion will cover only salient features of the use of those drugs used mainly as analgesics in the absence of inflammation.[42]

Mechanism of Actions

NSAIDs all inhibit prostaglandin synthesis, which explains their effectiveness in inflammatory states. Similar to aspirin, they inhibit both COX-1 and COX-2 to degrees that vary with individual agents. However, their effectiveness as analgesic agents may be related either to a direct peripheral or a central antinociceptive effect. Some of the newer NSAIDs are rather weak inhibitors of prostaglandin synthesis, yet they are effective analgesics.[43]

Adverse Effects

Major adverse effects associated with their use include gastrointestinal distress, hepatoxicity, blood dyscrasias, hypersensitivity reactions, and renal toxicity. Kidney disorders are among the most prominent of their adverse effects, with reversible renal insufficiency being the most common. Although the incidence of this complication is small, the elderly, especially those taking diuretics, are at risk.[44] Since these adverse effects are due to inhibition of COX-1, ideally those that selectively inhibit COX-2 would be preferable,

TABLE 5.10. Commonly Available Nonsteroidal Anti-Inflammatory Agents

	Trade	Analgesic Activity	Anti-Inflammatory Activity	Maximum Daily Doses mg
Propionic Acids				
Fenoprofen	Nalfron		+	1200
Flurbiprofen	Ansaid		+	200-300
Ibuprofen	Advil, Genpril, Haltran, Excedrin IB, Ibuprin, Medipren, Menadiol, Midol 200, Motrin, Nuprin, Pamprin, Rufen, Saleto, Trendar, Aches-N-Pain	+	+	2400
Ketoprofen	Orudis	+	+	300
Naproxen	Aleve**, Anaprox, Naprosyn	+	+	1250
Acetic Acids				
Diclofenac Sodium	Voltaren		+	200
Etodolac	Lodine	+	+	1200
Indomethacin	Indocin	+	+	150-200
Ketoralac	Toradol	+		120*
Sulindac	Clinoril		+	400
Tolmetin	Tolectin	+	+	1800
Anthracitic Acids				
Meclofenamate	Meclomen		+	400
Mefenamic Acid	Ponstel	+		1250
Nabumetone	Relafen		+	2000
Oxicans				
Piroxicam	Feldene	+	+	20

* By injection
** Relatively long-acting

whereas those that are more potent inhibitors of COX-1 should be avoided. Recent evidence suggests that piroxicam, indomethacin, and sulindac preferentially inhibit COX-1 as compared with COX-2, whereas nabumetone preferentially inhibits COX-2.[45] All of these drugs should be used cautiously, if at all, in persons with renal disease. Prior history of ulcer disease, use of corticosteroids, and heavy cigarette consumption are also risk factors.[45] Other adverse effects include dermatitis, headaches, hypersensitivity reactions, tinnitus, and bronchospasm in persons sensitive to aspirin.

Although the incidence of developing serious gastrointestinal complications while taking an NSAID is relatively low, nonetheless, current use of these has been associated with a fourfold greater risk than nonuse.[45] Persons at risk include those (1) over age 60, (2) also on steroids, (3) on large doses, (4) with a history of peptic ulcer disease, and (5) on long-term NSAID therapy. Persons at risk in need of NSAID therapy should be placed on misoprostol to decrease the chance of ulceration.

Drug Interactions

All NSAIDs exhibit an avidity to plasmas proteins, which may result in significant interactions with other drugs having a similar avidity. This is most important with respect to the oral anticoagulants, which are displaced from their binding sites by almost all of the NSAIDs. The interaction of drugs in this group is similar to that seen with aspirin, although it may vary in intensity with individual agents. The NSAIDs also cause inhibition of platelet aggregation. This is reversible, returning to normal when the drug is discontinued.

Of the NSAIDs effective in relieving pain not associated with inflammation, Ibuprofen is the most popular, and is readily available without a physician's prescription. Over-the-counter preparations, however, are at lower dosage than available by prescription. Approximately 200 mg of Ibuprofen are equal to 650 mg of aspirin or acetaminophen, with 400 mg equal to either of these drugs combined with codeine. Meclofenamate (Meclomen) and Mefenamic acid (Ponstel) are believed to be particularly effective in pain associated with menstruation. Ketoralac (Toradol) is an injectable drug found to be comparable in analgesic activity to 12 mg of intramuscular morphine in relieving postoperative pain.

Other Nonnarcotic Analgesics

Methotrimeprazine (Levoprome)

Levoprome is a phenothiazine derivative that can elevate the pain threshold as well as cause amnesia. Although its analgesic effect is believed to be comparable to morphine, associated sedative anticholinergic, antihistaminic and antiadrenergic effects may limit its use. It may interact with other drugs that depress the central nervous system as well as many antihypertensives. It is only available in injectable form, which limits use greatly.

Tramadol (Ultram)

Tramadol has been used as an analgesic in Germany for over two decades. In 1994, under the trade name Ultram, it became available as a non-scheduled analgesic. Tramadol is centrally acting, and although it exhibits some opioid activity by binding to the mu opioid receptors, it actually has a dual action. It not only displaces the endogenous opiates on the mu receptors, it also inhibits uptake of norepinephrine and serotonin. Tramadol's affinity to the opioid receptor is due mainly to the activity of its metabolite. Its ability to displace opiate drugs may result in withdrawal when given to someone who has been taking opiates. Similarly, since it does bind to the opiate receptor, the potential for dependence exists and serious adverse effects can occur if tramadol is given with a with MAO inhibitors.

Tramadol has been recommended for use in moderate pain at doses of 50-100 mg every four to six hours. Severe pain may require up to 100 mg doses. However, in clinical trials doses of 50 to 75 mg have been found to provide analgesia superior to codeine sulfate 60 mg, but not as effective as codeine-aspirin or codeine-tylenol combinations. Tramadol has certain advantages over both centrally and peripherally acting analgesics. Its bio-availability with oral use is higher than the opioids, and its analgesic effect is more sustained than combination analgesics.[48]

Tramadol can cause nausea, dizziness, and constipation in as many as one-quarter of the persons taking this medication. A decrease in dose is needed in the elderly as well as in persons with liver or renal disease. Respiratory depression is usually not seen unless given with other central nervous system depressants. Overdose is rare, and abuse, based on the European experience, is quite low. However, because of its action on the opioid receptor, it should not be used—or should be used quite cautiously—in persons with a history of opioid dependence.

SUMMARY

The newer NSAIDs with specific analgesic effects are equal to or better than aspirin or acetaminophen. Some also have longer durations of action, which allow for a lesser number of pills to be taken, improving patient compliance. Although generally well tolerated, toxicity similar to aspirin may be seen but is usually of lesser intensity. Under appropriate settings they have been quite effective in providing analgesia for mild to moderate pain without the need to progress to narcotic (opiate) drugs. In addition, when used in combination with narcotic agents, more effective analgesia at a lower dose of narcotic may be able to be achieved.

Finally, there is an individual variation to different NSAID's analgesic effectiveness, as well as to the potential for toxicity. There is also a considerable difference in cost that may vary by more than tenfold between the least and the most expensive (Table 5.11).[45] All of these factors should be taken into account when using these drugs to relieve pain. Recommendations for selecting a specific NSAID have been made, and these are quite helpful for patients and physicians alike (Table 5.12).

TABLE 5.11. Relative Average 30-Day Cost of Nonsteroidal Anti-Inflammatory Drugs

Less than $10
Aspirin—pain
Sodium salicylate—enteric
Aspirin—enteric
$10 to $30
Phenylbutazone (g), Ibuprofen (g)
Salsalate (g) (b)
$31 to $50
Indomethacin (g), Ibuprofen (b), Magnesium salicylate
$51 to $79
Sulindac (b), Meclofenamate (g), Phenylbutazone (b), Choline Magnesium Trisalicylate (b), Diclofenac (b), Tricosal (b), Trilisate (b)
$80 to $99
Naproxen (b), Indomethacin (b), Fenoprofen (g), Tolmetin (b), Meclofenamate (b)
Over $100
Piroxicam (b), Diflunisal (b), Ketoprofen (b), Fenoprofen (b)

Modified from reference 45
g = generic
b = brand name drug

TABLE 5.12. Suggestions for Selection of NSAIDs

Consider effective nonpharmacologic treatments as first line defense.

Initially use a drug that is a weak prostaglandin inhibitor or has no effects on prostaglandin synthesis.

Do not use more than one NSAID at a time.

Do not combine NSAID use with aspirin.

Start with lowest effective dose and increase slowly—not to exceed maximum recommended dose.

If inflammation is a prominent cause of pain, allow 1 to 2 weeks to assess effectiveness.

Always consider the least-expensive, most-effective agent.

The absence of a response to one NSAID does not preclude an analgesic response to another—even in the same class.

Do not use NSAIDs in persons at high risk for renal toxicity.

Avoid NSAIDs in persons on anticoagulants or with clotting disorders.

In persons at high risk for gastrointestinal effects: (1) consider use of misoprostal to prevent ulcers; (2) consider etodolac and nabumetone as drugs of choice; or (3) use meclofenamate or tolmetin with caution.

*Modified from references 45 and 47.

REFERENCES

1. Hall RCW, Gardner ER, Perl M. Psychiatric and physiological reactions produced by over-the-counter medications. *J Psychedelic Drugs,* 1978, 10:243–249.

2. Krantz JC, Jr. The rendezvous with pain and home remedies, with special reference to the origins of aspirin. *J Am Med Wom Assoc,* 1978, 33:223–224.

3. Leonards JR. The influence of solubility on the rate of gastrointestinal absorption of aspirin. *Clin Pharmacol Ther,* 1963, 4:476–479.

4. Leonards JR. Are all aspirins alike? *Aust NZ J Med,* 1976 (6 suppl.), 1:8–13.

5. Lanza FL, Royer GL Jr, Nelson RS. Endoscopic evaluation of the effects of aspirin, buffered aspirin, and enteric-coated aspirin on gastric and duodenal mucosa. *N Engl J Med,* 1980, 303:136–138.

6. Leonards JR. Presence of acetylsalicylic acid in plasmas following oral ingestion of aspirin. *Proc Soc Exp Biol,* 1962, 110:304–308.

7. Insel PA. Analgesic-antipyretics and anti-inflammatory agents: Drugs employed in the treatment of rheumatoid arthritis and gout. In: *The pharmacological basis of therapeutics,* 8th ed. Gilman AG, Rall TW, Nies AS, Taylor P (eds.). New York: Pergamon Press, 1990:638–681.

8. Bannwarth B, Demotes-Mainard F, Schaeverbeke T, Labat L, Dehais J. Central analgesic effects of aspirin-like drugs. *Fundam Clin Pharmacol,* 1995, 9:1–7.

9. Ferreira SH. Prostaglandins, aspirin-like drugs and analgesia. *Nature New Biol,* 1972, 240:200–203.

10. Smith MJH. Aspirin and prostaglandins: Some recent developments. *Agents Actions,* 1978, 8:427–429.

11. Miwa K, Kambara H, Kawai C. Exercise-induced anginas provoked by aspirin administration in patients with variant angina. *Am J Cardiol,* 1981, 47:1210–1214.

12. Alexander WD, Smith G. Disadvantageous circulatory effects of salicylate in rheumatic fever. *Lancet,* 1962, 1:768–771.

13. Thorsen WB, Jr, Western D, Tanaka Y, Morrissey JF. Aspirin injury to the gastric mucosa: Gastrocamera observations of the effects of pH. *Arch Intern Med,* 1968, 121:499–506.

14. Done AK, Temple AR. Treatment of salicylate poisoning. *Mod Treat,* 1971, 8:528–551.

15. Muther RS, Bennett WM. Effects of aspirin on glomerular filtration rate in normal humans. *Ann Intern Med,* 1980, 92:386–387.

16. Kimberly RP, Gill JR, Jr, Bowden RE, Keiser HR, Plotz PH. Elevated urinary prostaglandins and the effects of aspirin on renal function in lupus erythematosus. *Ann Intern Med,* 1978, 89:336–341.

17. Oyer JH, Wagner SL, Schmid FR. Suppression of salicylate-induced uricosuria by phenylbutazone. *Am J Med Sci,* 1966, 251:1– 7.

18. Yu TF, Gutman AB. Study of the paradoxical effects of salicylate in low, intermediate and high dosage on the renal mechanisms for excretion of urate in man. *J Clin Invest,* 1959, 38:1298–1315.

19. Hofmann LM, Krupnick MI, Garcia HA. Interactions of spironolactone and hydrochlorothiazide with aspirin in the rat and dog. *J Pharmaco Exp Ther,* 1972, 180:1–5.

20. Simon LS, Mills JA. Nonsteroidal anti-inflammatory drugs. Part 1. *N Engl J Med,* 1980, 302:1179–1185.

21. Collins E, Turner G. Maternal effects of regular salicylate ingestion in pregnancy. *Lancet,* 1975, 2:335–338.

22. Levin DL, Fixler DE, Morriss FC, Tyson J. Morphologic analysis of the pulmonary vascular bed in infants exposed in utero to prostaglandin synthetase inhibitor. *J Pediatr,* 1978, 92:478–483.

23. Stevenson DD, Lewis RA. Proposed mechanisms of aspirin sensitivity reaction. *J Clin Immunol,* 1987, 80:788–789.

24. Szczeklik A, Gryglewski RJ, Czerniawska-Mysik G. Clinical patterns of hypersensitivity to nonsteroidal anti-inflammatory drugs and their pathogenesis. *J Allergy Clin Immunol,* 1977, 60:276–284.

25. Vlasses PH, Nelson LA. Aspirin and mucosal injury (letter). *N Engl J Med,* 1980, 303:1122.

26. Lanza FL. Aspirin and mucosal injury (letter). *N Engl J Med,* 1980, 303:1122.

27. Mielants H, Verbruggen G, Schelstraete K, Veys EM. Salicylate-induced gastrointestinal bleeding: Comparison between soluble buffered, enteric-coated, and intravenous administration. *J Rheumatol,* 1979, 6:210–218.

28. Cohen A, Garber HE. Comparison of choline magnesium trisalicylate and acetylsalicylic acid in relation to fecal blood loss. *Curr Ther Res,* 1978, 23:187–193.

29. Schaller JG. Chronic salicylate administration in juvenile rheumatoid arthritis: Aspirin "hepatitis" and its clinical significance. *Pediatrics*, 1978, 62:916–925.

30. Hill JB. Salicylate intoxication. *N Engl J Med*, 1973, 288:1110–1113.

31. Hill JB. Experimental salicylate poisoning: Observations on the effects of altering blood pH on tissue and plasma salicylate concentrations. *Pediatrics*, 1971, 47: 658–665.

32. Black M, Raucy J. Acetaminophen, alcohol, and cytochrome P-450. *Ann Intern Med*, 1986, 104:427–429.

33. Facts and Comparisons. *Drug facts and comparisons*, 47th ed. St. Louis, MO, 1993.

34. Koch-Weser J. Acetaminophen. *N Engl J Med*, 1976, 295:1297–1300.

35. Sandler DP, Smith JC, Weinberg CR, Buckalew VM, Dennis VW, Blythe WB, Burgess WP. Analgesic use and chronic renal disease. *N Engl J Med*, 1989, 320:1238–1243.

36. Bennett WM, DeBroe ME. Analgesic nephropathy–A preventable renal disease (editorial). *N Engl J Med*, 1989, 320:1269–1271.

37. Boyer TD, Rouff SL. Acetaminophen-induced hepatic necrosis and renal failure. *JAMA*, 1971, 218:440–441.

38. McClain CJ, Kromhout JP, Peterson FJ, Holtzman JL. Potentiation of acetaminophen hepatotoxicity with alcohol. *JAMA*, 1980, 244:251–253.

39. Temple AR, Mrazik TJ. More on extended release acetaminophen. *N Eng J Med*, 1995, 333:1508.

40. Graudins A, Aaron CK, Linden CH. Overdose of extended release acetaminophen. *N Eng J Med*, 1995, 333:196.

41. Buchanan N, Moodley GP. Interaction between chloramphenicol and paracetamol. *Br Med J*, 1979, 2:307–308.

42. Beaver WT. Nonsteroidal antiinflammatory analgesics in cancer pain. In: Foley KM, Bonica JJ, Ventafridda V (eds.). *Advances in pain research and therapy*. New York: Raven Press, 1990:109–131.

43. McCormack K, Brune K. Dissociation between the antinociceptic and anti-inflammatory effects of the nonsteroid anti-inflammatory drugs. A survey of their analgesic efficacy. *Drugs*, 1991, 41:533–547.

44. Stillman MT, Schlesinger PA. Nonsteroidal anti-inflammatory drug nephrotoxicity. Should we be concerned? *Arch Inter Med*, 1990, 150:268–270.

45. Polisson R. Nonsteroidal anti-inflammatory drugs: Practical and theoretical considerations in their selection. *Am J Med*, 1996, (Suppl. 2A): 315–365.

46. Greene JM, Winickoff RN. Cost-conscious prescribing of nonsteroidal anti-inflammatory drugs for adults with arthritis. *Arch Intern Med*, 1992, 152:1995–2002.

47. Bjorkman DJ. Nonsteroidal anti-inflammatory drug-induced gastrointestinal injury. *Am J MED*, 1996, (Suppl 1A): 255–315.

48. Gibson TP. Pharmokinetics: Efficacy and safety of analgesia with a focus on Tramadol HC1. *Am J Med*, 1966, (Suppl. 1A): 475–535.

Chapter 6

Opioid (Narcotic) Analgesics I: Opioid Agonists

HISTORY

The history of the poppy begins in antiquity. Although the exact date of the first systematic cultivation remains unknown, seeds and capsules of poppies were found as early as the Stone Age in the area of lake dwellers.[1,2] In Mesopotamia (4000-3000 BC), the poppy was cultivated by the Sumerians in order to extract flower. Opium, however, has its origins from the Greek *opion*, meaning poppy juice. The Babylonian culture subsequently spread the cultivation of the poppy eastward to Persia and westward to Egypt.[3]

The medicinal value of the poppy as an hypnotic, a constipating agent, and an analgesic was first described in the Ebers Papyrus (1600-1500 BC).[5] Galen also praised opium's ability to relieve pain and suffering. In modern times, the eighteenth century marked the beginning of large-scale organized trade and importation of opium, which was most popular in the Orient. In the early part of the nineteenth century, Serturner in Germany separated meconic acid from opium, producing morphine from the alkaline base. In France in 1817, Robiquet isolated narcotine and subsequently codeine in 1832. By this time the use of opium and its products had become fashionable both in the United States and abroad. In fact, as described by Brecher, nineteenth century America could be described as a "dope fiend's paradise." The popularity of morphine and its derivatives for medicinal purposes, as well as for mood-altering properties, has continued unabated to the present.

CLASSIFICATION

The original terminology for morphine and related drugs was "opiate." Opiates were those drugs derived directly from morphine. The synthesis of chemically-related agents led to the term opioid, which medically is currently used to describe natural, semisynthetic, and completely synthetic derivatives with morphine-like actions. These consist of drugs that have actions similar (agonist) or opposite (antagonist) to morphine, drugs that have both effects (agonist-antagonist), substances produced by the body that have similar effects (endogenous), and the receptors in the body that serve as the sites of those drugs' action.

In common language, however, the term narcotic defines morphine and all of its derivatives, both natural and synthetic. Although initially used to define the sleep-producing effects of morphine (narcos = stupor), unfortunately, in common parlance, it has a pejorative connotation and often includes other mood-altering agents as well, such as cocaine and at one time barbiturates. It is the persistence of this negative image of narcotic that is often responsible for people receiving inadequate relief from their pain due to the fear of addiction. Since common usage still prevails, the term narcotic will be used to refer to the opiates and opioids interchangeably in an attempt to desensitize the reader to this negative image.

Currently available narcotics can be classified into three main groups: (1) the three naturally occurring opium alkaloids, (2) the semisynthetic opiates, and (3) the synthetic narcotic analgesics (Table 6.1). The opium alkaloids consist of the phenanthrenes containing morphine, codeine, and thebaine, and the benzylisoquinolines containing papaverine and noscapine.

Morphine, the prototype of narcotic analgesics, is the original derivative of the opiates and semisynthetic analgesics. Its actions are consistent and have been studied extensively. The following discussion concerning the properties of narcotic agents will refer to morphine unless otherwise stated.

GENERAL PHARMACOLOGIC PROPERTIES

Absorption, Biotransformation, and Excretion

Oral administration results in rapid absorption from the gastrointestinal tract or, if used as snuff or by smoking, the nasal mucosal membranes and the lung. When morphine or its congeners are administered subcutaneously or intravenously, a rapid onset of action occurs.[4] Morphine is concentrated in free or bound form in the tissues, most prominently in the liver, kidney, lung, spleen, adrenals, and thyroid. It readily crosses the placental membranes and can be identified in the fetal bloodstream, at times being responsible for respiratory depression or withdrawal symptoms in the newborn. Unlike heroin, however, the permeability of the blood-brain barrier to morphine is quite low.[5,6]

TABLE 6.1. Narcotic Analgesics

Drug	Trade name	Average dose mg[a]		Duration of action (Hr)	Relative potency[b]
		IM	Oral		
Morphine and derivatives					
Morphine	Astramorph PF, Duramorph, Infumorph 200, MS Contin, Roxanol, RMS	10[c]	60	4-5	1
Heroin		2-5		3-4	3-4
Hydromorphone	Dilaudid	1-2	7.5	4-5	6
Metopon	Metopon	3		4-5	3
Oxymorphone	Numorphan[d]	1		4-6	5-10
Various	Pantopon[d]	15		4-5	1
Codeine and derivatives					
Codeine		120	200	4-6	0.08
Hydrocodone	Hycodan[e]		5-10	4-5	4-5
Dihydrocodeine	DHC plus 9		16	4-5	1
Oxycodone	Roxicodone, Percodan[f], Percocet[g]	10	5 5	4-6 4-6	1
Morphinans					
Levorphanol	Levo-Dromoran	2	4	4-5	1
Phenylheptylamines					
L-alpha-acetylmethadol [i]	LAAM, or laam			48-72	
Methadone	Dolophine	10	20	4-6	3
Proxyphene	Darvon		65-120	4-6	0.04

TABLE 6.1 (continued)

Drug	Trade name	Average dose mg[a]		Duration of action (Hr)	Relative potency[b]
		1M	Oral		
Phenylpiperidines					
Diphenoxylate	Lomotil[h]				
Meperidine	Demerol	75	300	2-4	0.75
Sublimaze	0.1[i]			1-2	100
Fentanyl	Duragesic[k]	Varies		1-2	
				50-72	

Modified from Lasagna[68] and Jaffe and Martin[69].

[a]Dose is that producing the same effects equivalent to subcutaneous administration of 10 mg of morphine.

[b]In relation to morphine, equivalent of a potency of 1.

[c]Subcutaneous dose should be decreased in the presence of mitigating factors such as advancing age, anoxia, liver disease, and hypotension.

[d]Mixture of hydrochlorides of opium.

[e]Also contains homatropine.

[f]Also contains aspirin.

[g]Also contains acetaminophen.

[h]Also contains atropine sulfate.

[i]When used as trandermal patch 100 meal hr equivalent to morphine, 10 mg 1 m every 4 hours or 60 mg oral morphine every 4 hours.

[j]Used for maintenance in heroin addiction; initial dose 20-40 mg administered every 48-72 hours.

[k]Available in patches for transdermal administration every 72 hours.

126

Biotransformation is rapid, with a plasma half-life of approximately five hours, with tissue levels minimal at 24 hours. Excretion occurs mainly as the glucuronide (85 to 90 percent) or free morphine (5 to 10 percent), in the urine (90 percent), or in the enterohepatic circulation in the bile, with fecal elimination (8 to 10 percent). Excretion is rapid, with 90 percent occurring within the first 24 hours by glomerular filtration. Small amounts of normorphine and codeine have also been detected in the urine after administration of both heroin and morphine. Urinary metabolites may be detected for several days. It should be emphasized that on an individual basis inactivation rates of morphine may vary considerably by up to a factor of ten. This may be related to a slow release from tissues or absorption via the enterohepatic circulation.

Narcotics and the Central Nervous System

Opiate Receptors

The action of opiates on the central nervous system is complex and may ultimately result in either depression or stimulation, depending on the species studied, dose administered, site of action, and individual susceptibility. Although the existence of specific opiate receptors had long been hypothesized, it was not until 1973 when Pert and Snyder,[7] utilizing radioimmunoassay techniques, were able to measure opiate receptors in brain membranes directly. As discussed in Chapter 2, with the exception of the cerebellum, opiate receptor activity has been identified in all areas of the brain with the greatest concentration of opiate receptors is in the amygdala.[8]

The affinity of specific opiates for the receptor has, in general, paralleled their pharmacologic activity, with potent analgesics having a much greater receptor affinity than weaker agents. Exceptions, however, do exist. Narcotic antagonists (Chapter 7) *in vitro* show an affinity toward receptor binding similar to their corresponding agonist. *In vivo*, however, pharmacological effects of antagonists occur with much lower dosage than seen with the corresponding agonist.

Subsequent to opiate binding to receptors, a decrease in neuronal firing occurs, accompanied by an inhibition of normal sodium influx, which in turn results in a decreased affinity of opiates for the receptor sites. The incorporation of sodium into the receptor-agonist or antagonist media has been found to be a means of distinguishing between agonists and antagonists.[9,10] Concentrations of sodium similar to that found *in vivo* resulted in a higher receptor affinity for antagonists and a greatly decreased binding of agonists.

Receptor Types

As discussed in Chapter 2, there are currently believed to be five receptor types: mu (μ), delta (δ), sigma (σ), kappa (ϰ), and epsilon (ε) (Table 6.2).[11,12,13] Morphine and other opiates interact predominantly with the mu receptor, although kappa and delta receptors activity also exist, but to a lesser extent. Other opioid peptides have been observed to interact with the delta receptors, and the benzomorphans interact with both sigma and kappa receptors. Sigma receptors are believed to be involved in feelings of dysphoria, and in producing hallucinations. They have also been associated with stimulation of the respiratory and vasomotor systems.

The identification and functioning of the opiate receptors is a rapidly evolving field, and it is not at all unlikely that, in the near future, additional receptors will be identified, as well as the effects of various ions on their functioning. This will ultimately allow a more rapid ability to design newer analgesics with less side effects and perhaps a lesser chance of tolerance to develop to its analgesic effects.

It is believed that mu receptor activity is primarily responsible for morphine analgesia, as well as respiratory depression and euphoria. The narcotic agonist-antagonists pentazocine, butorphanol, and nalbuphine have a high

TABLE 6.2. Actions of Narcotic Agonists and Antagonists on Opiate Receptors

	Mu (μ)	Kappa (ϰ)	Delta (δ)	Epsilon (ε)	Sigma (σ)
Effects					
Analgesia	++	+	+/ −		
Euphoria	++				
Respiratory					
Depression	+				+
Sedation		+		+	+
Dysphoria					+
Hallucinations					
Stimulation					
Drugs					
Morphine	++	+	+		
Pentazocine	− /+	+			
Nalbuphine	−	+			
Butorphanol	+/ −	+			
Buprenorphine	+/ −	−			

+: agonist effect
−: antagonist effect
+/ −: partial agonist effect

affinity for the kappa receptors. The pure antagonists such as naloxone (Narcan) have no agonist activity and block the receptor from binding with agonist drugs.

Analgesia

In humans, morphine exerts a narcotic action characterized by analgesia, dysphoria, euphoria, somnolence, and, at times, respiratory depression (Table 6.3). The analgesia accompanying morphine is not associated with a loss of consciousness and may not be associated with decreased sensitivity to touch, sight, hearing, or impairment in motor or intellectual functioning. The relief of pain is accompanied by a marked feeling of tranquility, suggesting that morphine's principal action is on the affective components of pain rather than resulting from a change in pain threshold. The identification of opiate receptors has allowed for more definitive theories concerning the ways analgesia is produced (Table 6.4).

Effects on Limbic System

The paleospinothalamic tract presents an area of high density receptor activity. This pathway is responsible for a perception of dull, chronic pain that is well relieved by administration of opiates. The activation of the

TABLE 6.3. Effects of Morphine on the Central Nervous System

Effect	Manifestation
Analgesia	Increase in ability to tolerate pain
Dysphoria	Anxiety, fear, nausea, vomiting
Euphoria	Relief from pain, anxiety, and tension; positive feeling of pleasure
Mental clouding, somnolence	Change in mentation, inability to concentrate, apathy, lethargy, drowsiness, sleep
Respiratory depression	Decrease in respiratory rate, minute volume tidal exchange, irregular breathing, respiratory arrest
Stimulation of chemoreceptor trigger zone in medulla	Nausea and vomiting
Interference with hypothalamic function	Induction antidiuretic hormone release; inhibition of ACTH and gonadotropin release
	Hyperglycemia; disordered temperature regulation

TABLE 6.4. Possible Mechanisms of Opiate Analgesia

Activation of limbic system
Stimulation of descending serotonergic pathways
Increase in dopamine turnover
Suppression of dorsal horn nociceptive neurons

limbic system as part of the integrated response to pain may also be affected by opiates due to the high density of receptors.

Effects on Serotonin Pathways

Another hypothesis relates analgesia to the activation of descending serotonergic pathways.[14] As discussed in Chapter 2, serotonin (5-HT) is believed to play a prominent role in modulating the perception of pain. In animals, intracerebral ventricular injections of 5-HT can potentiate morphine analgesia. Inhibition of 5-HT synthesis is associated with diminished analgesia and a reduced capacity to develop dependence and tolerance.[15] Lesions of the nucleus raphe magnus—an area of high density of 5-HT—is accompanied by elimination of morphine analgesic activity that can be transiently restored by direct injection of 5-HT.

Effects of Noradrenergic Pathways

It has also been suggested that opiate analgesia may also be mediated by activation of descending noradrenergic pathways. Activation of noradrenergic (A$_2$) receptors inhibits nociception and has a synergistic (additive) effect on the opioid (mu receptor) analgesia.[16]

Effects on Dopamine Pathways

Cerebral dopamine metabolism is stimulated by narcotic analgesics, resulting in an increase in dopamine turnover that can be prevented by pretreatment with naloxone. Similarly, dopamine antagonists potentiate morphine analgesia. The effects of opiates on other neurotransmitters have been discussed in Chapter 2.

Alterations in Mood

At times, a feeling of drowsiness and euphoria may accompany morphine analgesia. The use of morphine in pain-free individuals, however, frequently is accompanied by dysphoria rather than euphoria, as well as fear, anxiety, nausea, and vomiting. At therapeutic doses, morphine may initially cause lethargy, somnolence, and mental clouding, resulting in an inability to concentrate. Slurring of speech or motor incoordination is unusual, although diminished physical activity is frequent. The absence of slurring of speech distinguishes the sedative effect of narcotics from those of hypnotic and sedative agents.[17,18] With chronic administration of morphine for pain relief, mental clouding soon resolves and cognitive and psychomotor functions are virtually unimpaired.[19]

Electroencephalographic (EEG) changes following morphine administration consist of high voltage, low frequency waves similar to those seen with natural sleep or low dose barbiturate administration.[20] Rapid eye movement (REM) phase of sleep and non-REM deep sleep phases are decreased, while non-REM light sleep and waking time are increased. Other opiates may be associated with differing EEG effects. Heroin has been associated with a biphasic EEG response that appears to correlate well with clinical descriptions of heroin-induced euphoria.[21] Chronic methadone administration is associated with a decrease in alpha and beta rhythms and an increase in theta rhythms. The clinical relevance of this remains to be determined.

Respiration

Respiratory depression at therapeutic doses routinely occurs primarily due to direct effect of morphine on the respiratory centers of the brainstem. This effect is able to be detected even with doses of morphine insufficient to produce sedation, and may be accompanied by irregular and periodic breathing. The time of maximum respiratory depression following morphine administration varies with the route of administration, occurring within seven minutes following intravenous, within 30 minutes following intramuscular, and within 90 minutes following subcutaneous administration. Normal functioning of the respiratory center can be seen within two to three hours following a morphine injection; however, respiratory function tests can reveal abnormalities for as long as four to five hours. Morphine depresses the response of the respiratory chemoceptors by elevating carbon dioxide tension and hydrogen ions, and inhibiting centers in the pons and medulla responsible for respiratory regularity. The diminished sensitivity to carbon dioxide may become important clinically in treatment of overdose reaction where hypoxia may be the only stimulus to respiration. Voluntary control of respiration is also affected, resulting in a decreased effort in breathing. An antitussive effect is prominent due to depression of the cough center.

Nausea and Vomiting

In contrast to the depressant effect that morphine exhibits on most brain centers, it directly stimulates the chemoreceptor trigger zones, frequently resulting in nausea and vomiting. This effect exhibits marked individual variation in both frequency and intensity, with chronic use at times associated with suppression of the vomiting center. It is of interest that the incidence of nausea and vomiting is greater in ambulatory patients than in persons who are recumbent. The emetic effect of morphine may be prevented by administration of a narcotic antagonist as well as phenothiazine derivatives.

Ocular Effects

Pupillary constriction (miosis), a consistent response to narcotics, frequently is used as a characteristic sign of opiate dependence. It should be emphasized that in a pharmacologic overdose of morphine resulting in anoxia, however, pupillary dilatation (mydriasis) will occur. Tolerance to miosis with continued use may also be observed.

Hypothalamic: Pituitary Axis

There have been many animal studies of the effect of morphine on the hypothalamic pituitary axis. Repeated morphine injections result in an inhibition of adrenocorticotropic hormone (ACTH), related to a corresponding decrease in 4-secretion of corticotropin releasing factor (CRF), with a subsequent decrease in adrenal cortical activity.[22] The diurnal release of corticosteroids is also altered. Withdrawal of morphine results in a rebound phenomenon with a marked increase in these hormones, which correlates with the abstinence syndrome. Chronic morphine administration results in a decrease in adrenal cortical function, but with time, tolerance to this effect may develop.

Morphine inhibits the secretion of thyroid stimulating hormone (TSH). Heroin- or methadone-dependent individuals are clinically euthyroid, although elevated serum levels of thyroxin (T4) and triiodothyronine (T3), probably secondary to increased levels of thyroxin binding globulin, have been noted.[22] Growth hormone secretion may increase with chronic morphine administration. Administration of morphine is also associated with a stimulation of antidiuretic hormone, with a corresponding decrease in urinary output. Tolerance to this effect occurs with normal levels of antidiuretic hormone observed in chronic narcotic users. Decreased urine output may also be related to morphine-induced hypotension, which is associated with a reduction in filtration rate when large doses of morphine are administered.

Cardiovascular System

Narcotics prescribed in therapeutic doses are associated with little effect on blood pressure, heart rate, or rhythm in the supine patient. Even in toxic doses resulting in respiratory depression, a significant effect on the vasomotor center is delayed so that hypotension seen late in the course of narcotic overdose is usually secondary to hypoxia. Physiologic response to gravitational shifts, however, are altered so that hypotension may occur on sitting or standing due to peripheral vasodilatation. Intravenous morphine has been demonstrated to cause significant arteriolar dilatation, manifested by a reduction in forearm vascular resistance as well as systemic vascular resistance.

The effect of morphine on heart rate is variable, although cardiac output is not significantly altered. Regional circulatory changes, with the exception of renal blood flow, which has been found to be decreased, are relatively unchanged. Cerebral vasodilatation, however, may occur in a pharmacologic overdose, secondary to carbon dioxide retention.

In patients with cardiac disease, especially acute myocardial infarction, the cardiovascular response to narcotic agents may be more attenuated. Decreases in oxygen consumption, cardiac index, left ventricular and diastolic pressure, and cardiac index have been found in persons with coronary artery disease. However, such patients are usually able to tolerate morphine analgesia without difficulty.

Administration of morphine to critically ill patients is associated with significant decreases in arterial pressure, heart rate, cardiac index, stroke index, and oxygen consumption similar in magnitude to that seen in cardiac patients.[23] The oxygen extraction ratio, however, remains relatively unchanged, suggesting the presence of a decreased oxygen demand rather than an inadequate oxygen delivery. This "hemodynamic sedation" in the absence of severe central nervous system depression is desirable and may explain the observed effectiveness of morphine in this setting.

These data suggest that morphine, when used appropriately, is a useful and safe drug in almost all patients, whether used as an analgesic agent or in the treatment of pulmonary edema, with alterations in the cardiovascular system being minimal. However, it should be emphasized that persons with right ventricular congestive failure (cor pulmonale) and hepatic dysfunction secondary to congestive change or to primary hepatic disease may be much more sensitive to standard doses of narcotics.

Gastrointestinal System

Morphine and other narcotics can reduce propulsive contractions of the intestines as well as inhibition of gastric, biliary, and pancreatic secretions.

This results in a decrease in motility and a delay in the passage of food through the stomach into the duodenum. Resting tone of smooth muscle of both small and large intestine is increased as is the tone of the ileocecal valve and the anal sphincter. Propulsive peristaltic movements are decreased. These effects all contribute to the constipation frequently associated with narcotic use.

Morphine-induced spasm of the sphincter of Oddi is associated with increases in biliary tract pressure, which may be clinically manifested as epigastric distress or even, on occasion, colic. Although the intensity of this effect is variable and may be of no clinical significance, when morphine is administered in biliary colic an exacerbation of pain may occur. Other narcotics, such as meperidine, are said to produce a lesser degree of spasm; however, the clinical relevance of this remains to be determined.

Tolerance to the gastrointestinal effects of narcotics develops slowly. Although these side effects are usually considered undesirable, narcotics may be a useful adjunct in individuals with bowel disorders associated with abdominal pain and diarrhea (Chapter 16).

The Peripheral Nervous System

Until recently it had been assumed the analgesic actions of the narcotics were solely due to the binding to opioid receptors in the central nervous system. Recently opioid receptors have been identified in the peripheral nervous system as well, with inflammation increasing their activity. Application of systemically ineffective doses of morphine in joint spaces has been associated with analgesia comparable to that seen with local anesthetics.[24] This analgesic effect that can be reversed by naloxone can persist up to 48 hours.

Other Organ System Effects

Morphine also increases tone and amplitude of contractions in the ureters, the bladder, and the vesicular sphincter. Clinically, this may appear as urinary retention, particularly in patients with enlarged prostates.

The effect of morphine on histamine release may be associated with local changes such as urticaria or dilatation of the small vessels of the skin. The augmentation in histamine secretion may be clinically relevant when morphine is administered to patients with a history of asthma.

MORPHINE AND ITS CONGENERS

Morphine

Morphine is available for oral use in both regular and timed release capsules, by injection, and as suppositories to relieve moderate to severe pain. Oral use of morphine is one-third to one-sixth as effective as parenteral use due to its inactivation during passage through the liver. The timed release form has been quite helpful in relieving chronic pain.

The use of morphine by injection for acute pain or as preoperative medication is quite effective. For reasons less than clear, most physicians still prefer the use of meperidine due to the misconception that this is a "less potent" narcotic. Morphine used epidurally to relieve chronic malignant pain has also been quite effective. Most recently, timed release morphine has been shown to be effective in providing relief from cancer pain without the encumbrance of frequent injections or reliance on taking pills every four to six hours.[25]

Dihydromorphinone

Dihydromorphinone (Dilaudid) is a semisynthetic derivative of morphine approximately six to eight times as potent. Absorption following oral administration is better than morphine, allowing its use both orally and parenterally. An analgesic effect can be demonstrated within 15 minutes of parenteral administration and within 30 minutes following ingestion. Analgesic doses of dihydromorphinone are associated with slightly less sedation, but a degree of euphoria and dependence quite similar to morphine.

Opium

Pantopon® is a mixture of all the alkaloids of opium in approximately the same proportions in which they are found naturally. Active ingredients, in addition to morphine, include codeine and papaverine. Its analgesic effect is directly proportional to its morphine content, although the other alkaloids may enhance both sedation and analgesia. Its dependency-producing potential is equal to that of morphine.

Tincture of opium and paregoric are used mainly as antidiarrheal agents, although at times they have been used to diminish withdrawal symptoms in infants born to narcotic-dependent women.

Oxymorphone

Oxymorphone (Numorphan) is a parenteral narcotic with a potency seven to ten times that of morphine. Its pharmacologic actions are quite similar.

Codeine

Codeine is a naturally occurring alkaloid of opium that, in contrast to morphine, is approximately two-thirds as effective orally as parenterally. Metabolism occurs chiefly in the liver, with excretion in the urine largely in inactive forms. Subcutaneous administration of 120 mg of codeine is approximately equal to 10 mg of morphine. Codeine is an extremely effective mild analgesic; however, dependence and withdrawal symptoms can occur on discontinuing the drug. The intensity of these syndromes is considerably milder than that seen with morphine. Codeine is of particular value in persons with pain due to chronic bowel disease associated with increased peristaltic activity and diarrhea. Codeine, in antitussive elixirs, as well as in combination with nonnarcotic analgesics, is probably the most frequently prescribed narcotics.

Heroin (Diacetyl Morphine)

Heroin is a derivative of morphine, approximately three to four times as potent. It is readily absorbed orally by mucous membranes in the nose as well as the gastrointestinal tract. Subsequent to injection, heroin is rapidly diacetylated at the three position to 6-monoacetyl morphine (MAM), which in turn is 6-diacetylated to morphine at a somewhat slower rate. Heroin disappears from the plasma rapidly, having a half-life of 2.5 minutes. Plasma levels of MAM reach peak values within five minutes. The decline in MAM levels is associated with the appearance of morphine, which reaches peak plasma levels at approximately 20 minutes, exceeding the concentration of both heroin and MAM within 40 minutes.[4,5] Although morphine is responsible for most of the pharmacological actions of heroin, both heroin and MAM are more lipid soluble and can rapidly pass through the blood-brain barrier. This may explain the great propensity for narcotic overdose associated with intravenous heroin use.

Heroin is an excellent analgesic, although studies comparing the oral effectiveness of heroin with morphine have been unable to find a significant difference. Investigational studies, comparing parenteral effects of morphine, heroin, and a saline placebo, also have found similar responses produced by the two drugs.[26] When morphine and heroin were administered to individuals with a history of narcotic addiction, the majority of addicts found morphine more pleasant than heroin. Heroin-induced euphoria did not occur more frequently.[27]

In this country, heroin remains unavailable as an analgesic agent, being a Schedule I drug to be used only for investigatory purposes. The feelings of many physicians concerning the superiority of heroin as an analgesic agent several years ago, resulted in an attempt to allow its use in the treatment of chronic pain syndrome. After considerable discussion and even legislative hearings, it was felt that the danger of diversion and potential for addiction outweighed its use as an analgesic agent, and it remained in Schedule 1. In fact, heroin in equianalgesic doses has little or no advantage over morphine in management of pain.

MORPHINANS

Levorphanol

Levorphanol (Levo-Dromoran) is a synthetic narcotic analgesic with a potency approximately four times that of morphine. It is relatively ineffective when given orally. Absorption is rapid following subcutaneous administration. Levorphanol's effects closely resemble morphine, with the exception that nausea and vomiting are less likely to occur. The relatively long half-life (12 to 16 hours) will result in its accumulation in tissues when administered constantly. Unless the dose is appropriately adjusted, central nervous system depression may occur.

PHENYLPIPERIDINES

Meperidine

The effects produced by meperidine (Demerol), the prototype of the phenylpiperidines, are quite similar to that of morphine. Meperidine is only one-quarter as effective an analgesic and exhibits a shorter duration of action, necessitating more frequent injections for relief of continuing pain. Unlike morphine, in large doses administration of meperidine may be associated with signs of central nervous system excitation, consisting of tremor, muscle twitches, and seizures. These excitatory effects may become apparent when the daily dose reaches 3 g and are unaffected by tolerance even after chronic use. Individuals with renal disease are at particular risk of these complications due to the accumulation of normeperidine, a toxic breakdown product of meperidine.

Absorption following ingestion of meperidine is good, with peak plasma concentrations occurring between the first and second hours. Approximately 40 percent of meperidine is bound to plasma proteins. Metabolism occurs predominantly in the liver, with hydrolysis to meperidinic acid or by N-demethylation and hydrolysis to normeperidinic acid and subsequent conjugation. Normeperidine, unlike meperidine, can cause stimulation of the central nervous system and, if it accumulates in the plasma, convulsions may occur. Similarly, if nalorphine is administered and meperidine is displaced from receptor sites, the increase in normeperidine may result in seizure activity, necessitating the use of a tranquilizing agent.

One of the main impediments to effective analgesia encountered with meperidine is the hesitancy of the physician to prescribe the drug as frequently as needed.[28,29] The relatively short action of this agent requires administration every two to three hours (Chapter 13). Yet in many instances, the meperidine is ordered at a less than optimal dose every four to six hours.

Meperidine is an effective analgesic best utilized when a shorter duration of analgesic action is required in an essentially healthy individual. Its effect on the cardiovascular system and the gastrointestinal tract are qualitatively similar to morphine, but less prominent. With meperidine, however, urinary retention is less frequent than that seen with morphine. It would therefore be a reasonable analgesic in individuals with prostatic hypertrophy and normal renal and cardiovascular function. In ambulatory patients, the use of meperidine may be associated with slightly higher incidence of dizziness, nausea, vomiting, and, at times, hypotension associated with palpitations and syncope.

Fentanyl

Fentanyl is a synthetic opiate approximately 80 to 100 times as potent as morphine. For a brief time, it was sold on the street as synthetic heroin (China White) and caused several fatal reactions. At high doses muscular rigidity and apnea may occur. At present, it is widely used in combination with anesthetic agents, as well as for postoperative analgesia. Since it is much more expensive than morphine, its routine use for postoperative analgesia is not warranted. Most recently a transdermal delivery system of Fentanyl was developed for management of chronic pain. Studies have revealed the Fentanyl patch to be quite effective in providing long-term analgesia.[30,31]

PHENYLHEPTYLAMINES

Methadone

Methadone was synthesized in Germany at the end of World War II. Over the next two decades, it received considerable attention in this country as an excellent drug for treatment of chronic intractable pain. The establishment of methadone maintenance as a therapeutic modality for the rehabilitation of heroin addicts resulted in a large number of persons being placed on chronic methadone therapy. Unfortunately, the use of methadone for maintenance therapy initially resulted in its removal for use as an analgesic. Until this action was ultimately reviewed, a considerable number of persons in severe pain were prevented from using this drug.

Methadone is a 6-dimethylamino-4-4 diphenyl-3-heptanone. Although its structure is markedly different from morphine, its actions are qualitatively quite similar. However, methadone: (1) is much more effective orally; (2) is slightly more potent on a milligram for milligram basis, when administered parenterally; (3) is associated with a greater sedative effect with repeated administration; (4) is able to provide consistent analgesia without the need for rapid dose escalation; and (5) is able to suppress acute withdrawal symptoms smoothly in narcotic-dependent persons due to its extended duration of action.

When administered orally, methadone is slowly absorbed from the gastrointestinal tract, with biotransformation in the liver beginning relatively early.[32] This results in a decrease in the initial rapid rise of plasma levels seen with other agents. The relatively long half-life and its widespread distribution to the tissues allows methadone to be slowly released into the blood as the circulating methadone is metabolized, resulting in constant blood levels and even analgesia. However, this will also result in increasing accumulation in the tissues over the first few days that methadone is administered. For this reason, the dose of methadone should be carefully monitored until a steady state develops to prevent oversedation and depression of the central nervous system.

Methadone is an excellent analgesic, providing relief from all types of pain in a manner comparable to that obtained by morphine. In contrast to morphine and other shorter-acting narcotics, however, methadone may be taken as infrequently as every six to eight hours without compromising analgesia. Tolerance develops slowly, allowing for a lesser need to increase dosage. The use of methadone in painful states will be discussed in Chapters 13 and 14.

Lα-Acetylmethadol

Lα-acetylmethadol (LAAM), a long-acting methadone initially developed as an analgesic agent in Germany, has recently been approved for use in maintenance therapy of narcotic addiction.[33] The onset of action of LAAM is slower (several hours) and its duration (two to three days) more prolonged than methadone. It can suppress withdrawal symptoms for as long as 96 hours with a single dose. Unlike methadone, its major metabolites, noracetyl methadol and normethadol, are pharmacologically active. Although initial enthusiasm for LAAM as a maintenance agent waned due to its possible toxic effects on the heart, more recently interest in this drug has been renewed. When used as a maintenance agent, an initial dose of 1.3 times that of the daily methadone dose is considered equivalent. Its long duration of action removes the need for take-home medication, thereby diminishing the chances of diversion.

Propoxyphene

Propoxyphene (Darvon), an ester of methadone, is a commonly prescribed analgesic medication. Indeed, various proprietary forms, alone or in combination with aspirin, phenacetin, or caffeine, are produced by 35 companies, making it one of the most commonly used analgesics. In 1978, the 312 million prescriptions written by physicians for propoxyphene placed it as the third most widely prescribed drug.[34,35] Dextropropoxyphene, the active isomer, provides analgesic effects similar to codeine, although its potency is felt to be approximately one-third as great.

Absorption, Biotransformation, Excretion

Propoxyphene is available as the hydrochloride or as Propoxyphene Napsylate (Darvon-N), alone or in combination with other analgesic agents. The hydrochloride is rapidly absorbed from the intestinal tract after oral or parenteral administration. Absorption is more rapid than that seen with the napsylate, although the differences in peak plasma concentrations between the two preparations are quite small. The drug is detected in the plasma following oral administration within one hour, peaks at two hours, and then slowly decreases, with a half-life of approximately 3.5 hours. Rapid hepatic metabolism of propoxyphene results in a low bioavailability, with only 18 percent of an oral dose reaching the systemic circulation unchanged.

Analgesic Effects

Clinically the analgesic effectiveness of propoxyphene is controversial. Although 65 mg are commonly considered to be equivalent to 30 mg of codeine, several studies have suggested that 35 mg of propoxyphene may be no more effective than placebo, with 90 to 120 mg being needed to provide an analgesic effect equivalent to 60 mg of codeine. Propoxyphene at a 65 mg dose has also been shown to provide less analgesic when compared to aspirin.[36,37] A combination of propoxyphene with aspirin or with acetaminophen has not been found to produce better analgesia than either aspirin or acetylaminophenalone administered alone.[38,39,40,42] Repeated doses of propoxyphene, resulting in an increasing plasma concentration, is associated with effective analgesia. The analgesic effects of 50 to 100 mg of the napsylate is equivalent to 1 mg of subcutaneously administered morphine, with 100 mg equivalent to 1 mg of oral methadone.[41]

Most physicians consider propoxyphene a relatively safe and effective analgesic agent. Although propoxyphene, in low doses, is not associated with serious adverse effects, it is a narcotic that binds to mu receptors and, when taken in larger doses, can induce both psychological and physical dependence as well as tolerance. Discontinuation of chronic propoxyphene therapy may result in withdrawal reactions. Physical dependence can be produced with as little as 500 to 800 mg/day of the hydrochloride or 800 to 1,200 mg of the napsylate salt.

Toxicity

Propoxyphene dependence has become a well-recognized phenomenon. According to the Drug Awareness Network (DAWN), which reports drug abuse incidents from diverse health care facilities, propoxyphene was the eighth most frequent substance of abuse in 1975, being responsible for 5 percent of deaths reported from medical examiners' offices.[43] The role of propoxyphene in drug abuse in England was even more prominent, and at one time was the leading cause of analgesic self-poisoning.[44] The increasing awareness of propoxyphene abuse resulted in its being placed in Schedule IV of the Controlled Substances Act in 1977. Two years later, the FDA was still sufficiently concerned and required that a warning of the risks of taking propoxyphene be placed in labeling for all products containing propoxyphene, as well as an information leaflet to be available for patients.[45]

Toxic reactions to propoxyphene are similar to other narcotics and include nausea, vomiting, and somnolence. Increasing doses may lead to respiratory depression, pulmonary edema, convulsions, coma, and ultimately, death. Cardiovascular reactions include ventricular bigeminy, which may progress to ventricular tachycardia. A national assessment of propoxyphene-related deaths noted cardiac arrest as the mode of demise to be almost as frequent as respiratory depression.[46] Treatment of overdose reactions is similar to that used in other narcotic overdose reactions and will be described below.

NARCOTIC COMBINATIONS

Codeine Derivatives: Hydrocodone and Oxycodone

Hydrocodone, related to oxycodone, is often used in combination with other drugs, including homatropine (Hycodan), as an antitussive as well as an analgesic in antipyretic mixtures (Chapter 5). Oxycodone, in combination with either aspirin (Percodan, Roxiprin) or acetaminophen (Percocet, Roxicet, Roxilox), is a frequently prescribed analgesic. It is approximately equal in potency to morphine and is as effective orally. Analgesic activity can be demonstrated within 10 to 15 minutes, peaking at 45 minutes, and persisting for three to six hours. It is also associated with a degree of dependence equivalent to that of morphine. Abrupt discontinuation will result in withdrawal.

In practice, its potential for addiction is probably greater than morphine, since it is promoted as a synthetic codeine derivative. Unwary physicians may prescribe this drug freely without realizing its dependency potential. Experience has shown that dependence to oxycodone is a very real phenomenon that is most frequently seen in persons under continuing medical care.

Phenylpiperidine Derivatives

Difenoxin and atropine sulfate (Motofen), and diphenoxylate and atropine sulfate (Lomotil, Lofene, Logen, LocoQuel, Lomate) are congeners of meperidine that are effective constipating agents. Although the risk of dependence with appropriate use of these drugs is low, high doses can result in dependence. In fact, in the 1970s Lomotil was used in several communities as a maintenance drug for the treatment of heroin addiction.

Loperamide (Imodium) is also a piperidine derivative that is an effective constipating agent. Although pleasurable effects have not been seen even with large doses, in the laboratory setting morphine dependent monkeys deprived of morphine have had withdrawal prevented by administration of high doses of Loperamide.

Brompton Cocktail

The use of narcotic and stimulant mixtures in an attempt to relieve pain predates this century, when Snow in 1896 reported the combined use of morphine and cocaine in persons with metastatic disease. The cocaine was felt to support a "positive attitude" while the morphine provided analgesic relief.[47] In the early twentieth century, this combination once again appeared as a postthoracotomy analgesic at the Brompton Hospital in London.[69] In addition to the morphine and cocaine, gin and honey were frequent additives.

In 1952, the use of this elixir became formalized when the Brompton Hospital printed its composition in a supplement to the National Formulary.[47,48,49] The original formula contained cocaine, alcohol, chloroform water, and syrup, in addition to heroin or morphine. At present, Brompton's is still widely used—not only in England, but also in this country—in the treatment of terminal cancer pain. The composition of this mixture, however, varies considerably. Heroin may be substituted for morphine. The alcohol content can vary greatly, with traditional spirits often substituted for absolute alcohol, and cocaine may be deleted with the addition of phenothiazine.

Recently, several studies have been undertaken to determine the effectiveness of Brompton's Mixture as well as the most appropriate ingredients. The effectiveness of a standard Brompton's Mixture compared to a solution of only morphine administered in a flavored aqueous solution, in a double blind crossover trial of 44 persons with intractable pain, found both mixtures to relieve pain in approximately 85 percent of the patients.[50] Subsequently, a study of 382 persons with terminal cancer confirmed cocaine to be unnecessary for analgesia.[51] The alcohol in the Brompton solution was effective in preventing contaminant growth while the solution was stored, with shelf time able to be increased without growth of fungi and yeasts. Little difference was demonstrated between pain relief afforded by heroin as compared to morphine.

The possibility of morphine-induced nausea often results in a routine prescription of chlorpromazine to patients receiving Brompton's. Although nausea may occur, it is unclear if this is due to the emetic qualities of morphine or to an individual distaste of other substances in the elixir, such as the alcohol or the syrup.

In summary, an elixir consisting of either morphine or heroin can be effective orally in relieving intractable pain. Additional ingredients added to suit individual taste may include the addition of small amounts of alcohol to prevent contaminant growth, or the use of juice or milk as a means to promote better patient acceptability.

Morphine-Amphetamine Combinations

In contrast to recent studies suggesting that the addition of cocaine to oral mixtures of narcotics adds little to the analgesic effect, simultaneous administration of dextroamphetamine and morphine has been shown to enhance morphine analgesia as well as diminish some of its undesirable side effects, with respect to respiration, pulse, and blood pressure.[52]

Patients receiving the dextroamphetamine-morphine combination were more alert and required less analgesia. It is suggested that 5 to 10 mg of dextroamphetamine administered in conjunction with morphine can provide pain relief equivalent to that obtained with 1.5 to 2 times the dose of morphine taken alone.

The use of this combination, however, is not without attendant risks. The potential for myocardial stimulation and arrhythmia prevents its use in cardiac patients. Urinary retention in the elderly might also be a problem due to the synergistic effect of these drugs on bladder motility.

OTHER CLINICAL EFFECTS ASSOCIATED WITH NARCOTIC USE

Dependence

All of the narcotic drugs can produce both physical dependence and tolerance with repeated use (Chapter 3). Even with sporadic use, psychological dependence may develop. This, in turn, may lead to more frequent use, with subsequent development of physical dependence.

However, the degree of physical dependence, the time required for it to develop, and the development of tolerance to specific drug effects vary greatly with individual agents. Dependence may be demonstrated by precipitation of withdrawal symptoms after administration of a narcotic antagonist as early as two to three days after therapeutic doses of morphine have been administered.[53,54] Naloxone has been able to precipitate mild withdrawal symptoms one week after ingestion of a single 40 mg methadone dose by former heroin addicts.

Tolerance

Intermittent use of narcotics for pain is associated with a slow developing tolerance to the analgesic effects even while used for relatively long periods. Continuing use, however, is associated with tolerance to respiratory depression, analgesia, sedation, vomiting, and euphoria. Tolerance may develop slowly or not at all with respect to miosis and constipation. Tolerance to the atropine-like actions of meperidine is minimal. Even when maintained on relatively high doses of meperidine, dilated pupils, increased muscular activity, or seizures can be observed.[55] A considerable degree of cross tolerance exists between narcotic agents, and on a dose equivalency basis any narcotic may be substituted for another without development of withdrawal symptoms.

It should be emphasized that both dependence and tolerance will occur when narcotics are used appropriately for relief of chronic pain. These are not contraindications to their use as analgesics. When the source of the pain is eliminated detoxification can occur (see below) with little difficulty. Even with long-term use of narcotics there have been no detrimental effects associated with dependence, providing the narcotics is taken appropriately.

Withdrawal

The characteristics and intensity of withdrawal symptoms vary greatly with specific agent, dosage, intervals between dosage, duration of use, and even one's psychological state. Patients who have received analgesic doses of narcotics for up to two weeks may be able to discontinue the drug with only mild symptoms, usually not attributed by either patient or physician to withdrawal. In most instances, the major complaint is slight irritability and difficulty in sleeping.

In contrast, an individual taking a narcotic primarily for its euphoric effect may develop withdrawal symptoms as soon as the scheduled time for the next dose has passed. It is, therefore, quite helpful to distinguish between those signs and symptoms considered to be oriented toward obtaining a narcotic drug (purposive) and those that can be objectively evaluated and are independent of the environment or psychological state of the patient (nonpurposive)

Signs and Symptoms

Purposive phenomena can appear quite early. The earliest symptom is anxiety, usually manifested by drug-seeking behavior, which in the clinical setting takes the form of immediate requests for additional analgesia. Purposive behavior usually reaches peak intensity by 36 to 72 hours following the last morphine injection. It can be modified greatly not only by the environment but also by the presence of a calm, sympathetic observer.

Nonpurposive symptoms appear 8 to 12 hours after the last morphine injection. The intensity of symptoms may be considered mild, moderate, marked, or severe (Tables 6.5 and 6.6).[56] Mild symptoms result from early autonomic hyperactivity, which may increase in intensity over the first day and then stabilize as the syndrome progresses. During this time, pupillary dilatation, loss of appetite, tremor, and the appearance of "gooseflesh" due to piloerecta stimulation will occur. At 16 to 18 hours, if a narcotic has not been administered, the individual may fall into a restless, tossing sleep for two to three hours called the "yen." On awakening, approximately 20 hours after the last dose, there is further evidence of withdrawal consisting of marked restlessness, deep breathing, fever, and insomnia. Hypertension is not infrequent, and complaints of chills alternating with flushing and intense perspiration may appear. Nausea and vomiting and diarrhea may appear in two-thirds of persons. Severe muscular spasms in the extremities, now infrequently

TABLE 6.5. Symptoms of Narcotic Withdrawal

Early	First 10 hours
Anxiety Sweating Rapid short respirations Slight rhinorrhea and lacrimation Dilated reactive pupils	
Late	10 hours to 14 days
Marked lacrimation and rhinorrhea Tachycardia Tremor Yawning Piloerection Nausea, vomiting, diarrhea Abdominal pain Fever Leukocytosis Elevation of blood pressure Diffuse muscle spasm	
Prolonged	10 days to several months
Irritability Fatigue Bradycardia Decrease in body temperature Persistent urinary catecholamine secretion Hyposensitivity of respiratory center to carbon dioxide	

TABLE 6.6. Intensity of Withdrawal Symptoms

Mild	Moderate	Marked	Severe
Anxiety	All mild signs	All moderate signs	All marked signs
Lacrimation	Loss of appetite	Fever	Vomiting
Rhinorrhea	Pupillary dilation	Hypertension	Diarrhea
Sneezing	Piloerection	Deep breathing	Abdominal pain
Sweating	Tremor	Nausea	Muscle spasms
Yawning			

seen, were responsible for the origin of the term "kicking the habit" describing heroin withdrawal.

The intensity of withdrawal varies greatly with the specific narcotic, as well as dose administered. In general, short acting narcotics tend to produce brief intense abstinence syndromes, whereas those drugs that are slowly eliminated produce mild withdrawal. With morphine and heroin, peak intensity is reached at 36 to 48 hours, continuing at a plateau for up to 72 hours and gradually subsiding over the next five to ten days. Withdrawal symptoms from meperidine usually develop within several hours after the last dose, reaching a peak within 8 to 12 hours and then declining over four to five days. Methadone withdrawal presents a syndrome that develops much more slowly without ever reaching the severity seen with morphine. Symptoms rarely occur before 48 hours after the last dose but can last for several weeks. Narcotic antagonists with agonist characteristics (Chapter 7) also can produce withdrawal symptoms varying in intensity with the specific agent.

Treatment

At any time during an acute withdrawal reaction, the administration of a narcotic agent in an appropriate dose will relieve all symptoms. In discontinuing narcotics prescribed for analgesia, it is important to remember that clinically significant withdrawal is unusual with short-term narcotic use. If, however, a person has been chronically maintained on narcotics on a continuous basis, abrupt discontinuation will result in withdrawal phenomena. When a narcotic is no longer needed for the treatment of chronic pain, it is, therefore, most appropriate to slowly taper the dose, rather than abruptly discontinuing it.

The Late Abstinence Syndrome

The intensity of the withdrawal syndrome slowly declines over a period of five to six weeks. This early syndrome, however, is followed by a secondary or protracted abstinence syndrome that may persist up to 12 months following cessation of drug use. This phase is characterized by a decrease in blood pressure, pulse rate, body temperature, and pupillary diameter, and is accompanied by persistent abnormalities in urinary secretion of catecholamines. There is a hyposensitivity to the respiratory stimulant effects of carbon dioxide as well as persistent behavioral modifications.

Detoxification

It should not be necessary for anyone taking narcotics under medical supervision or for those using illicit narcotics who seek medical assistance to ever experience withdrawal. Any narcotic will stop or prevent withdrawal symptoms and may be used in detoxification. One of the easiest and acceptable methods of detoxification is merely to taper the patient's current narcotic dose in decrements of 10 to 20 percent every two to three days until abstinence is achieved. Slowly tapering the analgesic narcotic has the advantage of assuring patient compliance without the necessity of introducing a new drug that might be associated with idiosyncratic side effects. However, the optimal way to detoxify someone who has been on narcotics for a long time is with a long acting narcotic, namely methadone.

Methadone in Detoxification

When one wishes to provide a smooth detoxification from chronic narcotic use, oral methadone hydrochloride is an excellent choice. There is no single regimen that can be considered the "only way" to detoxify. Personal experience has been to substitute an equivalent dose of oral methadone for the amount of narcotic being given on a daily basis, administering this methadone in divided doses every 8 to 12 hours. The daily dose then can be decreased approximately 10 percent every two to three days to allow for a smooth and uneventful detoxification.

An alternative methadone detoxification regimen, if it is not known whether dependence exists, would be to discontinue the narcotic and observe the patient's reaction. If withdrawal symptoms become prominent, 15 to 20 mg of methadone may be administered orally. At the end of four to six hours, if symptoms persist, an additional five to ten mg of methadone is administered. This process is repeated every six hours until signs and symptoms of withdrawal have abated. Once the patient has been stabilized on a constant methadone dose, this dose is administered every 8 to 12 hours for the next day. The total daily dose is then decreased by 10 to 20 percent every two to three days until detoxification is complete. If withdrawal symptoms appear, the rate of decremental dosage may be further slowed.

It should also be noted that the presence of associated medical problems may modify the detoxification procedure. Fever may change tolerance to opiates, requiring a slight increase in methadone dose. The presence of liver disease, associated with a decreased ability to metabolize narcotics, may result in a lower dose being needed.

Clonidine

As discussed in Chapter 3, opiate use is associated with a decrease in norepinephrine activity and turnover. A high density of opiate receptors has been identified in the locus coeruleus (LC), a major center of noradrenergic activity.[57,58,59,60,61] The narcotic antagonist naloxone can precipitate withdrawal when given to someone dependent on narcotics. Naloxone-precipitated withdrawal is accompanied by noradrenergic hyperactivity, suggesting that norepinephrine is the main neurotransmitter in the generation of withdrawal symptoms.

It has been hypothesized that chronic morphine administration results in a decreased synthesis of norepinephrine in the LC. In order to compensate for this, the cells increase their activity to maintain an acceptable level of norepinephrine in the body. Abrupt discontinuation of morphine results in "rebound" noradrenergic hyperactivity with subsequent withdrawal symptoms. Clonidine is an alpha adrenergic antagonist that can decrease neuronal firing in the LC, resulting in a marked decrease in norepinephrine release and turnover with a lessening of withdrawal symptoms (Table 6.7).

In an inpatient setting, the use of oral clonidine at 6 mcg/kg of body weight/day was associated with a significant decrease in signs or symptoms of opiate withdrawal, as compared to placebo with detoxification being complete after 14 days of decreasing clonidine doses.[57,58]

However, the use of clonidine is not unassociated with adverse effects. Systolic and diastolic blood pressures are significantly decreased, with an alteration of clonidine dosage due to hypotension required in approximately 50 percent of patients. Clonidine appears to be most effective when daily dose of narcotic is low. Individuals maintained on high doses of narcotics

TABLE 6.7. Use of Clonidine in Detoxification from Narcotics

Advantages	Problems
Abrupt discontinuation of narcotic possible	Hypotensive effect may limit ambulation
Detoxification can be readily accomplished within two weeks	Not as effective when high level of narcotic dependence exists
Able to reverse narcotic tolerance seen in chronic pain patients	Sedative action may limit use in high doses
Can be used without resulting in loss of work in those with job jeopardy	Potential "rebound" after long-term administration
Enhances physician/patient relationship by removing narcotic dose negotiations	In laboratory animals, behavioral changes reported
May be effective in relieving associated panic anxiety states	

must have their dose lowered prior to initiating clonidine therapy. The drug's sedative and hypotensive effects also limit its usefulness in an ambulatory setting.

In addition, the effect of clonidine on norepinephrine secretion may be time limited, making its use in slow detoxification difficult. The possibility of "rebound" effects, including behavioral changes, may also limit its widespread use.[59] Several observations have suggested that clonidine also has antinociceptive activity equal or slightly greater than that seen with morphine.[60] In human subjects, however, evidence of analgesic activity when clonidine was administered at standard therapeutic doses was not able to be demonstrated.[61] Most recently the use of clonidine with morphine in epidural anesthesia has been observed to double the duration of morphine analgesia without increasing its side effects.[62]

In summary, existing evidence suggests that clonidine may be a useful nonopiate means of detoxifying narcotic dependent persons. Its proclivity toward hypotension and its limited effectiveness in the presence of a high degree of narcotic dependence restrict its use to an inpatient setting.

Antianxiety Agents

The role of tranquilizers in detoxification remains controversial. It is possible to utilize tranquilizers and sedatives to allay the anxiety of discontinuing narcotic use. In the person chronically maintained on narcotics for pain, however, this procedure carries with it the risk of producing yet another form of dependence. Since tranquilizers and sedatives are relatively ineffective in relieving symptoms of narcotic withdrawal, the use of such agents cannot be recommended. Once detoxification has occurred, however, if the individual still appears to be somewhat anxious, short-term use of a mild tranquilizing drug may be appropriate.

Overdose Reactions

Etiology

An overdose due to narcotics administered in a medical setting should theoretically never occur. Unfortunately, overdose reactions are frequent (Table 6.8). The presence of hepatic dysfunction markedly reduces the ability to tolerate therapeutic doses of opioids. A usual dose in such instances may be associated with an overdose. The elderly are also particularly susceptible to overdose with narcotic drugs (Chapter 16), and adjustment of the dose may be necessary. When a narcotic is given subcutaneously to someone in shock, the normalizing of the blood pressure may be associated with an increased absorption from the tissues with a subsequent overdose. Whenever hypotension exists, intravenous route for administering narcotics should be used with the dose carefully monitored. The administration of an appropriate dose of narcotic, together with a sedative or tranquilizer, can result in an overdose reaction.

TABLE 6.8. Factors Associated with a Narcotic Overdose

Physician unawareness of equivalent narcotic doses
Routine prescription in the elderly
International dose manipulation by patient to achieve better analgesia
Presence of hepatic dysfunction
Presence of hypotension
Presence of respiratory impairment
Administration with other CNS depressant drugs or alcohol

Signs and Symptoms

The first major sign of narcotic overdose is depression of respiration. The respiratory rate is uniformly low, with apnea seen in severe cases. If the overdose is considerable, the patient may have a respiratory arrest. Hypoxia may lead to pulmonary edema due to impairment of pulmonary capillary permeability. Cardiovascular changes may be frequent due to the effects of hypoxia on arrhythmia formation. Hypotension, if present, is usually a late phenomenon. Acute pupillary constriction is present, except in severe hypoxia when dilatation may be noted. Urine formation is reduced due to decreased renal blood flow as well as the narcotic stimulant effect of antidiuretic hormone release. Death is almost always due to respiratory failure, frequently accompanied by convulsions. Other symptoms may be present, depending on the specific narcotic responsible for the overdose reaction. Seizures have been reported as part of meperidine and propoxyphene overdose.

Treatment

Initial treatment of narcotic overdose is similar to that of other respiratory depressant drugs (Table 6.9). Of immediate concern is the assurance of an open airway and provision of ventilation. Intubation or tracheotomy may be necessary. Immediate treatment with a narcotic antagonist, devoid of agonist activity, should be promptly instituted. The drug of choice is naloxone hydrochloride (Narcan). This drug is administered intravenously in doses ranging from 0.4 to 3 mg. In the presence of a narcotic overdose, a response is usually obtained within 30 to 50 seconds. This response consists of lightening of the comatose state, dilatation of the pupils, and a marked increase in respiratory rate and volume. If no response is seen after the administration of up to 5 to 10 mg of naloxone, it is more than likely that respiratory depressant effects are not due to a narcotic. Overdose

TABLE 6.9. Treatment of Narcotic Overdose

Maintain open airway
Artificial ventilation if needed
Administration of naloxone (0.4-3 mg) with continued administration as long as needed
Maintain hemodynamic state
Correct any metabolic abnormalities

reactions due to narcotic agonist-antagonist can also be alleviated by use of naloxone.

It should be emphasized that the duration of action of naloxone is two to three hours, whereas the depressant action of morphine may last for six to eight hours, and that of methadone for 24 to 72 hours. In treatment of narcotic overdose with naloxone, therefore, it is extremely important that periodic administration and careful observation occur in order to maintain consciousness. Continual administration of naloxone may be performed as indicated. Occasionally, the use of naloxone may be associated with hypoglycemia. This may become evident through the appearance of agitation. If hypoglycemia is present, this may be controlled by administration of 50 percent glucose intravenously.[63]

In summary, narcotic overdose is usually able to be rapidly diagnosed and treated. When overdose occurs in the hospitalized setting, institution of appropriate therapy in the absence of prolonged hypoxia should always result in a favorable outcome.

DRUG INTERACTIONS

Combinations of narcotic agents and other mood-altering drugs may result in a number of untoward reactions (Table 6.10).

Alcohol, Sedatives, and Tranquilizers

Concomitant consumption of alcohol or barbiturates and narcotics can intensify the narcotic's depressant action, often with fatal results, although the concentration of each individual agent may be sublethal. Diazepam has been observed to inhibit methadone metabolism, resulting in elevation in plasma methadone levels, with a greater potential for toxicity.[64] This is quite important to remember as diazepam is one of the drugs used most frequently with narcotics to allay anxiety.

Stimulants

As discussed earlier, concomitant administration of dextroamphetamine and morphine can potentiate morphine analgesia without enhancing the undesirable side effects of morphine analgesia.

Antipsychotic Drugs

The amount of narcotic required to produce a given level of analgesia can be reduced by administration of some of the phenothiazines (Chapter 10).

TABLE 6.10. Interactions of Narcotics with Other Drugs

Drug	Effect
Alcohol, Benzodiazepines, Barbiturates, Sedatives	Enhanced narcotic depressant effect[a]
Amphetamines	Potentiation of morphine analgesia without increasing toxic effects
Diazepam	Cardiovascular depression with high dose of fentanyl, alfentanil
	Prolongation and potentiation of methadone analgesia[b]
Droperidol	Hypotension when administered with fentanyl
Hydantoin	Decrease effects of meperidine and methadone
MAO inhibitors	Enhanced narcotic depressant effect
	With meperidine, can produce excitation syndrome, hyperpyrexia, and convulsions
Muscle relaxants	Prolongation of morphine-induced respiratory depression
Oral anticoagulants	May minimally prolong prothrombin time[b]
Phenothiazines	Enhanced narcotic depressant effect
	Reduction in amount of narcotic required for analgesia[c]
	Potentiation of hypotension
Rifampin	Decrease plasma methadone levels
Tricyclic	Enhanced narcotic depressant effect
	Potentiation of heroin toxicity and intensification of naloxone-induced morphine withdrawal[b]
	Potentiation and prolongation of methadone analgesia[b]

[a]Respiratory depressant effects prominent with acute administration.
[b]Effects documented only in laboratory animals.
[c]Effect variable. At times an antianalgesic effect may occur.

The respiratory depressant effect of these drugs, however, may be enhanced, and, although the degree of sedation is increased, at times an antianalgesic effect may occur requiring an increased amount of narcotics to produce satisfactory analgesia. Prolongation of morphine-induced respiratory depression has been reported with phenothiazines and monoamine oxidase (MAO) inhibitors.[65] The vasodepressor activity of the phenothiazines may result in an accentuation of the decrease in blood pressure that is seen in morphinized subjects. Concomitant use of meperidine and MAO inhibitors, in addition to respiratory depression, have also been associated with excitation, delirium, hyperpyrexia, and even convulsions.[66] Although the mechanism of this interaction has not been clarified, this effect appears to be specific for meperidine and not other narcotics.

Antidepressants

Several interactions between the tricyclic antidepressants and narcotic drugs have been reported in the laboratory setting.[67] An increase in morphine analgesia has been shown to occur in the rabbit treated with imipramine. Imipramine can also enhance meperidine- and morphine-induced respiratory depression, potentiate heroin toxicity, and intensify morphine withdrawal precipitated by naloxone. Desipramine has also been shown in the laboratory model to potentiate and prolong methadone analgesia by increasing the brain concentration of methadone as well as inhibiting metabolism of methadone in the liver.

Although the mechanism of these interactions has not been fully elucidated, it is more than likely that these drugs cause alterations in the metabolic pathways of the narcotic agents or in the concentration of neurotransmitters involved in producing opiate effects.

Other Interactions

A prolongation of morphine-induced respiratory depression may also occur with concurrent administration of skeletal muscle relaxants. Narcotic analgesics have also been reported to enhance the response to oral anticoagulants.[68] However, the clinical significance of this interaction has not been demonstrated, and it is unlikely that short-term administration of narcotics would have a detrimental effect. Chronic administration of narcotics to persons maintained on oral anticoagulants, however, should be followed by careful monitoring of prothrombin times.

SUMMARY

Narcotic agonists are effective analgesics in relieving mild to severe pain. It is important to remember, however, that in equianalgesic doses, these drugs are relatively interchangeable and the incidence of adverse effects quite comparable. Depending on the specific circumstance, the cause of the pain, its chronicity, and individual differences in response to a specific agent, one drug may be more preferable than another. Although continued use of these drugs will lead to dependence and tolerance, the primary concern with their use should remain effective relief of pain. Dependence should not become a clinical issue. The use of other agents in combination with other drugs, such as the NSAIDs, stimulants, and antidepressants may also provide effective analgesia at a lesser dose. The principle to using these agents will be discussed in considerable detail in Chapters 13 and 14.

REFERENCES

1. Lewin L. *Phantastica: Narcotic and stimulating drugs. Their use and abuse*. Wirth PHH (trans.). New York: Dutton, 1931.

2. Kritikos PG, Papadaki SN. The history of the poppy and of opium and their expansion in antiquity in the eastern Mediterranean area. *Bull Narc*, 1967, 19:17–38.

3. Brecher EM and the Editors of Consumer Reports. *Licit and illicit drugs*. Mount Vernon, NY: Consumers Union, 1972:3.

4. Spector S, Vesell E. Disposition of morphine in man. *Science*, 1971, 174:421–422.

5. Way EL, Kemp JW, Young JM, Grassetti DR. The pharmacologic effects of heroin in relation to its rate of biotransformation. *J Pharmacol Exp Ther*, 1960, 129:144–154.

6. Goldbaum LR, Whelton RL. Toxicologic investigation of sudden death in heroin addicts. Sixth International Meeting of Forensic Scientists. Edinburgh, Scotland, 1972:166.

7. Pert CB, Snyder SH. Opiate receptor: Demonstration in nervous tissue. *Science*, 1973, 179:1011–1014.

8. Bunney WE, Jr, Pert CB, Klee W, Costa E, Pert A, Davis GC. Basic and clinical studies of endorphins. *Ann Intern Med*, 1979, 91:239–250.

9. Pert CB, Pasternak GW, Snyder SH. Opiate agonists and antagonists discriminated by receptor binding in brain. *Science*, 1973, 182:1359–1361.

10. Pert CB, Snyder SH. Opiate receptor binding of agonists and antagonists affected differentially by sodium. *Mol Pharmacol*, 1974, 10:868–879.

11. Pasternak GW, Childer SR, Snyder SH. Opiate analgesia: Evidence for mediation by a subpopulation of opiate receptors. *Science*, 1980, 208:514–516.

12. Simon EJ. Opiate receptors and endorphins: Possible relevance to narcotic addiction. *Adv Alcohol Substance Abuse*, 1981, 1:13–31.

13. Snyder SH. Brain peptides as neurotransmitters. *Science,* 1980, 209:976–983.

14. Mayer DJ, Price DD. Central nervous system mechanisms of analgesia. *Pain,* 1976, 2:379–404.

15. Ho IK, Loh H, Way EL. Influence of 5,6 dihydroxy-tryptamine on morphine tolerance and physical dependence. *Eur J Pharmacol,* 1973, 21:331–336.

16. Pepeu G. Involvement of central transmitters in narcotic analgesia. In: Bonica JJ, Albe-Fessard DG (eds.). *Advances in pain research and therapy, Vol. 1.* New York: Raven Press, 1976: 595–600.

17. Beecher HK. *The measurement of subjective responses: Quantitative effects of drugs.* New York: Oxford University Press, 1959.

18. Hill HE, Haertzen CA, Wolbach AB, Jr, Miner EJ. The Addiction Research Center Inventory: Standardization of scales which evaluate subjective effects of morphine, amphetamine, pentobarbital, alcohol, LSD-25, pyrahexyl and chlorpromazine. *Psychopharmacologia,* 1963, 4:167–205.

19. Hanks GW. Morphine sans Morpheus. *Lancet,* 1995:652–653.

20. Fink M, Zaks A, Volavka J, Roubicek J. Opiates and antagonists. In: Clouet DH (ed.). *Narcotic drugs, biochemical pharmacology.* New York: Plenum Press, 1971: 452–477.

21. Volavka J, Zaks A, Roubicek J, Fink M. Electrographic effects of diacetylmorphine (heroin) and naloxone in man. *Neuropharmacol,* 1970, 9:587–593.

22. Cushman, P. Some endocrinological aspects of heroin addiction and methadone maintenance therapy. *Proceedings of 3rd Annual Conference on Methadone Maintenance.* Rockville, MD: National Institute of Mental Health, 1970: 140–149.

23. Rouby JJ, Eurin B, Glaser P. Hemodynamic and metabolic effects of morphine in the critically ill. *Circulation,* 1981, 64:53–59.

24. Ho ST, Wang JJ, Liaw WJ, Wong CS, Cherng CH. Analgesic effect of intra-articular morphine after arthroscopic surgery in Chinese patients. *Acta-Anaesthesiol-Sin,* 1995, 33:79–84.

25. Walsh TD, MacDonald N, Brueva E, Shepard KV, Michaud M, Zanes R. A controlled study of sustained-release morphine sulfate tablets in chronic pain from advanced cancer. *Amer J Clin Oncol,* 1992, 15:268–272.

26. Smith GM, Beecher HK. Subjective effects of heroin and morphine in normal subjects. *J Pharmacol Exp Ther,* 1962, 136:47–52.

27. Martin WR, Fraser HF. A comparative study of physiological and subjective effects of heroin and morphine administered intravenously in postaddicts. *J Pharmacol Exp Ther,* 1961, 133:388–399.

28. Marks RM, Sachar EJ. Undertreatment of medical inpatients with narcotic analgesics. *Ann Intern Med,* 1973, 78:173–181.

29. Charap AD. The knowledge, attitudes, and experience of medical personnel treating pain in the terminally ill. *Mt Sinai J Med,* 1978, 45:561–580.

30. Yee LY, Lopez JR. Transdermal fentanyl. *Ann Pharmacother,* 1992, 26: 1393–1399.

31. Herbst LH, Strause LG. Transdermal fentanyl use in hospice home-care patients with chronic cancer pain. *J Pain Symptom Management,* 1992, 7 (suppl.): S54–S57.

32. Martin WR, Jasinski DR, Haertzen CA, Kay DC, Jones BE, Mansky PA, Carpenter RW. Methadone — a reevaluation. *Arch Gen Psychiatry,* 1973, 28: 286–295.

33. Ling W, Klett CJ, Gillis RD. A cooperative clinical study of methadyl acetate. *Arch Gen Psychiatry,* 1978, 35:345–353.

34. Smith RJ. Federal government faces painful decision on Darvon. *Science,* 1979, 203:857–858.

35. Cushman P. Propoxyphene revisited. *Am J Drug Alcohol Abuse,* 1979, 6:245–249.

36. Moertel CG, Ahmann DL, Taylor WF, Schwartan N. A comparative evaluation of marketed analgesic drugs. *N Engl J Med,* 1972, 286:813–815.

37. Kay B. A clinical comparison of orally administered aspirin, dextropropoxyphene and pentazocine in the treatment of post-operative pain. *J Int Med Res,* 1974, 2:149–152.

38. Wang RIH, Sandoval RG. The analgesic activity of propoxyphene napsylate with and without aspirin. *J Clin Pharmacol New Drugs,* 1971, 11:310–317.

39. Moertel CG, Ahmann DL, Taylor WF, Schwartan M. Relief of pain by oral medications: A controlled evaluation of analgesic combinations. *JAMA,* 1974, 229:55–59.

40. Hopkinson JH, Bartlett FH, Jr, Steffans AO, McGlumphy TH, Macht EL, Smith M. Acetaminophen versus propoxyphene hydrochloride for relief of pain in episiotomy patients. *J Clin Pharmacol,* 1973, 13:251–263.

41. Jasinski DR, Pevnick JS, Clark SC, Griffith JD. Therapeutic usefulness of propoxyphene napsylate in narcotic addiction. *Arch Gen Psychiatry,* 1977, 34:227–233.

42. Analgesic Drugs Panel, National Research Council. *Drug efficacy study.* Washington, DC: National Academy of Sciences, 1969.

43. National Institute on Drug Abuse. Drug Abuse Warning Network (DAWN): *Phase II report.* Ambler PA: IMS America, 1974.

44. Treatment of dextropropoxyphene poisoning (editorial). *Lancet,* 1977, 2:542.

45. New warning on propoxyphene. *FDA Drug Bulletin,* 1979, 9(4):22–23.

46. Finkle BS, McCloskey KL, Kiplinger GF, Bennet IF. A national assessment of propoxyphene in postmortem medicolegal, investigation, 1972–1975. *J Forensic Sci,* 1976, 21:706–741.

47. The Brompton cocktail (editorial). *Lancet,* 1979, 1:1220–1221.

48. Kerrane TA. The Brompton cocktail. *Nurs Mirror Midwives J,* 1975, 140:59.

49. British National Formulary. London: British Medical Association, 1976: 272.

50. Melzack R, Mount BM, Gordon JM. The Brompton mixture versus morphine solution given orally: Effects on pain. *Can Med Assoc J,* 1979, 120:435–438.

51. Twycross RG. Effect of cocaine in the Brompton cocktail. In: Bonica JJ, Liebeskind JC, Albe-Fessard DG (eds). *Advances in pain research and therapy Vol. 3.* New York: Raven Press, 1979; 927–932.

52. Forrest WH, Jr, Brown BW, Jr, Brown CR, Defalque R, Gold M, Gordon HE. Dextroamphetamine with morphine for the treatment of postoperative pain. *N Engl J Med,* 1977, 296:712–715.

53. Wikler A, Fraser HG, Isbell H. N-allylnormorphine: Effects of single doses and precipitation of acute "abstinence syndromes" during addiction to morphine, methadone or heroin in man (post-addicts). *J Pharmacol Exp Ther,* 1953, 109:8–20.

54. Jaffe JH. Drug addiction and drug abuse. In Gilman AG, Rall TW, Nies AS, Taylor P (eds.). *Goodman and Gilman's the pharmacological basis of therapeutics,* 8th ed. New York: Pergamon Press, 1990:522–573.

55. Isbell H, White WM. Clinical characteristics of addictions. *Am J Med,* 1953, 14:558–565.

56. Himmelsbach CK. Clinical studies of drug addiction: Physical dependence, withdrawal and recovery. *Arch Intern Med,* 1942, 69:766–772.

57. Gold MS, Pottash ALC. Endorphins, locus coeruleus, clonidine, and lofexidine: A mechanism for opiate withdrawal and new nonopiate treatments. *Adv Alcohol Substance Abuse,* 1981, 1:33–52.

58. Gold MS, Kleber HD. A rationale for opiate withdrawal symptomatology. *Drug Alcohol Depend,* 1979, 4:419–424.

59. Lipman JJ, Spencer PSJ. Clonidine and opiate withdrawal (letter). *Lancet,* 1978, 2: 521.

60. Lipman JJ, Spencer PSJ. Further evidence for a central site of action for the antinociceptive effect of clonidine-like drugs. *Neuropharmacol,* 1979, 18:731–733.

61. Uhde TW, Post RM, Siever LJ, Buchsbaum MS. Clonidine and psychophysical pain (letter). *Lancet,* 1980, 2:1375.

62. Capogna G, Cellano D, Zanarillo A, Constanto P, Foresta S. *Reg Anesth,* 1995, 20:57–61.

63. Greene MH, DuPont RL. The treatment of acute heroin toxicity. In: Bourne, PG (ed.). *The treatment manual for acute drug abuse emergencies.* Rockville, MD: National Clearinghouse for Drug Abuse Information, National Institute on Drug Abuse, 1974:11.

64. Spaulding TC, Minium L, Kotake AN, Takemori AE. The effect of diazepam on the metabolism of methadone by the liver of methadone-dependent rats. *Drug Metab Dispos, Biol Fate Chem,* 1974, 2:458–463.

65. Evans-Prosser CDG. The use of pethidine and morphine in the presence of monoamine oxidase inhibitors. *Br J Anaesth,* 1968, 40:279–282.

66. Brownlee G, Williams GW. Potentiation of amphetamine and pethidine by monoamine oxidase inhibitors (letter). *Lancet,* 1963, 1:669.

67. Hansten PD. Tricyclic antidepressant interactions. In: Hansten PD (ed.). *Drug interactions, 4th ed.* Philadelphia: Lea & Febiger, 1979:257–263.

68. Lasagna L. The clinical evaluation of morphine and its substitutes as analgesics. *Pharmacol Rev,* 1964, 16:47–83.

69. Jaffe JH, Martin WR. Opioid analgesics and antagonists. In: Gilman AG, Rall TW, Nies AS, Taylor P (eds.). *Goodman and Gilman's the pharmacological basis of therapeutics*—8th ed. New York: Pergamon Press, 1990: 485–521.

Chapter 7

Opioid (Narcotic) Analgesics II: Opioid Agonist-Antagonists

INTRODUCTION

When an opioid's biochemical structure is modified by substitution of the methyl group attached to the tertiary nitrogen, the drug formed not only has less or no analgesic activity but, in addition, has actions that "antagonize" those of the original narcotic. These drugs are termed narcotic (opioid) antagonists. Although Pohl in 1915 initially recorded the ability of N-allylnorcodeine to reverse respiratory depression induced by morphine, it was not until 1951 that the clinical relevance of antagonists in the treatment of narcotic overdose was recognized. Over the next two decades, interest centered on developing antagonists devoid of any agonist or morphine-like effects. Only relatively recently has attention focused on the agonist effects of those drugs with the view toward developing antagonists with potent agonist activity able to be effective analgesics without the accompanying risk of physical dependence.[1]

Clinically, opioid antagonists are currently used for: (1) analgesia, (2) detection of opioid use, (3) treatment of acute opioid overdose, and (4) prevention of heroin-induced euphoria.

CLASSIFICATION

The opioid antagonists may be grouped into those with solely antagonist activity and those that also produce agonist effects in addition to their antagonist activity (Table 7.1).[2] This latter group can be further subdivided into agents predominantly antagonists (nalorphine type) and those predominantly agonists (morphine type). All of the narcotic antagonists, however, have the ability to reverse the antidepressant effects of morphine and

TABLE 7.1. Narcotic Antagonists

Generic name	Trade name	Derivative	Antagonist activity	Physical dependence liability	Equivalent analgesic Dose (mg)[c]
Buprenorphine	Buprenex Temgesic	Thebaine	17	+	0.3
Butorphanol	Stadol		1	+	2
Cyclazocine		Phenazocine	3.5	+	
Dezocine	Dalgan	Aminotetralin	0.5		10
Levallorphan	Lorfan	Levorphanol	3.7		
Nalbuphine	Nubain	Oxymorphone	0.25	+	10
Nalorphine	Nalline	Morphine	1	–	
Naloxone	Narcan	Oxymorphone	7	–	
Naltrexone[b]		Oxymorphone	17	–	
Pentazocine	Talwin Talacen	Phenazocine	0.02	+	30

[a]Ability to precipitate abstinence syndrome in morphine-dependent monkeys using nalorphine as a standard of 1.
[b]Naltrexone is the N-cyclopropyl-methyl congener of naloxone.
[c]Equivalent to morphine 10 mg 1.m.

related compounds, although the intensity of this reversal varies with specific agent. Narcotic antagonists with predominant agonist effects may actually suppress withdrawal in persons on low doses of morphine while precipitating withdrawal only in individuals maintained on high doses. These drugs act as an agonist at one receptor and an antagonist at another. Pentazocine, cyclazocine, nalorphine, and nalbuphine block the mu receptors while others such as buprenorphine are partial agonists.

PHARMACOLOGY

The discussion that follows of the pharmacologic properties of the narcotic antagonists will use naloxone and nalorphine as the prototypes unless otherwise specified. Following the general discussion, specific attention will be focused on those narcotic antagonists clinically used as analgesics (agonist-antagonists).

Absorption, Biotransformation, Excretion

Absorption from the gastrointestinal tract following oral administration of all the available pure narcotic antagonists is quite good. Nalorphine and naloxone, however, are so rapidly metabolized in the liver that oral use is ineffective. Naltrexone is also well absorbed and can retain its activity for up to 24 hours. Parenteral administration of naloxone and nalorphine is associated with a duration of action of approximately 30 minutes to 40 hours. Metabolism occurs mainly in the liver with conjugation to glucuronic acid.

Mechanism of Action

Opioid antagonists are presumed to compete with opioids for positions at receptor sites. This subject is discussed in detail in Chapters 2 and 6 and will only be summarized below. Antagonist binding to receptors may be more potent than opioids, with relatively small doses being able to reverse the effects of 10 to 100 times greater doses of narcotics. Nalorphine-type antagonists may produce analgesia but at doses that will be accompanied by adverse psychotomimetic effects. Other antagonists of the morphine-like type can produce analgesia unassociated with dysphoria.

Opioid antagonists have also been observed to antagonize analgesic effects induced by drugs other than opioids. Stress-induced analgesia can be reversed by naloxone. Reports have also documented the ability of naloxone to cause mild hyperalgesia.

It has been suggested that the relative ability of an opioid agonist-antagonist to produce analgesia may be predicted by the effect of sodium on its binding to receptors.[2] Sodium markedly increases the binding of opioid antagonists while decreasing the binding of pure agonists. The degree to which binding is decreased may indicate the prominence of the analgesic effect. This finding is of value in the development of narcotic antagonists that can be used as effective analgesics without high risk of producing dependency.

An alternative mechanism of action postulates the existence of two distinct receptor subpopulations consisting of high affinity and low affinity binding sites. High affinity binding sites are equated with analgesia, whereas binding to low affinity sites is associated with other known effects of opiates. Those antagonists with predominantly analgesic activity are thought to exhibit selectivity for high affinity sites, resulting in satisfactory analgesia without a potential for an overdose reaction.

Dependence, Tolerance, and Withdrawal

The use of any of the antagonists in an individual dependent on opioids will be associated with a withdrawal syndrome. Naloxone is the most potent of the antagonists, with 1 mg being capable of completely blocking the respiratory depressant effect of 25 mg of heroin.[3,4] Naloxone can also antagonize the adverse dysphoric effects of nalorphine and cyclazocine. Naloxone, unlike other antagonists, is completely devoid of agonist activity. Prolonged use produces neither dependence nor withdrawal on discontinuing the drug. Continued use of morphine-type antagonists will result in tolerance to both the agonistic and dysphoric effects. Once tolerance has developed, withdrawal symptoms will occur on discontinuing their use. Tolerance to the antagonistic effects, however, has not been noted.

ANALGESIC EFFECTS

Over the last decade considerable interest has focused on the use of narcotic agonists-antagonists as morphine substitutes to provide effective analgesia unaccompanied by a potential for abuse and physical dependency. Unfortunately, pentazocine, the first commercially available antagonist providing satisfactory analgesia, was subsequently demonstrated to have a definite abuse potential as well, causing a withdrawal syndrome of sufficient intensity to reinforce drug-seeking behavior.

Recently, several newly synthesized antagonists that have been demonstrated to provide potent analgesia have appeared. These antagonists, which will be briefly described below, all share several features in common (Table 7.2). With the exception of buprenorphine, they are relatively ineffective orally, with parenteral administration being required or preferred. Potent analgesia is achieved relatively rapidly with a much lesser intensity of respiratory depression and potential for abuse as compared to morphine. For this reason, these drugs are currently not subject to the Federal Controlled Substance Act. All of these agents, however, can produce physical dependence and, when discontinued after chronic use, a mild withdrawal syndrome. When administered to someone physically dependent on opioids, a withdrawal reaction can be precipitated. Individuals taking opioids for analgesia must, therefore, be detoxified prior to beginning use of these drugs. Due to the ability to produce a low degree of physical dependence, their use in persons with a history of opioid abuse should be carefully considered.

Although their depressant effect on respiration is considerably less than morphine, administration to persons with respiratory depression should be performed with caution. Similarly, concomitant use with tranquilizing agents should be avoided or be accompanied by a reduction in analgesic

TABLE 7.2. Common Characteristics of Newly Developed Analgesic Antagonists

Advantages	Precautions
Potent, relatively rapid analgesia	Most effective by parenteral use only
Respiratory depression less than with morphine	Use cautiously in persons with respiratory depression or when tranquilizers administered simultaneously
Low potential for physical dependence	Persons dependent on narcotic must be detoxified before use
Mild withdrawal after chronic use	Use cautiously in persons with history of narcotic abuse
Low potential for abuse	Use during pregnancy and in children under 18 years of age not yet established
Sedation without marked euphoria	Use cautiously in persons with ventricular dysfunction or coronary heart disease

dose. Similar to narcotics, their use should be restricted in persons with increased intracerebral pressure and with liver disease. The negative inotropic effect on cardiac muscle of most of these agents also precludes their use in individuals with cardiovascular disease.

AVAILABLE ANALGESICS

Pentazocine

The narcotic antagonist initially most frequently used as an analgesic was the benzomorphan derivative, pentazocine (Talwin), available since 1967 for the relief of moderate to severe pain.

Pharmacology

Absorption from the gastrointestinal tract following ingestion of pentazocine is good, with plasma levels appearing within one hour and peaking in up to three hours. Following intramuscular administration, peak plasma levels occur within 15 to 20 minutes, with a duration of action between three and four hours, although plasma levels can still be detected up to six hours.[4] The oral dose of pentazocine is approximately one-third to one-fourth as potent as the intramuscular dose, having a somewhat slower onset (one to three hours) but longer duration of action. Metabolic pathways occur predominantly in the liver through biotransformation with excretion predominantly through the kidney, with 60 percent eliminated within the first 24 hours. Metabolites represent the major excretory product, although some free pentazocine is also excreted.

The major effects of pentazocine on the central nervous system, smooth muscle, and gastrointestinal tract are similar to that of other narcotics, including analgesia, sedation, and respiratory depression. Approximately 20 to 30 mg of pentazocine parenterally is as effective as 10 mg of morphine. When administered orally, 50 mg of pentazocine are approximately equivalent to 60 mg of codeine. Larger doses of pentazocine have been associated with dysphoric effects, including hallucinations and other perceptual disturbances. At times these effects have been noted at dosages within the therapeutic range.[5] Therapeutic use of pentazocine has also been associated with nausea, drowsiness, dizziness and sweating, euphoria, and disorientation. The appearance of and the intensity of these symptoms vary considerably with individual susceptibility.

The cardiovascular response to pentazocine differs considerably from morphine.[11,12] Pentazocine produces elevations in plasma epinephrine and norepinephrine, with associated increases in both blood pressure and heart rate, suggesting caution in administrating this drug to persons with cardio-vascular disease.

Dependence and Withdrawal

Pentazocine was initially described as a nonnarcotic analgesic associated with a low risk of dependence. Physical dependence to pentazocine, however, has been demonstrated both in the laboratory setting as well as in clinical studies. On the sheet level, contrary to initial expectations, pentazocine use is strongly associated with dependence, with many cases of pentazocine addiction reported.[6,7] It is unfortunate that initially pentazocine dependence not only followed the medical use of this drug but occurred prominently in physicians and other health professionals.

Pentazocine has often been is used as an attractive alternative to heroin. Reports have described the injection of pentazocine and the antihistamine tripelennamine in a combination called "Ts and Blues."[8,9] The lack of physician awareness to the dependency-producing potential of pentazocine has resulted in prescriptions being the major source of inappropriate use.

Withdrawal symptoms following naloxone challenge can occur after daily administration of pentazocine for several weeks. The withdrawal syndrome is similar to that seen with opiates; however, it is much milder. The administration of pentazocine to someone currently maintained on a narcotic drug will result in the precipitation of withdrawal. This is quite important to remember as it is not an infrequent practice for a physician to prescribe pentazocine when pain is inadequately controlled by a narcotic. In many cases this has resulted in unrecognized mild withdrawal symptoms perceived by the patient and physician as an allergy to pentazocine (Chapter 13).

Toxicity and Overdose

Chronic use of pentazocine, even in a medical setting, has been associated with a number of complications, including cutaneous reactions, myopathy, and agranulocytosis.[10,11] The use of pentazocine in pregnancy has resulted in neonatal withdrawal.[12] Intravenous street injection of pentazocine is associated with all the complications seen in illicit heroin use. In addition, the crushing of the tablets prior to injection results in particles of cellulose and talc setting in the pulmonary arteries and lungs with pulmonary hypertension and granuloma formation.

Pentazocine overdose is manifested mainly by respiratory depression, which may be reversed by naloxone but not by agents with mixed agonist-antagonist activities, such as nalorphine. Treatment is quite similar to that of opiate overdose (Chapter 6). The increasing prevalence of abuse associated with pentazocine has resulted in this drug being placed in Schedule IV of the Controlled Substances Act.

Buprenorphine

Buprenorphine (Temgesic) is one of the newly synthesized opioid antagonist drugs exhibiting considerable analgesic effects. Buprenorphine is a derivative of thebaine, with an analgesic potency 25 to 40 times that of morphine but with an equivalent duration of action.[13] Metabolism occurs mainly in the liver, with excretion in the bile. Subjective effects of buprenorphine are quite similar to morphine but much longer in duration. Its antagonistic characteristics, approximately equivalent to naltrexone, can antagonize high doses of morphine for up to 24 to 36 hours. Its untoward effects are similar to that of morphine.

Analgesic Effects

Buprenorphine is an effective parenteral analgesic. Analgesic activity begins in 30 to 60 minutes and can last up to seven hours. In clinical trials assessing analgesic effectiveness of buprenorphine in painful states, 0.6 mg of buprenorphine as a single intramuscular dose relieved pain as effectively as 15 mg of morphine, with better pain relief being reported up to seven hours post injection. Intravenous doses of 0.3 mg have been reported to give a greater analgesia than 10 mg of morphine intravenously, lasting up to ten hours, and with continuous subcutaneous infusion has been shown to relieve patients with severe pain from cancer.[14]

Dependence, Tolerance, Withdrawal

The low level of dependence reported with buprenorphine has allowed prescription of this drug without any of the regulations that apply to dependency-producing narcotics. However, buprenorphine does produce a positive mood-altering effect that is reported by addicts to be similar to heroin, and its use can result in dependence and withdrawal.[15]

Abuse Potential

Since prescription of buprenorphine is not controlled, it is not surprising that reports of abuse have appeared in areas where this drug is readily available. In fact, in Edinburgh buprenorphine had become the primary drug of abuse by intravenous drug users as the purity of heroin declined, and by 1990 was more frequently used then all other narcotics.[16,17]

The agonist-antagonistic actions of buprenorphine suggested its value as an alternative to methadone maintenance. The potential of narcotic overdose with coexistent injections of heroin or other narcotic abuse is diminished, and the degree of physical dependence developing to buprenorphine is considered to be of minor consequence. Oral preparations of buprenorphine are presently being used as maintenance therapy.

Butorphanol

Butorphanol tartrate (Stadol, Dorphano), another newly synthesized agonist-antagonist analgesic, is a phenanthrene derivative with an antagonist activity approximately 1/40 that of naloxone, equal to that of nalorphine, and 30 times that of pentazocine.[18] Its agonist effects are quite good. Butorphanol administration can result in analgesia approximately five times that of morphine, 20 times that of pentazocine, and 40 times that of meperidine.[19]

Pharmacology

After oral administration, absorption from the gastrointestinal tract is complete, with peak plasma levels occurring within 1.5 hours. Circulation through the liver is rapid, however, so that the biologic availability approximates only 17 percent of that seen with intravenous administration.[20] Following intramuscular administration, analgesic activity appears within 30 minutes, with peak levels within one hour. Butorphanol exhibits a high degree of lipid solubility and is distributed extensively to lipid-rich tissues. It freely passes the placental membranes and has been identified in neonatal blood at 0.4 to 1.4 times the maternal serum concentration.[21] Metabolism occurs in the liver, with hydroxy-butorphanol being the main urinary metabolite. Biliary excretion accounts for approximately 14 percent of the parenteral dose. In the elderly, the plasma half-life may be increased by 25 percent.

Effects on Organ Systems

The effects of butorphanol on organ systems are more similar to pentazocine than to morphine.[22] Unlike the narcotic analgesics, however, increasing the butorphanol dose is not accompanied by a comparable increase in respiratory depression.[23] Changes in respiratory pattern, consisting of diminished tidal volume and bradypnea, do occur with increasing dosage. The duration of respiratory changes is dose related, with naloxone being capable of reversing all effects. The dose of naloxone required, however, is somewhat higher than needed to reverse the effects of pure agonists. Circulatory changes in healthy individuals given butorphanol appear to be clinically insignificant. However, the hemodynamic changes induced by intravenous administration are similar to those seen with pentazocine, although smaller in magnitude, yet suggest caution in prescribing it to persons with cardiac disease.

Analgesic Activity

Butorphanol has been found to be an effective analgesic agent in both open and blind studies in the relief of postoperative as well as chronic pain.[24,25] Butorphanol (2 mg administered intramuscularly) was found to provide equivalent analgesia to 10 mg of morphine, 40 mg of meperidine, and 40 mg of pentazocine. On oral administration, 8 to 16 mg of butorphanol appeared as effective as 60 mg of codeine and somewhat more effective than 50 mg of pentazocine.[19]

Toxicity

The most frequent side effect of butorphanol is drowsiness, with up to 40 percent of patients receiving the drug reporting a sedative effect. Changes in mood and psychotomimetic effects have also been reported, especially with higher doses.These symptoms include feelings of unreality and depersonalization, visual hallucinations, and distortions of body image. Approximately 1 to 2 percent of persons receiving the drug report nausea or vomiting. The use of butorphanol in persons currently dependent on narcotics is contraindicated due to its antagonistic properties.

Dependence and Withdrawal

Dependence will occur with continued butorphanol use, and stopping the drug after chronic use will result in a withdrawal syndrome within 24 hours, which may progress in severity for up to 48 hours. Administration of either nalorphine or naloxone will also produce typical withdrawal phenomena in persons chronically maintained on butorphanol.

Nalbuphine

Nalbuphine (Nubain) is a synthetic agonist-antagonist resembling both oxymorphone and naloxone. It is currently available only for parenteral use. The analgesic effect of 10 mg of nalbuphine is approximately equivalent to 10 mg of morphine, with the antagonist activity approximately one-fourth that of nalorphine.

Pharmacology

In humans, following an intramuscular injection of nalbuphine, peak plasma levels occur within one-half hour with a plasma half-life of up to five hours. In animal studies, peak plasma levels do not change after a single dose as compared to multiple doses, suggesting nalbuphine neither accumulates in the tissue nor affects enzyme induction to any great extent. Metabolism occurs in the liver, with fecal secretion of metabolites being the predominant excretory route. Urinary excretion accounts for approximately 7 percent.

Effects on Organ Systems

In general, nalbuphine shows pharmacologic properties similar to those of the other mixed agonists. The effects of nalbuphine on the cardiovascular system, however, are minimal.[26] In this regard it is quite similar to morphine, but different from pentazocine and butorphanol, which are associated with increases in pulmonary artery pressure and cardiac workload.[27]

Analgesic Activity

Clinical studies have demonstrated that nalbuphine is an effective analgesic (equivalent to morphine) in the relief of moderate to severe pain.[28] At equianalgesic doses, nalbuphine has a potency approximately three times that of pentazocine, with a lower peak effect and longer duration of action. Studies comparing nalbuphine with meperidine found a comparable analgesic effect with a longer duration of action and a lower incidence of nausea and vomiting.[29] Unlike other commercially available agonist-antagonists, the absence of adverse hemodynamic effects allows nalbuphine to be given to persons with cardiovascular disease. However, since nalbuphine appears to have no significant advantage over morphine, is considerably more expensive, and can only be given by injection, its use in the treatment of pain remains limited.

Toxicity

Adverse effects of nalbuphine are similar to those of other narcotic agonist-antagonists and may include hallucinations, feelings of unreality, and depersonalization. These reactions are less severe than those seen with pentazocine. In analgesic doses, nalbuphine depresses respiration in a manner similar to morphine. The depressant effect, however, is of shorter duration and, in contrast to morphine, is not appreciably intensified with administration of higher doses.

Dependence and Withdrawal

Although the abuse potential of nalbuphine is less than that of morphine, the subjective effects are similar.[30] Nalorphine and/or naloxone challenge in individuals chronically maintained on nalbuphine will result in an abstinence syndrome, indicating dependence. The degree of dependence is less than that seen with codeine or propoxyphene, approximately equal to pentazocine. The use of nalbuphine in individuals dependent on narcotics will result in withdrawal symptoms due to the drug's antagonist activity.

SUMMARY

Narcotic antagonists with agonist activity can provide effective analgesia, with some of the newer agents exhibiting a much greater potency than morphine.[31] Of these drugs, buprenorphine is probably the most useful in chronic pain, as it is relatively long-acting and effective sublingually or orally. Although the potential for dependence and for abuse is less than morphine, dependence will develop with chronic use. Furthermore, the mood-altering effects of these drugs prevents complacency concerning patient misuse. Since they are not controlled to the extent seen with pure narcotic agonists, it is more than likely that widespread prescribing will result in patterns of abuse similar to that seen with pentazocine. The greatest advantage of agonist-antagonists seems to be the small volume of solution injected to achieve satisfactory analgesia. This is of specific value to persons maintained on high doses of opioids requiring frequent injections of considerable volume.

REFERENCES

1. Hoskin PJ, Hanks GW. Opioid agonist-antagonist drugs in acute and chronic pain states. *Drugs,* 1991, 41:326–44
2. Snyder SH. Opiate receptors and internal opiates. *Sci Am,* 1977, 236:44–56.

3. Zaks A, Jones T, Fink M, Freedman AM. Naloxone treatment of opiate dependence. *JAMA,* 1971, 215:2108–2110.

4. Jaffe JH, Martin WR. Opioid analgesics and antagonists. In: Gilman AG, Rall TW, Nies AS, Taylor P (eds.). *Goodman and Gilman's the pharmacological basis of therapeutics,* 8th ed. New York: Pergamon Press, 1990, 485–521.

5. Byrd GJ, Kane FJ. Persistent psychotic phenomena following one dose of pentazocine. *Tex Med,* 1976, 72:68–69.

6. National Institute on Drug Abuse. *Drug abuse clinical notes: Pentazocine (Talwin) abuse increases.* Rockville, MD: Author, 1979: 1–7.

7. Parwatikar S, Gomez H, Knowles RR. Pentazocine dependency. *Int J Addict,* 1973, 8:87–98.

8. O'Driscoll WG, Lindley GR. Self administration of tripelennamine by a narcotic addict. *N Engl J Med,* 1957, 257:376.

9. Burton JF, Zawadski S, Wetherell HR, Moy TW. Mainliners and blue velvet. *J Forensic Sci,* 1965, 1:466–472.

10. Schiff BL, Kern AB. Unusual cutaneous manifestations of pentazocine addiction. *JAMA,* 1977, 238:1542–1543.

11. Marks A, Abramson N. Pentazocine and agranulocytosis (letter). *Ann Intern Med*, 1980, 92:433.

12. Goetz RL, Bain RV. Neonatal withdrawal symptoms associated with maternal use of pentazocine. *J Pediatr,* 1974, 84:877–888.

13. Mello NK, Mendelson JH. Buprenorphine suppresses heroin use by heroin addicts. *Science,* 1980, 207:657–659.

14. Kay B. A double-blind comparison of morphine and buprenorphine in the prevention of pain after operation. *Br J Anaesth,* 1978, 50:605–609.

15. Jasinski DR, Pevnick JS, Griffith, JD. Human pharmacology and abuse potential of analgesic buprenorphine: A potential agent for treating narcotic addiction. *Arch Gen Psychiatry,* 1978, 35:501–516.

16. LaVelle TL, Hammersley R, Forsyth A. The use of buprenorphine and temazepam by drug injectors (letter). *J Addict Dis,* 1991, 10(3):5–14.

17. Jasinski DR, Pevnick JS, Griffith JD. Human pharmacology and abuse potential of the analgesic buprenorphine: A potential agent for treating narcotic addiction. *Arch Gen Psychiatry,* 1978, 35:501–516.

18. Fuisz RE, Fuisz, RC. A clinical profile: Stadol (butorphanol tartrate). Bristol Lab 1978, 1:1–28.

19. Heel RC, Brogden RN, Speight TM, Avery GS. Butorphanol: A review of its pharmacological properties and therapeutic efficacy. *Drugs,* 1978, 16:473–505.

20. Vandam LD. Drug therapy: Butorphanol. *N Engl J Med,* 1980, 302:381–384.

21. Maduska AL, Hajghassemali M. A double-blind comparison of butorphanol and meperidine in labour: Maternal pain relief and effect on the newborn. *Can Anaesth Soc J,* 1978, 25:398–404.

22. Nagashima H, Karamanian A, Malovany R, Radnay P, Ang M, Koerner S, Foldes FF. Respiratory and circulatory effects of intravenous butorphanol and morphine. *Clin Pharmacol Ther,* 1976, 19:738–745.

23. Kallos T, Caruso FS. Respiratory effects of butorphanol. *Clin Pharmacol Ther,* 1976, 21:107.

24. Kliman A, Lipson MJ, Warren R, Noveck RJ, Caruso FS. Clinical experience with intramuscular butorphanol for the treatment of a variety of chronic pain syndromes. *Curr Ther Res,* 1977, 22:105–115.

25. Zeedick JF. Butorphanol-A new potent, parenteral analgesic. *Curr Ther Res,* 1977, 21:802–808.

26. Romagnoli A, Keats AS. Comparative hemodynamic effects of nalbuphine and morphine in patients with coronary artery disease. *Bull Tex Heart Inst,* 1978, 5:19–24.

27. *AMA Drug Evaluations,* 3rd ed. Littleton, MA: Publishing Sciences Group, 1977:366.

28. Beaver WT, Feise GA. A comparison of the analgesic effect of intramuscular nalbuphine and morphine in patients with postoperative pain. *J Pharmacol Exp Ther,* 1978, 204:487–496.

29. Stehling LC, Zauder HL. Double-blind comparison of butorphanol and meperidine in the treatment of postsurgical pain. *J Int Med Res,* 1978, 6: 306–311.

30. Jasinski DR, Mansky PA. Evaluation of nalbuphine for abuse potential. *Clin Pharmacol Ther,* 1972, 13:78–90.

31. Hanks GW. The clinical usefulness of agonist-antagonist opioid analgesics in chronic pain. *Drug and Alcohol Dependence,* 1987, 20:339–346.

Chapter 8

The Stimulants

INTRODUCTION

The use of stimulants, deeply rooted in the origins of organized societies, has survived and flourished through modern times. Stimulant use can be divided into four main categories: (1) prescribed, (2) nonprescribed over-the-counter (OTC) purchases, (3) illicit use, and (4) popular consumption of caffeine and nicotine.[1] The effects of all stimulants (Tables 8.1–8.4) have a considerable degree of overlap; however, nicotine is the only drug with no known medicinal value. Caffeine is consumed in beverages such as coffee, tea, and soft drinks, is chewed as Kola nuts, and is a prominent ingredient in OTC medications. Cocaine, available by prescription as a local anesthetic, is used illicitly for its mood-altering effects. Amphetamines and similar drugs, although frequently prescribed by physicians for a variety of disorders, also have a high "abuse" potential. Other stimulants used for attention deficit disorders (methylphenidate and pemoline) and occasionally narcolepsy are available by prescription only and are not commonly abused. Despite their extremely valuable therapeutic agents, their potential for misuse, habituation, and dependence is quite real.

A number of other stimulants (sympathomimetic drugs) are frequently combined in a variety of OTC analgesics, antitussives, or cold medications (Table 8.5). Toxic reactions to these drugs are similar to those seen with epinephrine and the amphetamines but are usually of a lesser magnitude. The phenylisopropylamines can readily cross the blood-brain barrier, however, and may be associated with considerable central nervous system activity. Chronic use and misuse of these medications may cause fatigue, depression, dizziness, and vasomotor disturbances. Diet aids (Table 8.6) are easily purchased at local pharmacies or supermarkets. Similar to other sympathomimetic drugs, their potential for misuse with the development of habituation or psychological dependence can occur.

This chapter will discuss only those stimulants that have been felt to have analgesic properties. Although the medical complications and dependency potential of nicotine have been well described, and the use of methyphenidate

TABLE 8.1. Commonly Used Stimulants

	Prescription required	OTC	Abuse potential	Illicit use	Frequent daily use
Amphetamine	+	−	+	+	±[a]
Caffeine	−	+	−	−	+
Cocaine	+	−	+	+	±[a]
Methylphenidate (Ritalin)	+	−	+	+/−	±[b]
Nicotine	−	+	+	−	+
Pemoline (Cylert)	+	−	+	−	+[b]

[a]Once dependence has been established.
[b]Used to treat attention deficit disorders.

TABLE 8.2. Commonly Prescribed Amphetamines

Generic	Trade name	Schedule[a]
Amphetamine sulfate[b]	Benzedrine	II
Dextroamphetamine sulfate[b]	Dexampex Dexedrine Diphylets	II
Ferndex	Oxydess	II
Span cap		I
Methamphetamine HCl	Desoxyn Methampex Obedrin-LA	II
Amphetamine mixtures	Amphaplex Biphetamine Delcobese Obetrol	II

[a]Controlled Substances Schedule
[b]Generic forms produced by various manufacturers

TABLE 8.3. Commonly Prescribed Anorexiants

Generic	Trade name	Schedule[a]
Benzphetamine HCl	Didrex	III
Phentermine HCl[b]	Adipex-P, Fastin, Obephen, Dapex, Phentrol, Ionamin, Obe-Nix 30, Zantryl	IV
Chlorphentermine HCl[b]	Pre-sate, Tyramine Chlorophane	III
Clortermine HCl	Voranil	III
Phendimetrazine tartrate[b]	Anorex, Bontril PDM, Dital, Dyrexan, Melfiat, Obalan, Prelu-2, Plegine, Rexigen Forte, Trimstat, Weightrol, Wehless	III
Diethylpropion HCl[b]	Tenuate, Tepanil	IV
Mazindol	Sanorex, Mazanor	III
Fenfluramine HCl	Pondimin	IV
Phenylpropanolamine	Acutrim, Control, Dexatrim Pre-Meal, Dex-A-Diet, Phenyldrine, Stay Trim, Spray-U-Thin, Unitrol	Non-prescription
Prenylpropanolamine Combinations	Appedrine, Dexatrim Plus, Grapefruit Diet Plan w/ Diadex	Non-prescription

[a]Controlled Substances Schedule
[b]Generic forms produced by various manufacturers

TABLE 8.4. Other Stimulants

Generic	Trade name	Schedule[a]
Caffeine	Ban, Caffedrine, Quick Pep, Tirend, No Doz, Vivarin	IV
Caffeine Combination Drugs	Arthritis Strength BC Powder. Excedrin, Bayer Select Headache Pain, Vanquish	
Benzoate		
Cocaine		II
Doxapram HCl	Dopram	
Methylphenidate HCl	Ritalin	II
Pemoline	Cylert	IV

[a]Controlled Substances Schedule

TABLE 8.5. Commonly Used Sympathomimetic Drugs

Ephedrine
Epinephrine
Ethylnorepinephrine
Isoetharine
Isoproterenol
Methoxamine
Phenylephrine
Phenylpropanolamine
Pseudoephedrine
Terbutaline

TABLE 8.6. Nonprescription Diet Aids

Acutrim
Appedrine
Control
Dex-A-Diet Plus
Dexatrim Pre-Meal
Grapefruit Diet Plan
Phenoxine
Prolamine
Phenyldrine
Slim-Mint
Stay Trim
Unitrol

and pemoline for attention deficit disorder is medically indicated (though, among some, controversial), these agents will not be reviewed.

AMPHETAMINES

Amphetamine was first synthesized in 1927. Since that time this drug and other related substances have proliferated to a remarkable degree (Table 8.2). The most commonly used amphetamines are *d*-amphetamine, *l*-amphetamine, and racemic mixtures of amphetamine and methamphetamine. Amphetamines have been recommended in treatment of obesity, depressive reactions, epilepsy, narcolepsy, parkinsonism, childhood hyperkinesia, and central nervous system depression caused by barbiturates (Table 8.7). They have also been prescribed to enhance alertness and to increase physical performance. A 1990 survey performed by the Massachusetts Psychiatric Society found that 47 percent of those psychiatrists who responded were currently treating patients with stimulants despite FDA stipulations that these drugs be used only to treat attention deficit hyperactivity disorder, narcolepsy, and with some amphetamines, obesity.[2] On the illicit market, the amphetamines are consumed in large quantities orally and, to a lesser degree, intravenously, alone or in combination with other drugs.

Patterns of Use

It is difficult to derive precise figures concerning the prevalence of amphetamine use. In 1962, the Food and Drug Administration (FDA) estimated that enough amphetamines were produced that year to supply

TABLE 8.7. Current Medical Uses of Amphetamines and Other Stimulants

Acquired Immune Deficiency Syndrome (AIDS)
Attention Deficit Hyperactivity Disorder
Analgesia (in conjunction with narcotic analgesics)
Chronic Fatigue Syndrome
Depressive states[a]
Hyperkinetic Syndrome of childhood
(minimal brain dysfunction)
Motion sickness
Narcolepsy
Obesity (short term)
Parkinsonism[a]
Urinary incontinence

Note: These drugs consist of dextroamphetamine (Dexedrine), methamphetamine (Desoxyn), methylphenidate (Ritalin).
[a]Usually tried only when other standard methods of treatment have failed.

the entire population of this country with 250 mg.[2] Approximately 50 percent of this amount was thought to be diverted to illicit use. The easy availability of this drug in the late 1960s has been amply demonstrated. An individual, through a $600 investment, was able to obtain from manufacturers more than one million amphetamine tablets, with a value of up to $500,000 on the black market. At that time, of the 19 companies filling these orders, nine asked for neither proof of licensure nor FDA registration.[2] Prior to the passage of the controlled drug laws, it is estimated that over eight billion 10 mg doses of amphetamine and methamphetamine were manufactured and prescribed in this country.[3]

Federal action to restrict amphetamine use have been accompanied by a marked reduction in physicians prescribing through limiting production quotas of pharmaceutical firms, as well as approved medical indications. Of most importance, however, was the placement of amphetamines in Schedule II of the Controlled Substance Act of 1971. A number of other stimulants used mainly as anorexians still remain in Schedules III and IV (Table 8.6).

Yet even after this legislation was enacted, patterns of abuse still were seen. In 1986, 25 percent of all Schedule II amphetamine and 33 percent of all Schedule II Preludin were found to be consumed in Pennsylvania, a state with only 4.8 percent of the country's population. Subsequent to action by the Drug Enforcement Agency, by 1989 the prescription rate of these drugs returned to a level proportionate to the state's population.[4]

More recent surveys have revealed a progressive decrease in the "past year" use of stimulants between 1988 to 1991 from 2.5 percent to 1.3 percent of the population.[5] Amphetamines ranked 17 out of 20 drugs mentioned in data collected on drug-related emergency room episodes reported nationwide with their use becoming firmly supplemented by a much more potent drug, cocaine, and its freebase, crack. However, recently in areas on the west coast, methamphetamine synthesized in illicit laboratories is appearing on the street, being chosen over crack due to its relatively long-lasting effects.

Pharmacology

The amphetamines comprise a group of noncatecholamine phenyliso-propylamines having potent central, as well as peripheral, sympathomimetic activity. They differ from the sympathetic amines, such as epinephrine, by having (1) a greater stimulating effect on the central nervous system, (2) a greater effectiveness after oral administration, and (3) a duration of action measured in hours rather than minutes. Phenmetrazine (Preludin) and diethylpropion (Tenuate), although not phenylisopropyla-mines, are considered amphetamine-like substances due to their marked similarities of action.

Amphetamines may be injected, taken orally, or absorbed through the nasal mucous membranes by "sniffing." Following oral ingestion, the amphetamines are readily absorbed from the intestinal tract and are distributed to most tissues, including the central nervous system. Peak effects can be seen within two to three hours following ingestion of a 10 mg dose. Inactivation occurs in the liver with excretion in bile and urine. Metabolism may be slow, with metabolites able to be detected up to two to three days. Urinary excretion is considerably affected by pH, with acidification of urine resulting in an increased elimination from the body.

The major effects of the amphetamines are felt to be mediated through direct and indirect release of norepinephrine, dopamine, or serotonin from nerve terminals, as well as preventing of their reuptake. At low doses the predominant effect is on the noradrenergic neurons. As the dose increases, dopamine and then serotonin (5HT) release are effected.

Effects on Organ Systems

Central Nervous System

Amphetamine is an extremely potent stimulator of the central nervous system, speeding up the reticular activating system and acting directly on the medial forebrain bundle.[6] These effects cause arousal, hypersensitivity, and a considerable high (euphoria), even when taken in low dosage. The intensity of the psychic effects, however, can be modified by several factors, including the personality of the user and the environment in which the drug is taken. Although amphetamine use is associated with enhanced mental activity and performance of unusual physical feats, such effects are not consistent and may be reversed with overdosage or continuous use. Prolonged use is usually accompanied by depression and fatigue. Unpleasurable (dysphoric) reactions to amphetamines, such as headache, dizziness, and vasomotor disturbances, may also occur.

Amphetamine use is accompanied by a marked stimulation of the medullary respiratory center of sufficient intensity to overcome the central depression caused by various tranquilizing drugs. Consumption of amphetamines in therapeutic doses, however, does not clinically affect respiration. The appetite suppressant activity of amphetamine is probably related more to a central action on the satiety center of the hypothalamus rather than an increase in metabolic rate. Tolerance usually develops with chronic use, preventing continuous weight reduction.[7]

Similar to other stimulants, large doses of amphetamines markedly increase oxygen consumption. Therapeutic doses, however, are accompanied by variable changes of small magnitude. As noted above, the weight loss experienced with amphetamines is related mainly to a direct effect on the satiety center rather than an increase in metabolism. Plasma concentrations of free fatty acids are increased with amphetamine use without any noticeable modification of carbohydrate utilization or blood glucose concentration.

Cardiovascular System

In humans, ingested amphetamine results in increases in both systolic and diastolic blood pressures. The blood pressure elevation is directly related to the dose of amphetamine administered, with the elevation in systolic pressure proportionately greater than in diastolic pressure.

Clinically, amphetamine ingestion or injection is followed by tachycardia, palpitations, flushing, sweating, and headache, although if the blood pressure increase is considerable, a reflex slowing of the heart may occur.

Continued administration results in a degree of tolerance so that a rapid heart rate or hypertension may not be prominent in chronic users.[7] Chronic intravenous use can result in flushing, palpitations, angina, severe hypertension, and even paradoxical hypotension, with circulatory collapse and seizures with extremely large doses.

Analgesic Activity

Since the 1930s, amphetamine has been known to enhance morphine analgesia in laboratory animals. The effectiveness of dextroamphetamine in increasing morphine analgesia in humans has also been demonstrated. A combination of these two drugs has been frequently reported to be associated with a much lesser incidence of undesirable morphine-related side effects, such as nausea, sedation, and respiratory depression.[8-10] However, use of this combination never received widespread clinical acceptance despite the evidence suggesting that the analgesic effectiveness of morphine could be increased by 50 to 100 percent when taken with 5 mg to 10 mg of amphetamines.

Undesirable side effects frequently seen with morphine, such as sedation and loss of alertness, are also diminished with this combination. Effects of amphetamine on blood pressure, pulse, and respiration were minimal and felt not to be clinically relevant. Simple tests of performance, such as tapping speed and arithmetic and symbol copying tests were found to be enhanced, suggesting that the patients were considerably more alert than they would have been with the same analgesic dose of morphine. This relationship between amphetamines and narcotics has been long recognized on the "street." Heroin users frequently inject amphetamine (speedballs) mixed with heroin to decrease the time of "going on the nod" to allow them to remain alert as the initial CNS depressant effects of heroin wear off.

The use of this combination in otherwise healthy patients recovering from surgery, however, has never become widespread. Perhaps this is related to the caveats that accompany its use. Patients recovering from bowel surgery might have problems with amphetamine-induced alterations in gastrointestinal motility as might orthopedic patients with respect to skeletal muscle spasm. The use of this combination in the elderly or in individuals with underlying heart disease might also be associated with untoward complications. Yet, in selected cases, amphetamine-morphine combinations may result in a relief of pain unassociated with undue sedation or respiratory depression.

Dependence, Tolerance, and Withdrawal

Amphetamines have always been considered to be associated primarily with psychological, rather than physical dependence. However, as discussed in Chapter 3, pragmatically this distinction is less than helpful. What is of importance is the observation that in the laboratory animal, chronic administration of amphetamines, similar to cocaine, will result in self-administration, with the animal frequently choosing the drug over food to the point of seizure and death secondary to its toxic effects.[11]

Clinically, abrupt withdrawal of amphetamines after chronic use is associated with a mild withdrawal syndrome consisting of nervousness and anxiety, followed by depression, lethargy, interpersonal withdrawal, and hunger. Sleep may be prolonged for up to 72 hours with increased REM sleep noted for almost two weeks.

Tolerance to the effects of amphetamines can develop and may be of considerable magnitude. Although tolerance has been reported with respect to most effects of the drug, several recent studies concerning amphetamine-induced anorexia have suggested that development of tolerance to appetite suppression may not invariably occur. Similarly, the use of amphetamines in narcolepsy has been associated with a relatively slow development of tolerance. The degree of tolerance in the chronic user, however, may be striking, with 1,000 to 1,700 mg of the drug able to be taken without untoward effects.

Toxicity and Overdose

Toxic effects of amphetamines are dependent on the: (1) pattern of drug use, (2) way the drug is taken, (3) existence of polydrug abuse, (4) degree of tolerance developed, (5) extent of underlying disease, and (6) conditions under which the drug is taken.

Signs and Symptoms

Acute pharmacologic overdose is not an infrequent phenomenon. Since individual tolerance to these agents varies considerably, severe toxic effects may be seen with dosages as small as 30 mg to 125 mg or, in chronic abusers, may not appear until more than 1,500 mg have been taken. In general, the toxic effects represent extensions of the therapeutic actions. Central nervous system effects may include restlessness, hyperactivity, talkativeness, euphoria, delirium, and acute psychotic reactions with suicidal or homicidal tendencies.

The ability of large doses of amphetamines to increase oxygen consumption, as well as to affect the thermal regulation centers in the hypothalamus, will often result in elevated temperatures (hyperpyrexia). This response places amphetamine users at risk when they perform strenuous exercises in hot weather. Cardiovascular effects, consisting of arrhythmias and hypertension resulting in intracranial hemorrhages, may occur. Hyperpyrexia, combined with hypertension, may be followed by convulsions associated with intracerebral or subarachnoid and subdural hemorrhages. Ultimately, hypotension with cardiovascular collapse and death can occur.

Toxic effects of chronic amphetamine use include marked weight loss associated with dermatitis. Psychotic reactions similar to schizophrenic states may be observed. Although clinically there have been few reports of amphetamine-induced myocardial disease, cardiomyopathy has been reported in a 45-year-old man without evidence of preexisting heart disease, who had been maintained on high-dose dextroamphetamine for seven years.[12] At postmortem examination, lesions similar to myocarditis associated with pheochromocytomas were found, suggesting a cardiomyopathy either directly related to excessive sympathetic activity or secondary to end-state amphetamine-induced chronic myocardiohypertrophy.

Chronic use of intravenous amphetamines is associated with all the complications seen with intravenous abuse of narcotic drugs. This includes hepatitis, bacterial or fungal endocarditis, pulmonary angiothrombotic granulomatosis, microangiopathic hemolytic anemia, and anaphylactic reactions. Some disorders are considered to be specifically related to amphetamines rather than heroin or other adulterants. They include intraarterial thrombosis, with clotting of small vessels in the brain and destruction of muscle tissue. The appearance of complications of chronic amphetamine abuse, however, occur in such a "contaminated" environment that it is difficult to separate specific amphetamine effects from other factors regarding illicit use.

Treatment

Treatment of amphetamine overdose should consist of restoring the temperature to normal and using sedatives to control seizures. The patient should be placed in a quiet environment so that agitation and environmental stimulation are minimal. In the presence of a marked psychotic reaction, appropriate use of the major tranquilizers may be effective. The phenothiazines, however, should be used cautiously, if at all, due to their ability to cause hypotension as well as cholinergic crisis.

It should be emphasized that alkalinization of urine will result in an increased tubular resorption of amphetamine and a marked decrease in urinary excretion of free amphetamine. For this reason, alkalinizing solutions should not be used in fluid replacement for amphetamine overdose or in treatment of toxic psychotic reactions.

COCAINE

Cocaine (benzoylmethylecgonine) is a naturally occurring alkaloid obtained from the leaves of erythroxylon coca, which comprise 0.5 to 1 percent of the plant's dry weight. It is a rather unique drug in that it is not only a local anesthetic but also a potent sympathomimetic and central nervous system stimulant. Unlike amphetamine, little tolerance appears to develop to cocaine, with some chronic users becoming hypersensitive to its effects.

Patterns of Use

At the present time, with the exception of its use as a local anesthetic, the prevalent use of cocaine is illicit; it is ingested by smoking, "snorting," or less frequently, by intravenous injection. Although street cocaine is relatively pure (80 to 90 percent) as compared to preparations of heroin, it is adulterated with a variety of substances, the most common being mannitol, glucose, and lactose. Other stimulants, such as caffeine and amphetamine, may be added to disguise the amount of cocaine present. Parenteral use, either alone or in combination with other illicit drugs, is associated with all of the previously mentioned complications accompanying intravenous amphetamine injection.

The magnitude of use of cocaine or its freebase form "crack" is impressive. The 1993 National Household Survey on Drug Abuse reported 23 million people to have used cocaine at some time during their lives with 2.1 million using cocaine that year.[13] Equally important, in minority communities, the violence associated with drug sales (mainly for cocaine) has escalated to the point where residents are afraid to be in the streets for fear of being stuck by stray bullets. Finally, the exchange of sex for cocaine or crack has led to transmission of the human immunodeficiency virus (HIV) with many users developing HIV infection, and ultimately the acquired immune deficiency syndrome (AIDS).

Pharmacology

When administered locally, cocaine is rapidly absorbed, with an onset action within minutes and a duration of action of up to two hours.[14]

Absorption through the intranasal route has a similar onset of action, with an effect detected within two to three minutes, peaking within 15 minutes. When taken orally, absorption occurs within 15 minutes. Intravenous injection will produce an effect within 15 to 30 seconds. Smoking crack or freebasing cocaine provides the quickest high with effects seen within 6 to 8 seconds. Intramuscular or subcutaneous administration is associated with somewhat limited absorption rate due to the vasoconstrictive action of the drug. Although cocaine is absorbed rapidly through mucous membranes, if ingested, hydrolysis occurs, with a marked decrease in gastrointestinal absorption. Nonetheless, effective plasma levels of cocaine can be seen within 30 minutes of ingestion.[15]

Detoxification occurring predominantly in the liver is rate limited. Elimination occurs in the urine within 24 to 36 hours mainly as the metabolite benzoylecgonine.[17] Less than 20 percent of the total absorbed dose may be eliminated unchanged in the urine. Similar to the amphetamines, excretion of the cocaine base is greatest in acidic urine and less in urine with a more alkaline pH. Although these metabolites were initially thought to be inactive, benzoylecgonine has now been shown to have vasoconstrictor activity and may be implicated in the sudden cardiac death seen after cocaine use. More recently a new metabolite has been identified. Cocaethylene found to be formed only in the presence of alcohol has been associated with cocaine-related deaths.[16]

Effects on Organ Systems

Central Nervous System

Cocaine is a potent stimulant of the central nervous system. Its cortical effects include an increased restlessness and excitement, at times accompanied by enhancement of mental prowess and lessened sense of fatigue. Motor activity may be unimpaired with low doses of cocaine; however, increasing doses may be accompanied by tremors and convulsive movements. The respiratory rate is increased and stimulation of the vasomotor adrenergic nerve endings occur, resulting in a potentiation of both excitatory and inhibitory responses of organs innervated by the sympathetic nervous system. Hyperpyrexia secondary to an increase in muscle activity, centrally induced vasoconstriction, or a direct effect of cocaine on the temperature regulatory center may be seen.[18]

Cardiovascular System

The experimental effects of cocaine on the heart have been well described. Small doses may actually result in a bradycardia secondary to vagal stimulation. However, in moderate or large amounts, a tachycardia, accompanied by elevated blood pressure, commonly occurs, which is dose related.[19] Frequently, an acute tolerance may occur whereby the heart rate and blood pressure may return to normal despite increasing levels of cocaine in the blood. In extremely large doses, sudden death may result due to a direct toxic effect on the myocardium or depression of the medullary centers with hypotension and respiratory arrest.

As the use of cocaine and crack exploded during the late 1980s, increasing reports of cocaine-related sudden death in young people without a previous history of heart disease appeared, as did reports of heart attacks. These complication often appear hours after using cocaine, suggesting that the metabolic products of cocaine may be responsible.

Analgesic Activity

Although cocaine is not an analgesic, it is a potent, widely used local anesthetic. Cocaine can block induction through sensory nerve fibers in extremely low concentrations. With higher concentrations, nerve trunks are affected.[21] Cocaine is unique among local anesthetics since it interferes with the uptake of norepinephrine, causing a sensitization to catecholamines. This has restricted its use with other anesthetics in fear of excessive stimulation of the central nervous system, especially in individuals with a known history of heart disease. The use of topical cocaine without any adverse effects on cardiovascular function, however, has been observed.[20]

Although cocaine's anesthetic qualities have been well established, its use as an effective analgesic agent either alone or in combination with other drugs remains to be clearly defined. Cocaine has been a primary ingredient in Brompton's Mixture for decades (Chapter 6). Recent studies, however, cast doubt on its ability to enhance analgesia, suggesting that an equal analgesic effect can be obtained in its absence.

Dependence, Tolerance, and Withdrawal

Psychological dependence is a common phenomena accompanying cocaine use. Monkeys allowed to choose between intravenous injections of cocaine and food will choose cocaine almost exclusively at the expense of caloric intake, resulting in weight loss, seizures, and ultimately death. Although chronic users may snort or inject large quantities of the drug without toxic effects, data concerning the development of tolerance with cocaine remain conflicting.[21, 22]

Toxicity and Overdose

Similar to the amphetamines, there is considerable variation with respect to the dose of cocaine considered to be toxic. Fatal oral doses have ranged from 800 to 1,430 mg., subcutaneous doses from 700 to 2,500 mg. Up to 300 mg of cocaine have been injected intravenously without adverse effects, whereas doses as low as 22 mg. administered subcutaneously, have resulted in severe toxic reactions.

Signs and Symptoms

Pharmacologic overdose reactions are characterized by a marked stimulation of the central nervous system (Table 8.8). Headache, dilated pupils, rapid heart rates, palpitations, hypertension, elevated temperatures, and rapid and irregular respiration are early signs. Abnormal heart rhythms, heart attacks, and strokes have also been observed. In severe cases, a progression of delirium, nausea, vomiting, irregular breathing, high fevers, convulsions, and even death may occur. In instances of overdose from street cocaine, death may be extremely rapid, secondary to an allergic (anaphylactic) reaction to contaminants mixed with the cocaine.

Individuals with preexisting medical conditions are at considerable risk of experiencing adverse effects. Persons with vascular disease or high blood pressure may have strokes or heart attacks. Those with diseases of the heart valves may experience irregular heartbeats, which may be life-threatening. Persons with seizure disorders, such as epilepsy, may experience convulsions with cocaine. Psychologic reactions in persons with underlying psychological difficulties have also been reported. The adverse effects of cocaine on the cardiovascular system have been observed to be more pronounced when coexisting use of marijuana, alcohol, or tricyclic antidepressants exist.

In addition to the actual pharmacologic effects of cocaine, use by injection exposes the user to a wide range of medical complications. These are similar to that seen with illicit injections of any substance, and are secondary to unsterile technique and introduction of contaminants in the drug directly into the bloodstream. They include infections of the lungs, liver, and heart, abscesses, and AIDS.

Treatment

Treatment of acute cocaine reactions is mainly supportive. Although drugs that block noradrenergic neuronal activity may be helpful, it is

TABLE 8.8. Acute Complications Associated with Cocaine Toxicity

Cardiovascular
    Cardiac Arrest—Ventricular Fibrillation
    Supraventricular Tachycardia
    Myocardial Infarction
    Hypertension
    Stroke
    Shock

Gastrointestinal
    Abdominal Pain
    Ischemic Bowel
    Gastric Ulcers
    Hyperthermia

Muscular
    Muscle death (Rhabdomyolysis)
    Muscle tenderness (Myalgia)

Neurologic
    Headache
    Seizures
    Hyperthermia
    Stroke
    Cerebral Hemorrhage
    Toxic delirious states

Renal
    Acute renal failure due to rhabdomyolsis

Respiratory*
    Pneumothorax
    Bronchospasm
    Pneumonias
    Tracheobronchitis
    Pulmonary Edema
    Alveolar Hemorrhage
    Tracheal burns

*Usually due to inhaling crack or snorting cocaine

important to use those agents that block all neuronal activity (alpha and beta blockers), such as Labetalol (Normodyne, Trandate) rather than only beta blockers, which may exacerbate cocaine's toxic effects. Calcium channel blockers may also be helpful. If central nervous system excitation predominates, use of a sedative or tranquilizing agent, such as diazepam, by intravenous or intramuscular route may be of value. The short duration of action of cocaine, combined with a relative lack of development of tolerance, suggests that, except in consumption of large doses, pharmacologic treatment is usually not necessary.

CAFFEINE

Caffeine-containing beverages have been consumed for centuries and are probably the most commonly used psychoactive substances. Although currently considered fairly innocuous and utilized by over 90 percent of the population, in the early twentieth century, dependence on caffeine was considered equal in severity to that of morphine or alcohol. At present, the most popular caffeine-containing drinks are coffee, tea, soft drinks, and cocoa. Caffeine is also found in maté and kola nuts.

Caffeine-Containing Beverages

Coffee beans contain 0.7 to 2 percent of caffeine as well as numerous other constituents, including carbohydrates, oils, proteins, ash, nonvolatile acids, and trigonelline. Roasting alters the constituents of over 90 percent of the water-soluble substance and volatilizes other products. Although minute amounts of vitamins are present in coffee, they are not felt to be of dietary importance with the possible exception of niacin. Tea contains approximately 2 percent caffeine and theophylline and tannic acid. The amount of caffeine actually consumed in coffee and tea is variable, depending on potency of brew (Table 8.9).[23] A random survey of caffeine beverages consumed at home found a lower and more variable caffeine content than previously realized. The mean caffeine content of coffee was 74 mg per cup (range 29 to 176 mg) and for tea, 27 mg per cup (range 8 to 91 mg).[24]

Pharmacology

Caffeine is one of the methylated xanthines. The other drugs in this group include theophylline and theobromine. All these agents have similar properties with respect to central nervous system stimulation, cardiac stimu-

TABLE 8.9. Approximate Caffeine Content of Common Beverages

	Caffeine Content mg/ cup[a]
Coffee	
Ground	85-190
Instant	30-100
Decaffeinated	3-5
Tea[c]	20-150
Cocoa[d]	5-30
Colas[b]	19-50
Chocolate[d,e]	1-35

[a]Six-ounce cup
[b]Eight- to twelve-ounce can
[c]Also contains approximately 1 mg theophylline
[d]Also contains approximately 250 mg theobromine
[e]Varies with type; bakers' chocolate has higher content than milk chocolate per ounce

lation, diuretic action, and smooth muscle relaxation. Of these, caffeine is the most potent central nervous system stimulant, whereas theophylline has a greater effect on the cardiovascular system and as a diuretic. Theobromine is the least potent. Caffeine may be consumed in prescribed medications, as OTC agents (Table 8.10), or in popular drinks. Theophylline is also prescribed for its pharmacologic actions. Theobromine consumption occurs as a constituent along with caffeine in cocoa and chocolate.

Regardless of route of administration, caffeine is readily absorbed; however, the rate of absorption from the intestinal tract may vary due to its low solubility in aqueous media. After oral administration, peak levels are reached in 1 hour, with an average half-life of 3.5 hours. Metabolism occurs in the liver. The half-life of caffeine in the plasma is between three to seven hours. However, in women in the last trimester of pregnancy or in persons on long-term oral contraceptives, the half-life may be doubled. On the other hand, in young children, the half-life is diminished. As with other drugs, genetic variations that influence the metabolic rate can exist.

Effects on Organ Systems

The methylated xanthines are believed to act by affecting the metabolism of cyclic nucleotides, the movement of intracellular calcium, and

TABLE 8.10. Caffeine-Containing Medications

	Caffeine Content mg
Anacin	32
Anodynes	34.4
APCs	32
Arthritis Strength BC	36
Amaphen with codeine	40
Bayer Select Headache Pain Relief	65
BC Powder	36
Bexophene Capsules	32.4
Buffets II	32.4
Caffedrine	200
Codalan	30
Coffee Break	200
Cope	32.4
Darvon Compound Pulvules	32.4
Dihydrocodeine Compound	30
Dristan with AF	16.2
Duradyne	15
Empirin with codeine	40
Ercaf	100
Esgic with codeine	40
Excedrin Extra Strength	65
Fiorinal with codeine	40
Histosal	30
Midol	32
No Doz	100
No Doz Maximum Strength	200
Phenetron	30
Pain Reliever Tablets	65
P-A-C Analgesic Tablets	32
Rid-A-Pain	32.4
Saleto	16
Tirend	100
Tri-Pain	16.2
Vivarin	200
Wigraine	100

blocking of adenosine receptors. As a result of these actions, they can affect the functioning of a variety of organ systems.

Central Nervous System

Caffeine stimulates all parts of the central nervous system. Cortical effects result in improved ability to concentrate, which is associated with a more sustained intellectual effort, and an increased activity for sensory stimuli. Motor activity is increased. This is usually seen at doses between 20 to 200 mgs.[24] As the dose of caffeine increases, adverse effects consisting of nervousness, hyperesthesia, and decreases in fine muscular coordination may be experienced. In high doses (200 to 800 mgs), caffeine stimulates vasomotor and respiratory centers in the medulla, as well as increases reflex activity at the level of the spinal cord. At one time those effects led to the recommendation to inject caffeine in people with tranquilizer or barbiturate overdose, especially in the presence of respiratory depression. Little objective evidence exists, however, to the clinical efficiency of caffeine or other stimulants in these conditions.

Cardiovascular System

The physiological effects of caffeine on the heart and circulation are complex relating to direct myocardial and vascular actions, as well as its actions on the medullary vasomotor centers.[25] Physiologically, all parts of the cardiovascular system may be affected.

Caffeine may have a stimulatory or an inhibitory effect on the heart, depending on the dose employed. The literature describing the cardiovascular effects of caffeine includes few double-bind trials with placebos and even fewer studies that truly separate coffee drinkers from the "caffeine naive." The administration of caffeine has been associated with palpitations, both rapid and slow heart rates, mild elevations of systolic and diastolic blood pressures, increased cardiac output, an increase or decrease in arterial venous oxygen difference, and an elevation in oxygen consumption.[26, 27]

Other Effects

Caffeine can increase the capacity for muscular work, but it does so at doses that also cause central nervous system stimulation. Its action on smooth muscle, however, is that of a relaxant.[28] The clinical importance of this action is minimal. The ability of both caffeine and theophylline to act as a mild diuretic, increasing urine flow is well-known. Similarly, heartburn is a recognized complication of excessive coffee consumption and felt to be related to the stimulation of both acid and pepsin secretion in the stomach.

Analgesic Activity

The methylxanthines have been used for a variety of medical conditions. In several their effectiveness is clear; in others less certainty exists (Table 8.11). Caffeine is a frequent component of OTC analgesic mixtures. Most often combined with aspirin or acetaminophen, caffeine is felt to exert a favorable influence on mood as well as enhance the analgesic effect. However, there has never been any compelling evidence in the literature to suggest that caffeine is either an effective analgesic or is able to enhance analgesic effects of other drugs. It is of interest that the amount of caffeine combined in these mixtures usually varies from 10 to 200 mg with few containing more than 30 mg whereas a cup of coffee may contain as much as 100 to 190 mg, with the average daily consumption of coffee drinkers estimated at 280 mg a day.

Dependence, Tolerance, and Withdrawal

Until recently there was little evidence to suggest that continued consumption of caffeine causes physical dependence. A study by Strain and associates demonstrated that caffeine can produce effects similar to other dependency-producing psychoactive substances.[29] Of 99 subjects in this study, 16 percent were caffeine-dependent, with 9 percent demonstrating signs of caffeine withdrawal. Habituation and psychologic dependence occur much more frequently, and a certain degree of tolerance may be demonstrated. It is a common experience that persons accustomed to drinking several cups of coffee in the morning will develop mild symptoms of anxiety and difficulty in concentration if the coffee is withheld.

TABLE 8.11. Current Medical Uses of the Methylxanthines

Asthma
Chronic obstructive lung disease
Apnea in premature infants
Increase alertness
Enhance analgesia*
Antagonize respiratory depression induced by drug overdose*

*Effectiveness not demonstrated

Headaches induced by withholding caffeine have also been demonstrated as have muscle aches.[30,31] The headaches began approximately 18 hours after caffeine intake ceased, peaked approximately three to six hours later, and lasted for at least 24 hours. It has been suggested that many persons diagnosed as having tension headaches may, in fact, be undergoing caffeine withdrawal. It is also conceivable, though far from proven, that intermittent intake of high levels of analgesics containing caffeine may result in a cycle of symptoms relieved by taking the analgesic with a progression to analgesic dependency. The considerable individual variation in sensitivity to caffeine, however, combined with the problems inherent in assessing subjective symptoms, make these findings difficult to evaluate.

Toxicity

Most of the serious toxic reactions to the methylxacthines occur with theophylline as this is the drug prescribed in pharmacologic doses for treatment of respiratory distress associated with asthma and chronic lung disease. In humans, actual overdose due to caffeine is extremely rare. Increasing caffeine consumption is associated with insomnia, restlessness, muscle twitching, and excitement, which can progress to delirium. Cardiovascular effects, such as arrhythmias, have been reported, with an age-related association demonstrated between frequency of ventricular premature contractions and coffee consumed. Habitual coffee drinkers can develop tachycardia and extra heartbeats by doubling their coffee intake. Although coffee at one time was implicated as a positive risk factor in development of myocardial infarction, this observation has not been able to be confirmed. Excess caffeine consumption may also give rise to a peptic ulcer diathesis in susceptible individuals. Not infrequently the development of heartburn associated with caffeine can be mistaken for cardiac symptoms with the attendant fear of an impending heart attack. Elimination of caffeine intake promptly provides relief.

DRUG INTERACTIONS

Amphetamine and cocaine both exert potent sympathomimetic effects. Concomitant use of either of these medications with antihypertensive drugs acting on the autonomic nervous system can be associated with interference of their antihypertensive action or, depending on the drug, precipitate acute hypertensive crises. Amphetamines in small doses have been shown to antagonize the antihypertensive effect of guanethidine. Their use with the monoamine oxidase (MAO) inhibitors can precipitate hypertension and intracerebral bleeding. Diazoxide is given by injection to lower extremely high blood pressure. It acts by exerting a direct dilating action on arterial musculature, which may be accompanied by an increased sympathetic discharge. A synergistic reaction may, therefore, occur with concomitant use of amphetamine or cocaine.

The use of cocaine in local anesthesia, associated with other local anesthetics containing epinephrine, may cause a marked tachycardia and hypertension. Although younger individuals can tolerate such effects fairly well, in the elderly patient, with or without cardiac disease, such a response may be quite detrimental. Epinephrine-containing anesthetic solutions in patients also receiving cocaine for topical anesthesia should be used quite cautiously, if at all, and with careful monitoring.

Interactions between the stimulants and other mood-altering drugs exciting autonomic or central nervous system effects may also occur. Concomitant use of the tricyclic antidepressants may diminish amphetamine effectiveness. Barbiturates have been reported to enhance the aggressive behavior seen following intravenous amphetamines. It has been suggested that amphetamines are less effective when taken with lithium carbonate.[32] Haloperidol and phenothiazines may also antagonize amphetamine-induced stimulation through interfering with its uptake into the neuron.[33] However, the clinical relevance of these observations is unclear.

Caffeine can enhance metabolism of various medications and correspondingly several drugs can also affect the time caffeine remains in the plasma.[34] Plasma half-life of caffeine is increased with concomitant use of oral contraceptives, the H^+ blocker cimetidine, disulfiram (Antabuse), and several antibiotics in the fluorquinolene group (Cipro, Noroxin, Floxin, Penetrex, and Maxaquin). Smoking tends to enhance caffeine metabolism increasing its elimination.

SUMMARY

Although the stimulants are frequently used as adjuncts to analgesia, with the exception of the amphetamines there is little evidence suggesting inherent analgesic activity in any of these drugs. Amphetamines can potentiate narcotic analgesia when used in acute pain. The associated effects of amphetamines, however, warrant careful consideration on an individual basis prior to their use. Cocaine's anesthetic qualities remain unquestioned. Its effectiveness as an adjunct to analgesia as when used in patients with neoplastic diseases, however, remains to be proven. Caffeine, the most widely consumed stimulant, is found in mild analgesics in concentrations approximately less than half one would obtain by drinking a cup of coffee with an analgesic devoid of caffeine. The rationale for its use in OTC medications is less than clear.

REFERENCES

1. Cole JO, Boling LA, Beake BJ. Stimulant drugs-medical needs: Alternate indications and related problems. In *Impact of prescription drug diversion control systems on medical practice and patient care* (NIDA Res Mono 131), J Cooper, DJ Czechowicz, SP Molinari, RC Peterson (eds.), Rockville, MD: NIDA, 1993, 89–108.

2. American Medical Association Committee on Alcoholism and Addiction and Mental Health. Dependence on amphetamines and other stimulant drugs. *JAMA*, 1966, 197:1023–1027.

3. Greene MH, Nightingale SL, DuPont RL. Evolving patterns of drug abuse. *Ann Intern Med*, 1975, 83:402–411.

4. Haislip GR. DNA diversion control systems, medical practice, and patient care. In *Impact of prescription drug diversion control systems on medical practice and patient care* (NIDA Res Mono 131), J Cooper, DJ Czechowicz, SP Molinari, RC Peterson (eds.), Rockville, MD: NIDA, 1993, 120–131.

5. Adams EH, Kopstein AN. The nonmedical use of prescription drugs in the United States. Ibid. p. 109–119.

6. Blundell JE, Leshem MB. Dissociation of the anorexic effects of fenfluramine and amphetamine following intrahypothalamic injection. *Br J Pharmacol*, 1973, 47:183–185.

7. Connell PH. Clinical manifestations and treatment of amphetamine type of dependence. *JAMA*, 1966, 196:718–723.

8. Ivy AC, Goetzl FR, Burril DY. Morphine-dextroamphetamine analgesia. *War Med*, 1944, 6:67–71.

9. Joshi JH et al. Amphetamine therapy for enhancing the comfort of terminally ill patients (PTS) with cancer. *Proc Am Soc Clin Oncol*, 1982, 1:C–213.

10. Forrest WH, Jr, Brown BW, Jr, Brown CR, Defalque R, Gold M, Gordon HE, James KE, Katz J, Mahler DL, Schroff P, Teutsch G. Dextroamphetamine with morphine for the treatment of postoperative pain. *N Engl J Med*, 1977, 296:712–715.

11. Pickens R, Thompson T. *Self-administration of cocaine and amphetamine by rats*. Report to NAS-NRC Committee on Problems of Drug Dependence, 1967.

12. Smith HJ, Roche AHG, Jausch MF, Herdson PB. Cardiomyopathy associated with amphetamine administration. *Am Heart J*, 1976, 91:792–797.

13. *National drug control strategy: Executive summary*. Washington, DC: The White House, 1995.

14. VanDyke C, Jatlow P, Ungerer J, Barash PG, Byck R. Oral cocaine: Plasma concentrations and central effects. *Science,* 1978, 200:211–213.

15. Fish F, Wilson WDC. Excretion of cocaine and its metabolites in man. *J Pharm Pharmacol,* 1969, 21 (Suppl.): 1355–1385.

16. Witkin JM, Katz JL. Preclinical assessment of cocaine toxicity: Mechanisms and pharmacotherapy. In *Acute cocaine intoxication: Current methods of treatment* (NIDA Res Mono 123), H Sorer (ed.), Rockville, MD: NIDA, 1992, 45–65.

17. Ritchie JM, Greene NM. Local anesthetics. In: Gilman AG, Rall TW, Nies AS, Taylor P (eds.). *Goodman and Gilman's the pharmacological basis of therapeutics,* 8th ed. New York: Pergamon Press, 1990: 319–331.

18. Resnick RB, Kestenbaum RS, Schwartz LK. Acute systemic effects of cocaine in man: A controlled study by intranasal and intravenous routes. *Science,* 1977, 195:696–698.

19. Fischman MW, Schuster CR, Resnekov L, Shick JF, Krasnegov NA, Fennell W, Freedman DX. Cardiovascular and subjective effects of intravenous cocaine administration in humans. *Arch Gen Psychiatry,* 1976, 33:983–989.

20. Fischman MW, Schuster CR, Krasnegov NA. Physiological and behavioral effects of intravenous cocaine in man. In: Ellingwood EM, Kilbey MM (eds.). *Cocaine and other stimulants.* New York: Plenum Press, 1977: 647–664.

21. Jaffe JH. Drug addiction and drug abuse. In: Gilman AG, Rall TW, Nies AS, Taylor P (eds). *Goodman and Gilman's the pharmacological basis of therapeutics,* 8th ed. New York: Pergamon Press, 1990: 522–573.

22. VanDyke C, Byck R. Cocaine 1884-1974. In: Ellingwood EG, Jr, Kilbey MM (eds.). *Cocaine and other stimulants.* New York: Plenum Press, 1977; 1–30.

23. Gilbert RM, Marshman JA, Schwieder M, Berg R. Caffeine content of beverages as consumed. *Can Med Assoc J,* 1976, 114:205 – 208.

24. Rall TW. Drug used in the treatment of asthma. In: Gilman AG, Rall TW, Nies AS, Taylor P (eds.). *Goodman and Gilman's the pharmacological basis of therapeutics,* 8th ed. New York: Pergamon Press, 1990: 618–637.

25. MacCornack FA. The effects of coffee drinking on the cardiovascular system: Experimental and epidemiological research. *Prev Med,* 1977, 6:104–119.

26. Polonovski M, Donzelot E, Briskas S, Doliopoulos TH. The comparative effects of coffee and soluble extracts of coffee on normal persons and on cardiacs. *Cardiologia,* 1953, 21:809–816.

27. Mathieu L, Hadot S, Hadot E. Cardiac repercussions of coffee drinking. *Actual Cardiol Angeiol Int,* 1962, 11:219–226.

28. White BC, Lincoln CA, Pearce W, Reeb R, Vaida C. Anxiety and muscle tension as a consequence of caffeine withdrawal. *Science,* 1980, 209:1547–1548.

29. Strain EC, Mumford GK, Silverman K, Griffiths RR. Caffeine dependence syndrome. Evidence from case histories and experimental evaluations. *JAMA,* 1994, 272:1043–1048.

30. Greden JF, Fontaine P, Lubetsky M, Chamberlin K. Anxiety and depression associated with caffeinism among psychiatric inpatients. *Am J Psychiatry,* 1978, 135:963–966.

31. Prineas RJ, Jacobs D, Crow R, Blackburn H. Coffee, tea and VPB. *Circulation,* 1977, (Suppl. III):15.

32. Flemenbaum A. Does lithium block the effects of amphetamine? A report of three cases. *Am J Psychiatry,* 1974, 131:820–821.

33. The Medical Letter on Drugs and Therapeutics. Haloperidol. *Med Lett,* 1967, 9:70–72.

34. Mitoma C, Sorich TJ, II, Neubauer SE. The effect of caffeine on drug metabolism. *Life Sci,* 1968, 7:145–151.

Chapter 9

Barbiturates, Nonbarbiturate Hypnotics, and Minor Tranquilizers

INTRODUCTION

Although barbiturate-hypnotic use has been consistently decreasing since the early 1960s, the prescription of the benzodiazepines since this time has been nothing short of phenomenal. In 1967, psychotropic drugs represented 17 percent of the 1 billion prescriptions written by physicians, with chlordiazepoxide and diazepam (Valium) accounting for almost one-third of psychotropic drugs.[1] By 1972, over 70 million prescriptions were written for these two agents at a cost to the public of approximately $200 million. In 1980, worldwide sales of diazepam were purported to reach $350 million. In 1987, of the top 50 drugs prescribed nationally, five were benzodiazepines (Xanax, Halcion, Valium, Ativan, and Tranxene).

Abuse or misuse of sedatives, hypnotics, or minor tranquilizers remains considerable. In 1976 barbiturates accounted for almost 51 percent of suicides in four large metropolitan cities. Subsequent to this finding, barbiturate overdose has been increasingly replaced by benzodiazepine overdose.[1] In a nationwide survey of 1,265 facilities, including emergency rooms, crisis centers, and medical examiners' offices, diazepam was found to be the first or second drug of abuse noted in all drug abuse contacts.[2] Unfortunately, in up to 60 percent of cases, the diazepam was initially obtained through a physician's prescription. The risk of physician misuse of the benzodiazepines can be illustrated by the agreement of the pharmaceutical industry to include a statement in the indications section of promotional literature advising against routine prescription for managing the daily stresses of living.

For the purpose of this discussion, these agents will be classified following their pattern of use as: (a) hypnotics and sedatives, and (b) anxiolytics or minor tranquilizers.

HYPNOTICS AND SEDATIVES

The agents in this category comprise a large group of chemically unrelated substances, including alcohol, which is capable of inducing sedation and sleep with small doses and varying degrees of amnesia or anesthesia with larger quantities (Table 9.1). Prolonged and uninterrupted use of these agents can result in both physical and psychological dependence. Unless otherwise stated, the information presented will refer to the barbiturates, the most extensively studied of these drugs.

Although chloral hydrate, first synthesized in 1832, is the oldest of the hypnotic and sedative agents, subsequent to the introduction of the first hypnotic barbiturate barbital (Veronal) in 1903, barbiturates have become the commonly accepted prototype, and until recently, have been the most frequently used.[3] Barbiturates may be classified by duration of action and plasma half-life into long-acting, short-to-intermediate-acting, and ultra-short-acting drugs (Table 9.2).

Pharmacology

After oral administration, absorption is dependent on lipid solubility of the particular agent as well as the dissolution of the drug in the intestinal lumen. The short-acting lipid soluble barbiturates in the form of sodium salts are absorbed more rapidly than long-acting barbiturates, which have a lesser affinity for lipids and are administered as free acids. The slow absorption rate of the long-acting barbiturates makes these agents less likely to be used for "highs" by those specifically seeking a mood-altering experience. Distribution is widespread. The half-lives of the barbiturates used as hypnotics and sedatives, such as pentobarbital, phenobarbital, and secobarbital, may be as long as 120 hours depending on the specific agent. Other hypnotics such as methyprylon and ethchlorvynol have considerable shorter half-lives of four to six hours.[4,5] Biotransformation of the barbiturates occurs mainly in the liver. Nonmetabolized barbiturates are excreted unchanged in the urine over a period of several days. Barbital metabolism differs from other barbiturates, with urinary excretion representing the major route of elimination.

Effects on Organ Systems

Nervous System

Barbiturates depress activity in almost all excitable tissues. Clinically, the response to barbiturates may include sedation, euphoria, or anesthesia, depending on specific drug and dose administered.[6] The effects of central nervous system depression may vary from sleep to coma, depending on (1) dose, (2) barbiturate administered, (3) underlying excitability of the

TABLE 9.1. Classification of Sedative and Hypnotic Drugs

Generic name	Trade name	Schedule[a]
Antihistamines		
Hydroxyzine hydrochloride	Atarax	
Hydroxyzine pamoate	Vistaril	
Azaspirodecanedione		
Buspirone	Buspar	
Barbiturates		
Benzodiazepines		IV
Estazolan	ProSom	IV
Flurazepam hydrochloride	Dalmane-2	
Quazepam	Doral	IV
Temazepam	Halcion	IV
Chloral derivatives		
Chloral hydrate[b]	Aquachloral, Noctec, Somnos	IV
Chloral betaine	Beta Chlor	IV
Triclofos sodium	Triclos	
Ethchlorvynol	Placidyl	IV
Bromides	Sedamyl	
Carbamates		
Meprobamate[b]	Miltown, Neurate-400, Tranqui-tab, Traumep, Equanil, Mepriain, Saronil Neuramate, Robamate Bamate, Bamo, Canqui, Coprobate	IV
Ethinamate	Valmid	
Tybamate	Solacen, Tybatran	
Imidazopyridine		
Zolpidem	Ambien	
Paraldehyde[c]	Paral	IV
Phenothiazines		
Propiomazine	Largon	
Piperidinedione derivatives		
Glutethimide[b]	Doriden, Rolathimide	II
Methyprylon	Noludar	III
Quinazalones		
Methaqualone	Quaalude, Sopor	II
Methaqualone Hydrochloride	Parest, Somnfac	II
Scopolamine and/or Methapyrline	Sleepeze, Mr. Sleep, Sominex, Nytol	
Ureides		
Acetylcarbromal	Paxarel	

[a] Controlled Substances Schedule

[b] Other benzodiazepines used primarily as minor tranquilizers are listed in Table 9.3.

[c] Generic brands produced by various manufacturers

TABLE 9.2. Classification of Barbiturates

Drug	Trade Name	Action	Half-life (Hrs)	Schedule[a]
Phenobarbital[b]	Pheno-Squar Solfoton Luminal	Long	80-120	IV
Mephobarbital	Mebaral	Long	11-67	IV
Amobarbital[b]	Amytal	Intermediate	16-42	II
Aprobarbital	Alurate	Intermediate	14-34	III
Butabarbital[b]	Butisol	Intermediate	34-42	III
Pentobarbital[b,c]	Nembutal	Short	15-48	II
Secobarbital[b,c]	Seconal	Short	15-40	II
Talbutal	Lotusate	—	—	II

[a]Refers to Controlled Substances Schedule
[b]Generic brand also produced by various manufacturers
[c]Sodium salt also exists

central nervous system, and (4) route of administration. Certain areas, such as the reticular activating system (RAS), are exceedingly sensitive to the depressant effect of the barbiturates.[7] When applied directly to peripheral nerves, barbiturates may exhibit a local anesthetic action, decreasing the rate in rise of amplitude of the action potential accompanied by a slowing of conduction.

The sedative effect of barbiturates is accompanied by a decrease in REM sleep, which may return to normal as tolerance develops. Withdrawal is accompanied by a rebound in REM activity. A postsedative effect may occur manifested by distortions of mood and impairments of judgmental motor skill. Alternatively, these aftereffects may be mainly excitatory.

Respiratory System

The respiratory center is quite sensitive to barbiturates. Both respiratory rhythm and drive are affected. Therapeutic doses of barbiturates cause a decease in alveolar ventilation and a slight increase in alveolar carbon dioxide tension accompanied by a decrease in arterial oxygen saturation. As the dose is increased, the hypoxic stimulus to respiration is diminished, with the respiratory center ultimately becoming insensitive to carbon dioxide. At this point, respiration is maintained on an hypoxic stimulus. Administration of oxygen without providing ventilatory support will, therefore, result in respiratory arrest.

Cardiovascular System

Clinically, barbiturates produce minimal changes in the cardiovascular system unless the person is critically ill and hemodynamically unstable.[8] Depression of the medullary vasomotor center usually occurs with relatively little effect on the baroreceptors and autonomic nervous system. This results in a slight decrease in cardiac output with increased peripheral resistance and a maintenance of arterial pressure—unless high doses are injected. Vascular flow and volume in the extremities are increased, and there is a decrease in cerebral blood flow with a fall in cerebral spinal fluid pressure.

Other Organ System Effects

Barbiturates may decrease smooth muscle tone in the gastrointestinal tract, ureter, urinary bladder, and uterus. However, this is of clinical relevance only when prescribed in large doses or during intravenous anesthesia. Renal effects of barbiturates include a slight depression in sodium and glucose reabsorption by direct action on tubular cells, and a stimulation of antidiuretic hormone secretion. The net effect on renal function may vary depending on dose. In large doses, especially when accompanied by hypotension, there is a decrease in urine flow. Acute barbiturate poisoning with accompanying hypotension may ultimately result in renal failure.

Barbiturates exert marked effects on hepatic enzyme systems. This may interfere with other drugs metabolized in the liver (see Drug Interactions) through either a competitive inhibition of the microsomal system or an increase in enzyme activity secondary to increase in enzyme content.

Analgesic Activity

Prior to the development of the benzodiazepines, barbiturates were most frequently used for treatment of anxiety. When used without analgesics, barbiturates and related drugs cannot relieve pain without impairing consciousness. In the presence of severe pain, the sedative or soporific effects may even be inhibited. In small doses, barbiturates have been shown to have a hyperanalgesic effect, increasing the reaction to painful stimuli.[9] The explanation for this hyperanalgesic activity is unclear but may be related to the depressant effect of barbiturates on the neuronal systems responsible for releasing the neurotransmitter serotonin.

The use of barbiturates and nonbarbiturate sedatives, therefore, will not promote analgesia, and if used in combination with narcotics, may potentiate central nervous system depression. Their use in the relief of pain is therefore contraindicated. Unfortunately, these drugs can cause euphoria similar to morphine, and despite the ineffectiveness of these drugs in relieving pain, all too frequently, a person with chronic pain will take one or more sedative-hypnotics. It is quite important to be aware of their dependency-producing qualities as well as the best way to manage withdrawal and overdose reactions.

Dependence, Tolerance, and Withdrawal

Chronic use of the hypnotic drugs is associated with both psychological and physical dependence. The severity of physical dependence may vary depending on dose administered and frequency of ingestion. Tolerance develops with chronic administration of barbiturates or nonbarbiturate hypnotics. Although the degree of tolerance can be considerable, the tolerance-toxicity ratio is quite low. Acute intoxication can, therefore, occur with only slight increases in dosage above the tolerance threshold. A considerable degree of crosstolerance exists between all hypnotics and nonhypnotic sedatives, with the substitution of any one of these drugs being able to present or diminish withdrawal symptoms.

Abrupt discontinuation of high doses of barbiturates will result in a characteristic and a severe withdrawal syndrome. Barbiturate withdrawal is potentially more dangerous than that of narcotics and if not treated may be fatal. Treatment of barbiturate withdrawal is based on slowly reducing the maintenance dose of the drug. Similar to the concept of methadone detoxification in narcotic withdrawal, it is best to use a long-acting barbiturate, such as phenobarbital. The use of phenobarbital provides for less fluctuation in barbiturate levels and is usually unaccompanied by the euphoria seen with the shorter-acting barbiturates.

In general, a daily dose of phenobarbital is calculated by substituting 30 mg of the drug for each 100 mg of the short-acting barbiturate.[10] A person should be stabilized for one to two days on this equivalent phenobarbital dose prior to beginning withdrawal. The presence of toxic syndromes such as slurred speech, nystagmus, or ataxia usually indicates too high an initial phenobarbital dose, which requires this dose to be decreased by 30 to 50 percent. Alternatively, if discomforting signs of barbiturate withdrawal appear, such as tremors or hyperreflexia, the daily dose should be increased. The appearance of major signs of withdrawal, such as seizure activity, can be avoided by an intramuscular injection of phenobarbital. Once the daily dose of phenobarbital has been stabilized, a slow withdrawal at approximately 10 percent a day can be instituted. As with detoxification from most dependence-producing drugs, the challenge is not successful detoxification but rather the development of a therapeutic regimen to prevent relapse.

An alternate procedure is to use a benzodiazepine such as chlordiazepoxide at an initial dose less than that needed to produce intoxication. This dose is maintained for 36 to 48 hours and then tapered at 10 percent per day. It should be remembered, however, that the challenge with dependency-producing drugs is not successful detoxification but rather the development of effective regimens to prevent relapse.

Toxicity and Overdose

Barbiturate and nonbarbiturate hypnotic overdoses are recognized phenomena in emergency rooms, most often resulting from deliberate suicide attempts. The lethal dose can very considerably depending on (1) the drug ingested, (2) individual tolerance, (3) presence of polydrug abuse, and (4) time course of ingestion. Symptoms are primarily referable to a marked depression of the central nervous system, and in extremely large doses, to cardiovascular dysfunction.

Signs and Symptoms

Although mild intoxication may resemble the alcoholic state, as intoxication proceeds in severity, hypoxia and respiratory acidosis will appear.

Irregular (Cheyne-Stokes) breathing may be present, accompanied by a marked diminution in respiratory volume.

Cardiovascular changes induced by barbiturate overdose include hypotension and depression of myocardial function. In severe overdoses, especially in the elderly, a severe shock-like state that is associated with lowered body temperatures may occur at times.[11]

Dermatological changes such as sweat gland necrosis and superficial bullous lesions have also been described. These findings may not be specifically related to a barbiturate effect but may result from positional changes.

Treatment

The general principles involved in the treatment of central nervous system depressant overdose are the same regardless of agent involved. These measures include (1) maintenance of an open airway, (2) artificial respiration, if needed, (3) maintenance of circulation (closed chest massage if peripheral pulses are absent), and (4) institution of an intravenous infusion to maintain adequate hydration. Dehydration and shock associated with reduced intravascular volume or vascular collapse may occur. Adequate hydration and careful monitoring of intake and output are essential until consciousness is resumed.

Analeptics or stimulants have been shown to be relatively ineffective in depressant overdose and, in addition, may be associated with adverse effects. Gastric lavage should not be performed if the patient is seen more than six hours after ingestion and, if seen earlier, deferred until cardiovascular stability has been obtained and airway patency is ensured with an inflated endotracheal tube. Dialysis may be warranted depending on the severity of the intoxification as well as the specific agent responsible.[12]

Although it may be very difficult to initially identify the specific drug responsible for an overdose, toxic reactions to several nonbarbiturate sedatives do present with some distinctive features. Glutethimide (Doriden) overdose results in a coma, usually of long duration. Symptoms consist of hypotension, papilledema, apnea, and pulmonary edema. Plasma glutethimide levels and the clinical course are usually not well correlated. In addition to supportive measures, hemodialysis and hemoperfusion have been shown to be helpful.[13]

Methaqualone overdose has also been associated with of toxic cardiovascular effects of acute heart failure.[14]. Meprobamate (Equanil, Miltown, Meprospan) poisoning may be accompanied by severe hypotension, usually adequately managed by plasma expanders and mild vasoconstrictors, unless myocardial failure is present, making fluid loading hazardous.[15]

It should be emphasized that synergistic effects due to ingestion of several hypnotic-sedatives may be especially hazardous. Alcohol is the drug most frequently used in combination with other hypnotics. Recently a chloral hydrate-alcohol interaction has been observed. Patients maintained on chloral hydrate have been found to develop anginal symptoms associated with marked vasodilation after consuming small amounts of alcohol.[16]

Summary

In summary, most patients admitted with overdose from central nervous system depressants will be able to recover with supportive therapy. If the responsible drug is predominantly excreted by the kidneys, forced diuresis may be quite helpful. If adequate attention is given to maintenance of respiration and circulation, the prognosis is good, providing therapy is instituted early enough to preclude the presence of any permanent cerebral damage secondary to anoxia.

BENZODIAZEPINES

Since the introduction of chlordiazepoxide (Librium) into clinical medicine in 1960, other benzodiazepine derivatives have appeared (Table 9.3). At present, the three most commonly prescribed benzodiazepines are chlordiazepoxide (Librium), diazepam (Valium), and flurazepam (Dalmane). These drugs are widely used for the treatment of anxiety, for muscle relaxation, as anticonvulsants, and as soporifics (hypnotics) having replaced the barbiturates and other hypnotics (Table 9.4). Flurazepam, specifically packaged as a hypnotic, comprises 53 percent of all hypnotics prescribed.[17]

Pharmacology

The benzodiazepines are widely distributed in tissues. After oral administration of diazepam, peak blood levels are noted within several hours, with a half-life of one to two days. Tissue accumulation is preferential in lipid-rich organs such as the brain. Cumulative dose effects may occur. Metabolism results in only small amounts of free and conjugated compounds being excreted in the urine. Some of the metabolites are pharmacologically active and may be responsible for the "day after" effect seen with the use of hypnotic benzodiazepines.[18] Excretion is biphasic, with a rapid phase seen within two or three hours followed by a slow decay over the next several days. The half-life of these drugs varies from 20 to 50 hours.

In normal individuals, the plasma half-life of the benzodiazepines increases with advancing age (Chapter 16). The presence of hepatic disease

TABLE 9.3. Benzodiazepine Derivatives[a]

	Speed of Onset	Duration of Action
Antianxiety		
Alprazolam (Xanax)	Intermediate	Short
Chlordiazepoxide[b] (Librium, Mitran, Reposams-10, Libritabs)	Intermediate	Intermediate
Clonazepam (Klonopin)	Intermediate	Intermediate
Clorazepate (Tranxene)	Fast	Long
Diazepam[b] (Valium, Valrelease, Dizac)	Fast	Intermediate/Long
Halazepam (Paxipam)[c]	Intermediate	Short
Oxazepam (Serax)	Intermediate	Short
Lorazepam (Ativan)	Intermediate	Short
Prazepam (Centrax)	Slow	Long
Sedatives, Hypnotics		
Estazolam (ProSom)	Intermediate	Intermediate
Flurazepam (Dalmane)	Fast	Long
Quazepam (Doral)	Intermediate	Long
Temazepam (Restoril)	Intermediate	
Triazolam (Halcion)	Fast	Short

[a] All commonly prescribed benzodiazepines are classified as schedule IV drugs.
[b] Generic brands produced by various manufacturers.
[c] Defined by half-life: Short = under 20 hours; Intermediate = under 50 hours; Long = 50–100 hours.

TABLE 9.4. Indication for Benzodiazepines

Acute Treatment of Agitated Psychosis
Anesthetic Agent During Surgery
Anxiety
    Short-Term—Acute
    Generalized Anxiety Disorder
Epilepsy
Insomnia
Muscle Disorders
Panic Disorders

may be associated with the prolongation of diazepam's half-life of approximately twofold, accompanied by a twofold decrease in total plasma clearance. The reduction is of clinical importance when diazepam is given to persons with liver disease, especially if administered with other drugs that compete with diazepam for a common metabolic pathway.

Seventy percent of the oral diazepam dose is excreted in the urine, with 9 to 10 percent undergoing fecal excretion. Urinary excretion is in the form of conjugated metabolites, primarily glucuronides with oxazepam conjugates predominating.

Benzodiazepines maybe classified as short-, intermediate-, or long-acting depending on their half-life in the body. Whether all benzodiazepines are therapeutically similar in equivalent doses is controversial. It is, however, accepted that the use of short-acting benzodiazepines in high doses for long periods is associated with more severe withdrawal when discontinued.

The metabolites of chlordiazepoxide and diazepam are pharmacologically active, whereas those of nitrazepam and oxazepam are inactive. This is clinically relevant since the latter agents may be used as hypnotics with relatively little sedation persisting after one day. Chlordiazepoxide and diazepam, although capable of producing sleep in sufficient dosage, will retain a sedative effect for longer than 24 hours, with cumulative effects occurring on repeated administration.

Prazepam and clorazepate are two of the longer-acting benzodiazepines. Both drugs are essentially completely transformed into the pharmacologically active substance desmethyl diazepam.[19] The half-life of desmethyl diazepam in humans may be as long as 200 hours, which allows these drugs to be used as once daily for effective anxiolytic actions. Biotransformation of prazepam proceeds more slowly than with clorazepate. This may be beneficial in patients where a rapid absorption would be associated with untoward central depression.

Lorazepam has a half-life intermediate between diazepam and oxazepam. Although absorption following intramuscular injection is rapid and complete, it is relatively slow. Restricted tissue distribution results in a more prolonged amnestic effect. This is in contrast to diazepam and chlordiazepoxide, the two commonly utilized parenteral benzodiazepines that have quite rapid decline in plasma concentrations as well as variable absorption following intramuscular injection.

Effects on Organ Systems

Central Nervous System

The use of radioimmunoassay techniques has enabled the identification of high-affinity binding sites for benzodiazepines in brain tissue with two receptor sites being identified. These drugs effect gamma-aminobutyrate (GABA) neurotransmission.

Cardiac and Respiratory Function

When taken orally the benzodiazepines have minimal respiratory effects. Their use as preanesthetic agents is associated with a slight depression of ventilation. This may be significant in persons with chronic obstructive lung disease. When used in narcotics or administered intravenously, respiration arrest can occur.

The benzodiazepines can influence cardiac function through centrally mediated effects on the nervous system, but in doses used clinically, these effects are minimal. However, when used as preanesthetic agents, slight decreases in blood pressure and increases in heart rate can occur.[20]

Analgesic Activity

The benzodiazepines are frequently prescribed as adjunctive therapy for patients in pain. At times they may be the sole drug used when anxiety is felt to be the predominant cause of symptoms despite animal and clinical studies having failed to demonstrate any consistent direct analgesic properties of benzodiazepines. Although the use of these drugs in combination with morphine and acetaminophen has at times been associated with potentiation of analgesia, these findings, have not been consistently confirmed.[21]

The postulated effectiveness of the benzodiazepines, especially diazepam as a muscle relaxant, has led to their frequent prescription for low back pain. Noncontrolled studies have suggested that diazepam may be of benefit, either through its anxiolytic or muscle relaxant effect. Relief of pain has been reported in 70 percent of patients even in the presence of structural disorders such as disc lesions, spasm-induced fractures, or rheumatoid arthritis. Controlled studies, however, have resulted in less consistent findings. Diazepam has been found to be more effective than other muscle relaxants in several studies, with chlordiazepoxide more effective than placebo. Other investigators, however, have failed to show any advantage of the benzodiazepines over placebo or aspirin. One of the limitations in the use of these drugs for muscle spasms is the sedation that often accompanies their use. At times this effect may limit the use of benzodiazepams in muscular disorders.

Adjunctive use of benzodiazepines in pain and anxiety associated with myocardial infarction has been reported to be of value. Hackett and Cassem, in a comparison of chlordiazepoxide and amobarbital in coronary care patients recovering from myocardial infarction, found those patients given chlordiazepoxide to require analgesia less often and in smaller doses than those receiving amobarbital.[22]

In summary, although benzodiazepines have not been shown to exert specific analgesic activity, their short-term use for treating painful states, especially where anxiety is prominent, may be of value. Chronic use, however, has not been definitely shown to be effective and, in addition, carries with it the development of both psychological and physical dependence. Prescription of these drugs for long-term use should, therefore, be avoided if possible.

Dependence, Tolerance, and Withdrawal

Continued use of all central nervous system depressants, including the benzodiazepines, can be associated with habituation, dependence, tolerance, and withdrawal. The intensity of these phenomena relates to the characteristics of the specific drug, the dose administered, and the duration of administration. For those benzodiazepines with long half-lives, withdrawal may not appear for more than a week after discontinuing use.

Although some investigators have felt that prolonged use of extremely high doses of benzodiazepines is necessary for the development of dependence (300 to 5,600 chlordiazepoxide or 80 to 120 diazepam per day), dependence can occur at much lower doses.[23-25] Withdrawal symptoms on high doses of chlordiazepoxide (100 to 600 mg per day) may occur within four to eight days after the drug is discontinued. Initial symptoms are mild, consisting of apprehension, anxiety, insomnia, and dizziness. These symptoms may progress to nausea, vomiting, fever, postural hypotension, muscle twitches, hallucinations, and psychoses. Severe symptoms are identical to that seen with other drugs in the alcohol-barbiturate group.

Dependence and withdrawal in persons maintained on low therapeutic doses of benzodiazepines are less easy to document but are being described with increasing frequency in up to 40 to 50 percent of persons on short-term therapy and in up to 100 percent of persons in chronic therapy. One of the problems in recognition of the symptoms of mild withdrawal is that such symptoms may be indistinguishable from those of the anxiety state promoting the initial prescription. When this factor is considered, the incidence of withdrawal can decrease to 5 percent with short-term use and no more than 50 percent with long-term use.[26] Benzodiazepine dependence, however, should be considered whenever repeated episodes of headache or dysphoria are associated with discontinuation of drug use. These findings are of special importance when such symptoms are unrelated to the initial anxiety reaction.

Although there is no certain way to prevent the development of psychological or physical dependence to the benzodiazepines, the chances of dependence developing can be markedly diminished by short-term use. This is especially true with respect to the use of flurazepam for insomnia associated with pain or the use of diazepam for low back pain. Prolonged use of these agents will not only result in the potential for dependence but also in a progressive decrease in their effectiveness. To minimize the chances of withdrawal after prolonged use, a slow tapering of the dose over several weeks might be helpful.

Rebound

When short-term therapy with benzodiazepines is suddenly discontinued or the dose tapered too rapidly, return of initial symptoms may occur with accelerated intensity. This phenomenon, termed "rebound," can occur in up to 50 percent of persons. Symptoms will usually subside within a week and may not require treatment. However, a slow tapering of the drug will provide relief.

Toxicity and Overdose

Not unexpectedly, the major toxic reactions to the benzodiazepines are drowsiness and muscular incoordination, resembling alcoholic intoxication. Paradoxical stimulation and increase in hostility may rarely occur associated with marked changes in affect. These reactions may be more prominent with triazolam (Halcion) than with other benzodiazepines.[27] Adverse reactions have been reported in approximately 11 percent of persons receiving chlordiazepoxide and 7 percent receiving diazepam, with oversedation being the most frequent finding.[28] Daytime muscular incoordination following flurazepam use has also been reported. Unusual reactions, such as allergic responses, dermatitis, and agranulocytosis, have been observed. Menstrual abnormalities associated with anovulatory cycles may occur and gynecomastia has also been observed.

Serious sequela due to overdose with benzodiazepines are rare although suicidal attempts are quite frequent. For several years, the Drug Abuse Warning Network (DAWN) recorded diazepam as the most frequent drug identified in suicide attempts. In a study of 1,239 fatal cases associated with diazepam ingestion, the role of diazepam in causing death was felt to be minimal, with actual cause of death being attributed to other drugs ingested.[30] Treatment of actual overdose is similar to that of the hypnotics and sedatives, with maintenance of cardiovascular function and respiratory support being of prime importance.

Recently, the benzodiazepine receptor antagonist flumazenil (Mazicon) has become available for treatment of benzodiazepine overdose or to reverse the sedative effects of benzodiazepines after anesthesia. Flumazenil has a relatively short half-life of 15 minutes and is rapidly cleared by the liver and excreted in the urine. Although intravenous flumazenil has been shown to be effective in improving the level of consciousness is persons who have had an benzodiazepine overdose, its use is not without risk. The use of flumazenil has been associated with increase in symptoms of central nervous system stimulation and can cause seizures in persons on benzodiazepine for epilepsy or when tricyclic antidepressants have been taken and overdose is present. It is also consistently effective in reversing benzodiazepine-induced respiratory depression or respiratory depression in a mixed-sedative overdose.

BUSPIRONE

Buspirone (Buspar) is a recently developed antianxiety agent, unrelated to the benzodiazepines, that acts as an antagonist on the 5-hydroxytryptamine receptors. It is reported to cause minimal sedation and have little potential for abuse and dependence. However, its most frequent side effects include dizziness and light-headedness of sufficient intensity to result in 10 percent of persons in a chemical trial discontinuing its use.

HYDROXYZINE

Hydroxyzine (Atarax, Anxanil, Vistaject, Hydroxacen, Hyzine-50, Quiess, Rezine, Vistacon, Vistaquel, Vistaril) is an antianxiety agent, chemically unrelated to either the sedative-hypnotic drugs or the phenothiazines.[31-33] It has been found to be effective in relieving anxiety and in higher doses is an effective hypnotic. The circulatory effects of this drug are minimal although electrocardiographic alterations similar to those seen with the tricyclic antidepressants and the phenothiazines have been reported. It has been demonstrated that the use of hydroxyzine with 8 mg of morphine can enhance morphine analgesia.[31] Although increased sedation was noted with this combination, it was felt not to be clinically significant.

Hydroxyzine at a dose of 100 mg has been demonstrated to reduce analgesia equivalent to that of 8 mg morphine, suggesting that the combination of these two agents might result in a more effective analgesic state without the increased risk of respiratory depression or undue sedation.

ZOLPIDEM

Zolpidem (Ambien) is a drug chemically unrelated to the benzodiazepines that, nonetheless, binds to the benzodiazepine receptors in the central nervous system. It is an effective hypnotic. However, it is considerably more expensive than several of the currently available agents.[34]

DRUG INTERACTIONS

Many of the hypnotics, sedatives, and minor tranquilizers are known to influence the hepatic endoplasmic reticulum (HER) of the liver, with barbiturates having the most prominent effects (Table 9.5). In general, the direction of the enzymatic response is both frequency- and dose-related. Chronic administration of barbiturates and other sedatives will result in enzymatic induction, whereas acute administration of large doses may cause an inhibition of enzymatic activity. Concomitant administration of these agents with other drugs whose metabolism is dependent on the HER can result in drug interactions that may be of clinical importance. An interaction between barbiturates and benzodiazepines may also occur at the level of the benzodiazepine receptor. Pentobarbital has been shown to enhance GABA-induced receptor affinity to diazepam as well as potentiate diazepam binding to receptor sites.[35] When used with digoxin or phenytoin, benzodiazepine may increase serum levels of both drugs with a potential for toxic reactions.

Interactions with Other Mood-Altering Drugs

The potentially hazardous effects of drinking and consuming sedative drugs are well known. When taken simultaneously, synergistic respiratory

TABLE 9.5. Selected Drug Interactions of Barbiturates and Benzodiazepines

Drug	Barbiturates	Benzodiazepines
Alcohol	Synergistic respiratory depressant activity with acute administration	Synergistic respiratory depressant activity with acute administration
Cimetidine	No reported chemical effect	Increased effect
Diphenylhydantoin (DPH)	Increase in plasma DPH levels	Increase in plasma DPH levels
Disulfiram		Increased effect
Isoniazid	No reported effect	Increased effect
Ketoconazole	No reported effect	Increased effect
Levodopa	No reported effect	Decreased levodopa effect
Metoprolol	No reported effect	Increased effect
Monoamine oxide inhibitors	Increased effect	No clinical effect
Oral anticoagulants	Decrease in anticoagulant effect[a]	Minimal clinical effect
Oral contraceptives		Increased effect
Phenothiazines	Decrease in plasma levels	No reported clinical effect
Probenecid		Increased effect
Propoxyphene		Increased effect
Propranolol	Decrease in propranolol effect	Increased effect
Quinidine	Decrease in quinidine serum half-life	No reported clinical effect
Rifampin		Decreased effect
Tricyclic antidepressants	Decrease in antidepressant effect	Increase in anticholinergic symptoms
Smoking		Decreased effect
Valproic acid	Increased effect	Increased effect

[a]Potential for serious bleeding when barbiturate therapy is discontinued.

depressant activity is likely to occur. Similarly, central nervous system depression will be enhanced if any of the individual drugs in this group are taken simultaneously.

The use of barbiturates with therapeutic doses of the tricyclic antidepressants has been associated with a decrease in antidepressant activity.[36] The use of barbiturates in tricyclic overdose has been associated with a potentiation of adverse effects and is therefore contraindicated.[37] Additive depressant effects and an increase in anticholinergic symptoms have also been reported with continued use of chlordiazepoxide and the tricyclics. Unlike barbiturate-tricyclic interactions, however, serious adverse effects are rare.[36] If convulsions present as a manifestation of tricyclic antidepressant overdose, a benzodiazepine such as diazepam is the preferred agent for treatment of this complication.[36]

Plasma levels of phenothiazines have been shown to decrease and urinary excretion of phenothiazine increases in patients simultaneously given barbiturates. This effect is believed to be secondary to the induction of hepatic enzymes responsible for phenothiazine metabolism. The clinical significance of this interaction remains to be defined.

Barbiturates, when administered with a variety of other agents, may decrease their efficacy. These drugs include acetaminophen, cortisteroids, Digoxin, Doxycycline, beta blockers, Metronidazole, Phenmetrazine, Quinidine, Rifampin, and the oral anticoagulants.

Anticoagulants

Hypnotic-sedative drugs can interact with several medications routinely prescribed to persons with cardiovascular disease. Clinically, the interactions of most importance involve the oral anticoagulants.

Barbiturates

Of all the sedatives, the barbiturates have the most prominent effect on metabolism of the coumarin derivatives. Concurrent barbiturate administration may necessitate the doubling of the anticoagulant dosage in order to maintain the desired prothrombin time. This interaction occurs with all barbiturates, although phenobarbital exerts the most potent effect.[38] Dicumarol absorption from the intestine is inhibited by heptabarbital administration, whereas it is little affected by the other barbiturates.[39]

The main importance of this interaction, however, is the propensity for hemorrhage when the sedative is discontinued, rather than the initial difficulty in establishing adequate levels of anticoagulants. Microsomal enzyme activities usually return to normal within two or three weeks following cessation of barbiturate therapy. If an adjustment in warfarin dosage is not made, the potential for serious hemorrhage exists.

Chloral Hydrate

Chloral hydrate interacts with warfarin in a somewhat complex manner. During early therapy with both agents, a major metabolite of chloral hydrate (trichloracetic acid) accumulates in the plasma and, having a higher affinity for plasma albumin, displaces warfarin. This results in an increase in unbound plasma warfarin and enhancement of anticoagulant action. With time, however, hepatic enzyme induction occurs with an increased rate of warfarin metabolism and inhibition of anticoagulation. Although these interactions have been pharmacologically documented, recent studies have questioned their importance.[40,41]

Benzodiazepine

Interactions between the oral anticoagulants and the benzodiazepines appear to be of little clinical importance; more carefully designed studies are needed.[42]

Antiarrhythmics

Induction of the hepatic microsomal system by barbiturates can affect the metabolism of quinidine, diphenylhydantoin (DPH), and lidocaine. The serum half-life of quinidine may diminish by an average of 50 percent with concomitant use of these agents.[43] Similarly, an increase in DPH blood levels to toxic concentrations has also been reported, although clinically this interaction may show individual variation.[44] Several reports have also appeared in the literature describing an increase in DPH levels with concomitant administration of benzodiazepines. Although this interaction may also be of clinical importance, the paucity of published data is inconclusive; further investigation is warranted. Lidocaine metabolism can also be affected in a similar manner.[45]

Antihypertensives

Interaction at a metabolic level has been reported with barbiturate administration and the simultaneous use of alpha-methyldopa[46] and monoamine oxidase inhibitors.[47] The clinical importance of these reactions, however, has not been demonstrated.

Cimetidine

An interaction between cimetidine and diazepam has recently been described.[48] Concomitant use of these two drugs will result in an elevation of diazepam blood levels as well as a decreased rate of excretion of both diazepam and its active metabolite desmethyl diazepam. This is associated with increased sedation and potential for toxicity. Similarly, chlordiazepoxide clearance has also reported to decrease with concomitant administration of cimetidine.[49]

Digitalis

A lowering of plasma digitoxin levels and a diminished digitoxin half-life have been reported in persons maintained on digitoxin and given phenobarbital. Concomitant use of these two drugs is also associated with an acceleration of conversion of digitoxin to digoxin.[50] Although the interaction does not uniformly occur, concomitant use of digitoxin and phenobarbital should be avoided.

REFERENCES

1. American Medical Association Committee on Alcoholism and Addiction and Council on Mental Health. Dependence on barbiturates and other sedative drugs. *JAMA*, 1965, 193:673–677.

2. Cooper JR. *Sedative-hypnotic drugs: Risks and benefits*. Rockville, MD: National Institute on Drug Abuse, Dept. of Health, Education, and Welfare, 1977.

3. Harvey SC. Hypnotics and sedatives. In: Goodman LS, Gilman A. (eds). *The pharmacological basis of therapeutics*, 6th ed. New York: Macmillan, 1980: 339–375.

4. Jaffe J. Hypnotic and sedative agents. In: Jarvik ME (ed). *Psychopharmacology in the practice of medicine*. New York: Appleton Century Crofts, 1977: 327–342.

5. Freudenthal RI, Carroll FI. Metabolism of certain commonly used barbiturates. *Drug Metab Rev*, 1973, 2:265–278.

6. McClane TX, Martin WR. Subjective and physiologic effects of morphine, pentobarbital and meprobamate. *Clin Pharmacol Ther*, 1976, 20:192–198.

7. Weakly JN. Effect of barbiturates on "quantal" synaptic transmission in spinal motor-neurones. *J Physiol (London)*, 1969, 204:63–77.

8. Andersen TW, Gravenstein JS. Cardiovascular effects of sedative doses of pentobarbital and hydroxyzine. *Anesthesiol*, 1966, 27:272–278.

9. Dundee JW. Alterations in response to somatic pain associated with anaesthesia. II. The effect of thiopentone and pentobarbitone. *Br J Anaesth,* 1960, 32:407–414.

10. Wesson DR, Smith DE. Managing the barbiturate withdrawal syndrome. In: Bourne PG (ed.). *Acute drug abuse emergencies.* New York: Academic Press, 1976:99–104.

11. Thorstrand C. Cardiovascular effects of poisoning by hypnotic and tricyclic antidepressant drugs. *Acta Med Scand Suppl,* 3:1–34.

12. Schreiner GE, Teehan BP. Dialysis of poisons and drugs: Annual review. *Trans Am Soc Artif Intern Organs,* 1971, 17:513–544.

13. Chazen JA, Cohen JJ. Clinical spectrum of glutethimide intoxication. Hemodialysis reevaluated. *JAMA,* 1969, 208:837–839.

14. Pascarelli EF. Methaqualone abuse, the quiet epidemic. *JAMA,* 1973, 224:1512–1514.

15. Blumberg AG, Rosett HL, Dobrow A. Severe hypotensive reactions following meprobamate overdosage. *Ann Intern Med,* 1959, 51:607–612.

16. Sellers EM, Carr G, Bernstein JG, Sellers S, Koch-Weser J. Interaction of chloral-hydrate and ethanol in man II: Hemodynamics and performance. *Clin Pharmacol Ther,* 1972, 13:50–58.

17. Institute of Medicine, Division of Mental Health and Behavioral Medicine. *Sleeping pills, insomnia and medical practice* (report of a study). Washington, DC: National Academy of Sciences, 1979.

18. Tallman JF, Paul SM, Skolnick P, Gallagher DW. Receptors for the age of anxiety: Pharmacology of the benzodiazepines. *Science,* 1980, 207:274–281.

19. Greenblatt DJ, Shader RI. Prazepam and lorazepam, two new benzodiazepines. *N Engl J Med,* 1978, 299:1342–1344.

20. Rao S, Sherbaniuk RW, Prasad K, Lee SJ, Sproule BJ. Cardiopulmonary effects of diazepam. *Clin Pharmacol Ther,* 1973, 14:182–189.

21. Grotto M, Sulman FG. Interaction of analgesic effects of psychopharmaca. *Arch Int Pharmacodyn Ther,* 1967, 170:257–263.

22. Hackett TP, Cassem NH. Reduction of anxiety in the coronary-care unit: A controlled double-blind comparison of chlordiazepoxide and amobarbital. *Curr Ther Res Clin Exp,* 1972, 14:649–656.

23. Hollister LE, Motzenbecker FP, Degan RO. Withdrawal reactions from chlordiazepoxide ("Librium"). *Psychopharmacologia,* 1961, 2:63–68.

24. Abernathy DR, Greenblatt DJ, Sharder RI. Treatment of diazepam withdrawal syndrome with propranolol. *Ann Intern Med,* 1981, 94:354–355.

25. Roy-Burne PP, Hommer D. Benzodiazepine withdrawal: Overview and implications for treatment of anxiety. *Amer J Med,* 1988, 84:1041–1052.

26. Rickels K, Case WG, Schweizer EE, Swenson C, Fridman R. Low-dose dependence in chronic benzodiazepine users: A preliminary report on 119 patients. *Psychopharmacol Bull,* 1986, 22:407–415.

27. Lasagna L. The Halcion story: Trial by media. *Lancet,* 1980, 1:815–816.

28. Miller RR. Drug surveillance utilizing epidemiologic methods: A report from the Boston Collaborative Drug Surveillance Program. *Am J Hosp Pharm*, 1973, 30:584–592.

29. Moerck HJ, Magelund G. Gynecomastia and diazepam abuse. *Lancet*, 1979, 1:1344–1345.

30. Finkle BS, McCloskey KL, Goodman LS. Diazepam and drug-associated deaths: A survey in the United States and Canada. *JAMA*, 1979, 242:429–434.

31. Beaver WT. Comparison of morphine, hydroxyzine, and morphine plus hydroxyzine in postoperative pain. In: *Hospital practice special report: recent studies on the nature and management of acute pain*. New York: HP Publishing, 1975: 23–28.

32. Forrest WH. Bioassay of morphine and morphine plus hydroxyzine in postoperative pain. In: *Hospital practice special report: recent studies on the nature and management of acute pain*. New York: HP Publishing, 1975.

33. Momose T. Potentiation of postoperative analgesic agents by hydroxyzine. In: *Hospital practice special report: Considerations in management of acute pain*. New York: HP Publishing, 1977: 22–27.

34. Zolpidem for insomnia. *Med Lett Drugs Ther*, 1993, 35:35–36.

35. Skolnick P, Moncada V, Barker JL, Paul SM. Pentobarbital: Dual actions to increase brain benzodiazepine receptor affinity. *Science*, 1981, 211:1448–1450.

36. Silverman G, Braithwaite R. Interaction of benzodiazepines with tricyclic antidepressants. *Br Med J*, 1972, 4:111.

37. Crocker J, Morton B. Tricyclic antidepressant drug toxicity. *Clin Toxicol*, 1969, 2:397–402.

38. MacDonald MG, Robinson DS. Clinical observations of possible barbiturate interference with anticoagulation. *JAMA*, 1968, 204:97–100.

39. Aggeler PM, O'Reilly RA. Effect of heptabarbital on the response to bishydroxycoumarin in man. *J Lab Clin Med*, 1969, 74:229–238.

40. Udall JA. Warfarin-chloral hydrate interaction. *Ann Intern Med*, 1971, 74:540–543.

41. Griner PF, Raiss LG, Rickles FR, Wiesner PJ, Odoroff CL. Chloral hydrate and warfarin interaction: Clinical significance. *Am Intern Med*, 1971, 74:540–543.

42. Breckenridge A, Morme M. Interactions of benzodiazepines with oral anticoagulants. In: Garatini S, Mussini E, Randell LO (eds.). *Benzodiazepines*. New York: Raven Press, 1973:647–654.

43. Data JL, Wilkinson GR, Nies AS. Interaction of quinidine with anticonvulsant drugs. *N Engl J Med*, 1976, 294:699–702.

44. Diamond WD, Buchanan RA. A clinical study of the effect of phenobarbital on diphenylhydantoin plasma levels. *J Clin Pharmacol New Drugs*, 1970, 10:306–311.

45. Dunbar RW, Boettner RB, Haley JV, Hall VE, Morrow DA. The effect of diazepam on the antiarrhythmic response to lidocaine. *Anesth Analg*, 1971, 50:685–692.

46. Kaldor A, Juvancz P, Demeczky M, Sebestyen K, Polotas J. Enhancement of methyldopa metabolism with barbiturate. *Br Med J*, 1971, 3:518–519.

47. Sjöqvist F. Psychotropic drugs (2): Interaction between monoamine oxidase (MAO) inhibitors and other substances. *Proc R Soc Med,* 1965, 58:967–978.

48. Klotz U, Reimann I. Delayed clearance of diazepam due to cimetidine. *N Engl J Med,* 1980, 302:1012–1014.

49. Desmond PV, Patwardhan R, Schenker S, Speeg KV, Jr. Cimetidine impairs elimination of chlordiazepoxide (librium) in man. *Ann Intern Med,* 1980, 93: 266–268.

50. Hutcheon DE. Cardiovascular drug interactions. *J Clin Pharmacol,* 1975, 15:129–134.

Chapter 10

The Major Tranquilizers

The major tranquilizers, antipsychotic, or neuroleptic drugs (Tables 10.1 and 10.2) are utilized mainly in the treatment of psychoses. However, these drugs have a variety of other effects, including the ability to potentiate analgesia, as well as prevent vomiting. Since several of these agents are prescribed as adjuncts to control pain, the major groups of neuroleptics will be briefly reviewed.

PHENOTHIAZINES

Of this group of drugs, the phenothiazines had been among the most widely used in medical practice. With the arrival of butyrophenones (Haldol) and other neuroleptics, however, the use of phenothiazines has diminished. Chlorpromazine (Thorazine) can be considered the prototype of this group.

Pharmacology

The absorption of these drugs from the gastrointestinal tract is influenced by many factors, including individual variability, dose, presence of food in the stomach, and simultaneous use of antacids. However, once absorbed, their biological effects may persist for up to 24 hours and, depending on the drug, their metabolites may be detected in the urine for months after they have been stopped.[1]

Metabolism occurs in the liver, with excretion of metabolites in both urine and feces. Chlorpromazine and other phenothiazines can cause an induction of the hepatic microsomal system, which can effect not only its own breakdown but also result in interactions with other drugs metabolized by this system.

TABLE 10.1. Commonly Utilized Phenothiazines

Phenothiazines	Trade Name[b]
Alphatics[a]	
chlorpromazine[b]	Thorazine, Ormazine
promazine[b]	Sparine, Prozine-50
triflupromazine	Vesprin
Piperazines[a]	
acetophenazine	Tindal
fluphenazine	Prolixin, Permitil
perphenazine	Trilafon
prochlorperazine[b]	Compazine
trifluoperazine	Stelazine
Piperidines[a]	
mesoridazine	Serentil
thioridazine	Mellaril
Methotrimeprazine	Levoprome

[a] Refers to substitution of the side group on position 10 of the three-ring structure of the phenothiazines.
[b] Generic preparations may be made by various manufacturers.

Effects on Organ Systems

Central Nervous System

The phenothiazines affect all areas of the central nervous system through their ability to block postsynaptic dopamine receptors interfering with dopamine-mediated neurotransmission. It is believed that the phenothiazines bind both the D_1 and D_2 receptors whereas haloperidol binds selectively to D_2 sites. It is the avidity of a drug to bind to the D_2 receptor site that is felt to correlate best with its activity as a neuroleptic.[1] These drugs can also block alpha adrenergic receptors, and such blockage is responsible for the hypotension often accompanying their use.

The behavioral effects of the phenothiazines vary, depending on their administration to normal or psychotic individuals. Acute administration of chlorpromazine results in sedation accompanied by a marked showing of mentation as well as a decrease in spontaneous motor activity and response to external stimuli. The antipsychotic effects of the drug take considerable time to fully develop. Most frequently there is a loss of emotional response and

TABLE 10.2. Other Major Tranquilizers

Other Antipsychotic Agents	Trade Name[a]
Butyrophenones	
haloperidol	Haldol
Dibenzodiazepines	
clozapine	Clozaril
Dibenzoxazepine	
loxapine	Loxitane
Dihydroindolone	
molindone	Lindone, Moban
Rauwolfia alkaloids[b]	
deserpidine	Harmonyl
reserpine[a]	Serpalan, Serpasil
Thioxanthenes	
chlorprothixene	Taractan
thiothixene	Navane
Benzisoxazole	
risperidone	Risperdal
Diphenylbutylpiperidine	
pimozide	Orap

[a] Generic preparations may be made by various manufacturers.
[b] Used in psychotic states of agitation only when other agents are not able to be tolerated.

initiative. Agitation is markedly reduced as is aggressive behavior. Although tolerance to its sedative effects develops with continuing use, their antipsychotic effects are not associated with tolerance.

Chlorpromazine can increase reticular brainstem activity. Vasomotor reflexes are depressed as is the chemoreceptor trigger zone responsible for the vomiting reflex. It is this property that allows the use of these drugs with agents to treat nausea and vomiting. Autonomic nervous system effects include a blocking of alpha adrenergic and cholinergic receptors, as well as inhibition of serotonin (5-HT) activity. Clinically, this results in hypotension and diminished gastric secretion, intestinal motility, sweating, and salivation.

Cardiovascular System

The actions of phenothiazines on the cardiovascular system are complex, relating to the direct effects on the heart and vascular system as well as indirect actions mediated through the autonomic and central nervous systems. The autonomic effects of chlorpromazine result in reflex tachycardia and vasodilation accompanied by hypotension. Chronic administration has been associated with the development of cardiomegaly, congestive failure, and refractory arrhythmias. Paradoxically, chlorpromazine has also been demonstrated to have coronary vasodilator activity equal to and at times greater than that seen with papaverine and nitroglycerin. An antiarrhythmic effect on the heart, similar to that of quinidine, has also been reported.[2,3,4,5]

Hypotension

Hypotension may occur following parenteral administration of chlorpromazine. This is most pronounced when rising from a lying or seated position (orthostatic). The hypotension may be secondary to either centrally mediated pressor reflexes or an adrenergic blockade. The ability of phenothiazines to serve as effective alpha blockers assumes importance in the treatment of chlorpromazine-induced hypotension. The use of an agent with both α and β receptor activity, such as epinephrine, might result in an "unmasking" of β effects with an associated worsening of the hypotension. For this reason, only sympathomimetic drugs with α activity should be administered.

Hypotension is more frequent with chlorpromazine and thioridazine and less so with piperazine derivatives. Oral doses may also be related to a mild hypotensive reaction, which may resolve with time as tolerance develops.[6] Orthostatic changes, however, may persist for long periods, especially in the elderly. Hypotension has been found to be significantly related to smoking, the dose of chlorpromazine administered, and the initial level of diastolic blood pressure.[7] The incidence of hypotension in nonsmokers was 10 percent, light smokers (21 cigarettes per day) 8 percent, and intermediate smokers (21 to 40 cigarettes per day) 5 percent. No hypotension was seen in heavy smokers. The reasons for the relationship remain to be clearly defined but may be related to the ability of nicotine to stimulate the microsomal enzyme system.

Electrocardiographic Changes

Although several of the phenothiazines have been reported to have a stabilizing effect on cardiac rhythm, electrocardiographic (ECG) changes can occur in persons on phenothiazines, with the degree of abnormality being dose-related. The most frequent asymptomatic alterations seen are repolarization abnormalities resembling those produced by quinidine. In one study, only 32 percent of persons on Mellaril 150 to 400 mg per day had normal

ECGs.[8] Similar changes have been noted with chlorpromazine (Thorazine), trifluoperazine (Stelazine), mesoridazine (Serentil), and fluphenazine.[9,10,11] The percentage of abnormal electrocardiograms was found to differ considerably with the specific phenothiazine used. Thioridazine, combined with chlordiazepoxide, was found to give the lowest incidence of abnormal records (31 percent), whereas fluphenazine, combined in oral and intramuscular form, resulted in the greatest percentage (91 percent) of abnormal records.[12]

The presence of first degree atrioventricular block with conduction delay, nonconducted premature atrial beats, and atrial flutter with varying block and ventricular arrhythmias has also been reported in persons receiving thioridazine therapy.[13,14] Although most of these arrhythmias have appeared in patients receiving extremely high doses of thioridazine (1,500 to 3,600 mg), arrhythmias in patients receiving lower doses (less than 800 mg per day) have also been reported.

Sudden Death

Over the past 13 years, reports of sudden, unexplained death in persons receiving phenothiazine have appeared in the literature, implicating a fatal arrhythmia as the cause of death.[15,16,17] The clinical relevance of ECG alterations in producing sudden death secondary to fatal arrhythmias has not been clearly defined. It must be emphasized that cardiac patients in psychiatric institutions will be expected to have an incidence of sudden death due to their cardiac disease independent of the prescription of phenothiazine or other psychotropic agents. A review of 1,932 consecutively monitored psychiatric inpatients could not relate the appearance of serious cardiac effects of any specific drug, although the incidence of these adverse effects was clearly higher in persons with cardiac disease (19 percent versus 1.3 percent).[18] Mechanisms for sudden death in patients maintained on phenothiazines can be easily hypothesized. Prolongation of QT interval increases the duration of the ventricular vulnerable period. This is associated with the propensity for ventricular premature beats to lead to ventricular fibrillation.

Other Organ System Effects

Chlorpromazine can inhibit secretion of antidiuretic hormone and diminish the release of corticotropin-releasing hormone and growth hormone. Other endocrinological alterations, including lactation and breast engorgement in women and gynecomastia in men, secondary to elevation of prolactin levels, have also been observed. Chlorpromazine-induced hepatic microsomal activity affects not only its own metabolism, but also results in interactions with other drugs metabolized by this system. Jaundice, resembling that seen with extrahepatic obstruction, may occur. Hematologic disorders, the most serious being agranulocytosis and aplastic anemia, have also been reported.

Analgesic Activity

The widespread effects of the phenothiazines on the central nervous system, associated with their known interactions with noradrenergic and dopaminergic receptors, have led to the hypothesis that these agents can provide analgesia independent of any neuroleptic effect. Successful treatment of central pain with chlorpromazine has been reported.[19,20] These studies, however, were neither controlled nor blinded. When such studies were performed, neither primary analgesic activity nor an enhancement of morphine analgesia could be well documented.[21,22]

Other studies have reported effective analgesia utilizing phenothiazines alone or in combination with tricyclic antidepressants in persons with refractory diabetic peripheral neuropathy and neuromuscular disease.[23-25] Combinations of fluphenazine and amitriptyline were reported to relieve pain within five days. A double-blind study comparing fluphenazine with placebo in 50 patients with tension headache, found daily doses of fluphenazine to diminish both duration and severity of headache significantly as compared to placebo. There was also a significant decrease in the amount of analgesic needed during fluphenazine treatment. Approximately 70 percent of patients considered fluphenazine to be markedly superior to placebo.[26]

These studies suggest that some of the phenothiazines may be helpful in relief of refractory pain. However, more controlled trials are necessary prior to recommending their routine use.

Combinations of phenothiazines with narcotics, although possibly associated with a reduced requirement of the narcotic agent, can cause hazardous drug interactions. The ability of the phenothiazines to block noradrenergic activity can result in circulatory depression and orthostatic hypertension, which may potentiate the adverse effects of narcotics. The administration of the phenothiazines in acute pain may also be associated with sedation, making their use for ambulatory patients quite difficult.

Methotrimeprazine

Methotrimeprazine (Levoprome) is a phenothiazine derivative specifically marketed as an injectable analgesic for moderate to severe pain.[27] Analgesia, comparable to that produced by morphine, occurs primarily by elevating the pain threshold, although its amnestic effect may also facilitate pain relief. It is also a potent sedative with considerable central nervous system depressant activity and, therefore, should be used cautiously.

A maximum analgesic effect believed to be equivalent to morphine and meperidine is usually produced within 20 to 40 minutes after intramuscular injection of 10 to 20 mg of methotrimeprazine. The duration of analgesia is approximately four to six hours. Dependence and withdrawal have not yet been reported. Parenteral use is accompanied by all of the adverse effects seen with other phenothiazines, with orthostatic hypotension being most prominent. Its use in the elderly and in patients with heart disease should be carefully monitored and considered only when these individuals are refractory to standard analgesics.

Promethazine

Promethazine (Phenergan) is a phenothiazine that is a histamine antagonist with prominent sedation and antiemetic effects. Clinically, Phenergan is used by injection with parenteral narcotics to enhance analgesia during postoperative pain and is available in liquid form in combination with codeine as an antitussive for cough.

Dependence, Tolerance, and Withdrawal

There are no reports of addiction, physical dependence, or withdrawal with the use of phenothiazines. Tolerance to the sedative effects may occur with continued use. Abrupt discontinuation of phenothiazines, however, has at times been accompanied by insomnia and muscular discomfort.

Toxicity and Overdose

In addition to the toxic effects of phenothiazines described above, acute administration of large amounts of phenothiazines or chronic consumption of these agents may be associated with additional sequelae.[28] Chronic high-dose phenothiazine treatment may be associated with increasing pigmentation in the skin, cornea, lens, and retina. Tardive dyskinesia is not an infrequent occurrence, especially in the elderly. Jaundice, secondary to a hypersensitivity reaction, as noted earlier, may occur during the first month of therapy. Although usually reversible, chronic hepatic damage may occur.

Treatment of phenothiazine overdose is mainly supportive, directed toward therapy of cardiovascular complications. These drugs are highly bound to plasma proteins. Although elimination by diuretics may be enhanced, conventional dialysis techniques are usually ineffective. Since the anticholinergic effects of phenothiazines result in a delayed gastric emptying time, gastric lavage, even some time after ingestion, may be effective in removing considerable amounts of the drug.

Neurologic complications, such as hypothermia and seizure activity, should be managed appropriately. Extrapyramidal symptoms can be diminished by use of antiparkinsonian medications. However, since these agents also have anticholinergic effects, they should be used only when extrapyramidal signs are severe.

The presence of ventricular arrhythmias should be managed in a manner similar to quinidine-induced ventricular tachycardia. Lidocaine, which enhances conduction velocity in myocardial fibers, may be effective if re-entrant excitation secondary to depressed conduction velocity is the precipitant cause of the arrhythmia. The successful use of lidocaine may result in an underlying sinus node dysfunction, such as sinus bradycardia or sinus arrest with a slow idioventricular response. In such cases, pacemaker insertion becomes mandatory.

If present, hypotension, in the absence of an arrhythmia as a precipitating cause, may be treated with intravenous fluid administration. Too-rapid replacement may result in precipitation of acute pulmonary edema and myocardial failure in the face of direct depressant effect of phenothiazines on the myocardium. Pressor agents, without significant B receptor activity (norepinephrine, methoxamine), may also be used. Agents with primary beta activity (epinephrine) are contraindicated. With adequate treatment, mortality in the absence of serious underlying disease should be low.

Drug Interactions

The phenothiazines may induce the hepatic endoplasmic reticulum, affecting metabolism of other drugs detoxified by this system. The alpha adrenergic blocking activity of the phenothiazines may also result in clinical drug interactions when administered with sympathomimetic agents (Table 10.3).

Mood-Altering Drugs

Combination with alcohol may result in a synergistic, central nervous system depressant effect. Metabolism of the tricyclic antidepressants has been shown to be inhibited, whereas the use of barbiturates and phenothiazines is associated with an acceleration of phenothiazine metabolism due to the more

TABLE 10.3. Selected Drug Interactions of Phenothiazines

Drug	Effect
Alcohol	Synergistic respiratory depressant effect
Alpha-methyldopa	Exacerbation of hypertension
Amphetamines	Decrease in stimulant effect
Antacids with aluminum	Decrease absorption
Atropine	Increase in anticholinergic effect
Barbiturates	Decrease in phenothiazine half-life
Diphenylhydantoin	Enhanced antiarrhythmic effect
Guanethidine	Exacerbation of hypertension
Lithium	Potentiation of phenothiazine-induced hypoglycemia, lowering plasma phenothiazine levels
Meperidine	Excessive sedation and hypotension
Phenytoin	Varying phenytoin blood levels
Propranolol	Enhancement of hypotensive effect
Quinidine	Enhanced antiarrhythmic effect[a]
Sympathomimetic drugs	Increased plasmacatecholamine levels[b]
Tricyclic Antidepressants (TCA)	Increased serum TCA levels
Valproic Acid	Increased serum levels

[a] When phenothiazine overdose may result in depression of myocardial contractility.

[b] Use with agents having both alpha and beta receptor activity, e.g., epinephrine, can enhance beta activity with resulting toxicity.

potent enzyme-inducing properties of barbiturates.[29] Hyperglycemia, known to be associated with both lithium and chlorpromazine administration, might potentially be accentuated with concomitant use of these drugs. Concomitant use with amphetamines may interfere with amphetamine uptake into the adrenergic neuron, with a subsequent decreased effect.

Cardiovascular Agents

Use of phenothiazines with sympathomimetic drug results in a dose-dependent increase in plasma norepinephrine and epinephrine levels. Concomitant use with agents having both α- and β-receptor activity, such as epinephrine, might result in an unmasking of β-effects with resulting adverse reactions.

Antihypertensives that act on the adrenergic neuron, such as guanethidine and alpha-methyldopa, when administered concomitantly with phenothiazines, may be associated with an exacerbated hypertensive response that may be of clinical importance.[30,31,32] Conversely, the use of phenothiazines and propranolol may be associated with an enhancement of propranolol-induced hypotension.

The use of quinidine or diphenylhydantoin (DPH) in the presence of phenothiazines may also be associated with a potentiation of antiarrhythmic action of either drug.

BUTYROPHENONES

Pharmacology

Haloperidol, the prototype of the butyrophenones, in an effective alternative to the phenothiazines as an antipsychotic agent. It resembles the piperazine group of phenothiazines in its activity and is readily absorbed from the gastrointestinal tract, concentrated in the liver with excretion in bile and urine. Haloperidol can be detected in the body weeks following ingestion, and therefore, its effects may be cumulative.

The clinical use of haloperidol is accompanied by a less prominent sedative effect than chlorpromazine, although other central nervous system effects are quite similar. Its action on the autonomic nervous system is also less intense. Extrapyramidal side effects are frequent during the first several days of therapy. Concurrent administration of artane is usually sufficient to prevent this reaction. Administration of haloperidol has not been associated with any detrimental cardiovascular effects. However, tachycardia and transient hypotensive reactions can occur.[33,34] Other systemic reactions similar to those seen with the phenothiazines have been reported.

Analgesic Activity

Haloperidol has been observed to potentiate the effects of both anesthetics and narcotics.[35] Clinically, combinations of haloperidol and tricyclic antidepressants have been found to be effective in providing analgesias.[36] Haloperidol given to psychiatric patients also complaining of chronic pain has resulted in a marked decrease in pain in some instances to the extent that narcotics were no longer required.[37] The effectiveness of haloperidol as an analgesic, however, remains to be more clearly demonstrated.

Drug Interactions

Since haloperidol is metabolized in the liver, it is possible that an interaction may occur with concomitant use of drugs similarly metabolized. The use of anticholinergic drugs and haloperidol should be avoided. Its action on the central nervous system may result in an interference with amphetamine when both drugs are administered simultaneously. Enhanced toxicity has also been associated with concomitant use of lithium and methyldopa. The clinical importance of these interactions remains to be defined.

SUMMARY

The neuroleptics, with the exception of methothimeprazine (Levoprome) have consistently not been found to be primary analgesics. Promethazine (Phenergan) can enhance morphine analgesia, relieve anxiety, and diminish postoperative nausea. It is therefore prescribed with opioids in surgical patients. Promethazine in combination with codeine is also used in liquid form as a mild antitussive for cough.

REFERENCES

1. Baldessarini RJ. Drugs and the treatment of psychiatric disorders. In: Gilman AG, Rall TW, Nies AJ, Taylor P (eds.). *Goodman and Gilman's the pharmacological basis of therapeutics,* 8th ed. New York: Pergamon Press, 1990: 328–435.

2. Ebert M, Shader R. Cardiovascular effects by psychotropic drug side effects. In: Shader R, DiMascio A (eds.). *Psychotropic drug side effects: Chemical and theoretical perspectives.* Baltimore: Williams and Wilkins, 1963: 152.

3. Alexander CS. Cardiotoxic effects of phenothiazine and related drugs. *Circulation,* 1968, 38:1014–1015.

4. Shamsi MA, Kulshrestha VK, Dhawan KN, Bhargava KP. Correlation of chemical structure of phenothiazines with their coronary dilator and antiarrhythmic activities. *Jpn J Pharmacol,* 1971, 21:747–754.

5. Alexander CS, Nino A. Cardiovascular complications in young patients taking psychotropic drugs. *Am Heart J,* 1969, 78:757–769.

6. Carlsson C, Denker SJ, Grimby G, Haggendal J. Circulatory studies during physical exercise in mentally disordered patients I: Effects of large doses of chlorpromazine. *Acta Med Scand,* 1968, 184:499–509.

7. Swett C, Cole JO, Hartz SC, Shapiro S, Slone D. Hypotension due to chlorpromazine: Relation to cigarette smoking, blood pressure, and dosage. *Arch Gen Psychiatry,* 1977, 34:661–663.

8. Graupner KI, Murphree OD, Meduna LJ. Electrocardiographic changes associated with the use of thioridazine. *J Neuropsychiat,* 1964, 5:344–350.

9. Backman H, Elosuo R. The effect of neuroleptics on electrocardiogram. *Acta Med Scand,* 1968, 183:543–547.

10. Dillenkoffer RL, Gallant DM, Phillips JH. Electrocardiographic evaluation of mesoridazine (Serentil). *Curr Ther Res Clin Exp,* 1992, 14:71–72.

11. Quitkin F, Rifkin A, Klein D. Very high dosage vs. standard dosage: Fluphenazine in schizophrenia. A double-blind study of nonchronic treatment-refractory patients. *Arch Gen Psychiatry,* 1975, 32;1276–1281.

12. Holden M, Itil T. Electrocardiographic changes with psychotropic drugs. In: Wheatley D (ed.). *Stress and the heart.* New York: Raven Press, 1977: 87–96.

13. Fowler NO, McCall D, Chou TC, Holmes JC, Hanenson JB. Electrocardiographic changes and cardiac arrhythmias in patients receiving psychotropic drugs. *Am J Cardiol,* 1976, 37:223–230.

14. Landmark KH. Cardiac effects of phenothiazines. *Nord Med,* 1970, 83:617–620.

15. Leestma JE, Koenig KL. Sudden death and phenothiazines: A current controversy. *Arch Gen Psychiatry,* 1968, 18:137–148.

16. Peele R, Von Loetzen IS. Phenothiazine deaths: Critical review. *Am J Psychiatry,* 1973, 130:306–309.

17. Swett CP, Jr, Shader RI. Cardiac side effects and sudden death in hospitalized psychiatric patients. *Dis Nerv System,* 1977, 38:69–72.

18. Margolis LH, Gianascol AJ. Chlorpromazine in thalamic pain syndrome. *Neurology* (Minneapolis), 1956, 6:302–304.

19. Bonica JJ. Symptomatic therapy of cancer pain. In: Bonica JJ, Loesser JD, Chapman CR, Fordyce WE. *The management of pain,* 2nd ed. Philadelphia: Lea & Febiger, 1990:423.

20. Houde RW. On assaying analgesics in man. In: Knighton RS, Dumke PR (eds.). *Pain.* Boston: Little-Brown and Company, 1966.

21. Keats AS, Telford J, Kurosu Y. "Potentiation" of meperidine by promethazine. *Anesthesiol,* 1961, 22:34–41.

22. Merskey H, Hester RA. The treatment of chronic pain with psychotropic drugs. *Postgrad Med J,* 1972, 48:594–598.

23. Davis JL, Lewis SB, Gerich JE, Kaplan RA, Schultz TA, Wallin JD. Peripheral diabetic neuropathy treated with amitriptyline and fluphenazine. *JAMA,* 1977, 238:2291–2292.

24. Taub A. Relief of postherpetic neuralgia with psychotropic drugs. *J Neurosurg,* 1973, 39:235–239.

25. Hakkarainen H. Fluphenazine for tension headache: Double-blind study. *Headache,* 1977, 17:216–218.

26. Drug facts and comparisons. Drug information. St. Louis: Facts and Comparisons, Inc., 1995, 1236.

27. Foley KM. Analgesic drug therapy in cancer pain: Principles and practices. *Med Clin Am,* 1987, 71:207.

28. Davis JM, Bartlett E, Termini BA. Overdosage of psychotropic drugs: A review. Major and minor tranquilizers. *Dis Nerv System,* 1968, 29:157–164.

29. Gram LF, Overo KF. Drug interaction: Inhibitory effect of neuroleptics on metabolism of tricyclic antidepressants in man. *Br Med J,* 1972, 1:463–465.

30. Westervelt FB, Jr, Atuk NO. Methyldopa-induced hypertension (letter). *JAMA,* 1974, 227–557.

31. Fann WE, Janowsky DS, Davis JM, Oates JA. Chlorpromazine reversal of antihypertensive action of quanethidine. *Lancet,* 1971, 2:436–437.

32. Carlsson C, Dencker SJ, Grimby G, Haggerendal J, Johnsson G. Hemodynamic effects of thiothixene and chlorpromazine in schizophrenic patients at rest and during exercise. *Int J Clin Pharmacol Biopharm,* 1976, 13:262–268.

33. Aman MG, Werry JS. The effects of methylphenidate and haloperidol on the heart rate and blood pressure of hyperactive children with special reference to time of action. *Psychopharmacologia,* 1975, 43:163–168.

34. Ban TA. *Psychopharmacology.* Baltimore: Williams and Wilkins, 1969.

35. Kocher R. Use of psychotropic drugs for the treatment of chronic severe pain. In: Bonica JJ, Albe-Fessard DG (eds.). *Advances in pain research and therapy.* Vol. I. New York: Raven Press, 1976: 579–582.

37. Cavenar JO, Jr, Maltebie AA. Another indication of haloperidol. *Psychosomatics,* 1976, 17:128–130.

Chapter 11

The Antidepressants

INTRODUCTION

The antidepressants comprise a wide variety of drugs (Table 11.1) prescribed most frequently to alleviate anxiety associated with depression or to treat primary depression. They are also used to relieve depression accompanying other disorders, such as cancer or severe debilitating conditions. Antidepressants are increasingly being used as a primary drug to treat a variety of painful states, often providing considerable relief. In general their effects are believed to be due to their ability to block uptake of neurotransmitters in the brain, notably serotonin and norepinephrine; they also affect pre- and postsynaptic receptors. The newer antidepressants, which selectively inhibit serotonin uptake (Prozac, Paxil, and Zoloft), are currently used most frequently for depression, while the tricyclics are often used as analgesic agents—especially for neuropathic pain. The following discussion will briefly review the available antidepressants and their use as analgesics.

TRICYCLIC ANTIDEPRESSANTS

The tricyclics are widely used for the treatment of depression although other less well-documented indications for their use have been recognized (Table 11.2). Their effectiveness is reflected by the observation that as early as 1973 U.S. physicians wrote over 24 million prescriptions for these agents alone or in combination with other drugs.[1] The widespread acceptability of the tricyclics has also been accompanied by a greater realization of their adverse effects, including the potential of toxicity due to self-poisoning.

PHARMACOLOGY

Imipramine, synthesized in 1848 is considered the prototype of these agents. Generically, the term tricyclics is applied to all agents in this group

TABLE 11.1. Antidepressant Drugs

Group	Trade Name
Tricyclics	
Amitriptyline	Elavil, Endep, Enovil
Amoxapine	Asendin
Clomipramine	Anafranil
Desipramine	Norpramin, Pertofrane
Doxepin	Adapin, Sinequan
Imipramine	Janimine, Tofranil
Nortriptyline	Aventyl, Pamelor
Protriptyline	Vivactil
Trimipramine	Surmontil
Aminoketone	
Bupropion	Wellbutrin
Bicyclic	
Fluoxetine	Prozac
Sertraline	Zoloft
Tetracyclic	
Maprotiline	Ludiomil
Triazolopyridine	
Trazodone	Desyrel, Trazodone
Monoaminoxidase Inhibitors (MAO-I)	
Isorcarboxazid	Marplan
Phenelzine	Nardil
Tranylcypromine	Parnate
Phenylpiperidines	
Paroxetine	Paxil
Phenylpiperazines	
Nefazodone	Serzone

containing a linkage of two benzene rings to form a third central ring. Those drugs with three substituents on the nitrogen atom of the aminopropyl side chain are termed tertiary amines (e.g., imipramine, doxepin, and amitriptyline) and those with two substituents are secondary amines (e.g., desipramine, protriptyline, and nortriptyline).

TABLE 11.2. Current Use of Tricyclic Antidepressants

Depression
Enuresis
Adjunctive therapy with analgesics
Obsessive-compulsive phobias
Cataplexy associated with narcolepsy
Minimal brain damage and hyperkinesis in children
Neuropathic pain

Mechanism of Action

The tricyclic antidepressants act by preventing the reuptake of serotonin (5-HT) and norepinephrine (NE) at noradrenergic and serotonergic neurons, thereby raising the concentration of NE and 5-HT at the receptor sites. This activity is selective, with little or no effect being noted at dopamine receptors, with the exception of imipramine.[2]

This adrenergic potentiation can be eliminated or even reversed when high doses of tricyclics are administered.[3,4] In addition, when tricyclics are administered concomitantly with sympathomimetic agents acting indirectly on the noradrenergic neurons, uptake of these drugs is prevented, which results in an antagonism of the intended drug action.[5,6] The effect of direct-acting sympathetic agents, however, is enhanced by tricyclics since the increased concentration of NE at the receptor site would cause a diminished NE uptake.

The tricyclics have also been demonstrated to have anticholinergic effects. Dry mouth, blurred vision, urinary retention, and constipation may occur, varying with the individual drugs and a person's preexisting medical conditions. Amitryptline exerts the most potent anticholinergic effects and desipramine the least. Several of the newer antidepressants, such as trazodone and fluoxetine, have minimal anticholinergic side effects.

Absorption, Biotransformation, and Excretion

The tricyclics are quickly absorbed from the gastrointestinal tract after oral administration. Imipramine is rapidly distributed and metabolized by N-demethylation to form desmethylimipramine (DMI), which is also subsequently further metabolized. Both imipramine and DMI are fat soluble and readily cross the blood-brain barrier. Protein binding is considerable, with over 90 percent of amitriptyline and its active metabolite nortriptyline present in plasma in the bound state. Since metabolism occurs primarily in the liver, plasma levels can be increased by concomitant administration of drugs that inhibit the hepatic enzyme systems. Clinically, there also appears to be a genetically determined individual variation in steady-state plasma concentrations of tricyclics after single dose administration. A standard dose of 150 mg of amitriptyline can result in an interpatient variation of up to thirtyfold in the steady-state plasma concentration.[7]

Excretion is relatively rapid with 40 percent of a radioactive dose of imipramine appearing in the urine within 24 hours, and 70 percent excreted within 72 hours. Fecal excretion accounts for only a small portion.[8]

Effects on Organ Systems

Central Nervous System

A single administration of a tricyclic antidepressant usually neither stimulates nor relieves depression. Sedation may occur, frequently being accompanied by a decrease in motor performance. Continued administration over time results in antidepressant activity. Administration of tricyclics may be associated with considerable side effects due mainly to their anticholinergic activity (Table 11.3). Tachycardia is also common, representing a direct action of the drug on the adrenergic neuron. The intensity of anticholinergic and adrenergic side effects vary considerably with individual tricyclics.

TABLE 11.3. Autonomic Side Effects of Tricyclic Therapy

Blurred vision
Constipation
Delayed ejaculation
Dry mouth
Epigastric distress
Sweating
Tachycardia
Urinary hesitancy

Respiratory System

When given in therapeutic doses, a minimal effect on respiration is observed. Respiratory depression may occur, however, with tricyclic overdose.

Cardiovascular System

Clinically, the use of tricyclics has been associated with an increased heart rate (tachycardia) and alterations in blood pressure that vary with the specific tricyclic, the person's age, the time of measurement, and the presence of preexisting cardiac disease. Administration of therapeutic doses of tricyclics to depressed persons without evidence of cardiac disease can increase the heart rate, with minimal changes in blood pressure. No relationship exists between plasma levels and the resulting tachycardia. Significant orthostatic changes following administration of nortriptyline in healthy young adults was not demonstrated. A peripheral vasodilatory effect of the tricyclics has also been reported with use of high doses and may be of clinical importance in overdose reactions.[9-11]

The administration of tricyclics to the elderly, especially those with cardiovascular disease, is associated with clinically important orthostatic hypotension dependent on the specific tricyclic administered.[12] Doxepin has been associated with a lower incidence of hypotension and tachycardia than amitriptyline. Both of these agents are less likely to produce orthostatic changes than imipramine. Maprotiline (Ludiomil), a trazodone (Desyrel), and fluoxetine (Prozac) are considered to be associated with the least adverse hemodynamic effects. Existing evidence regarding the efficacy of one agent over the other in the elderly or cardiac patient remains inconclusive.

Asymptomatic electrocardiographic changes in persons on tricyclics are frequent. These changes, consisting of prolongation of the QT interval, widening of QRS complexes, and ST and T wave changes, similar to those seen with the phenothiazines, have been noted in up to 20 percent of persons.[13-16] Other complications in patients with cardiac disease include congestive heart failure and myocardial infarction. In most instances, these events have been associated with tricyclic poisoning rather than appropriate clinical use.

Other Effects

Confusional states have been noted with the use of tricyclics especially in the elderly. This may be of concern when other drugs having anticholinergic activity are simultaneously administered. Weight gain following initiation of tricyclic therapy is a well-recognized phenomenon. Whether this is a direct result of the drug or due to an alleviation of the depression is difficult to determine.

ANALGESIC ACTIVITY

The effects of tricyclic antidepressants on biogenic amines suggest that these drugs may have a role in treating pain in which neurotransmitter hyperactivity predominates. In this setting the perception of and the reaction to pain may be modulated by factors other than acute physiological or anatomical insults, with psychological components often being prominent (Chapter 4). Their effectiveness in relieving pain may be related to their (1) antidepressant activity relieving accompanying anxiety and depression, (2) ability to exert a direct analgesic action, and (3) potentiation of the analgesia activity of other drugs.

Animal Models

Laboratory evidence indicating a specific analgesic action of tricyclic antidepressants has not been impressive but those drugs with the selective ability to block 5-HT uptake have been shown to potentiate morphine analgesia.[17] The administration of clomipramine and morphine over several days was associated with a significantly greater degree of tolerance in animals given both drugs, whereas prolonged administration of morphine and maprotiline resulted in less tolerance. It is of interest that the development of a lesser degree of tolerance was associated with a greater degree of analgesic activity. This suggests a possible therapeutic advantage in the combination of morphine and a tricyclic antidepressant that specifically inhibits norepinephrine uptake to delay the development of morphine tolerance.

Clinical Studies

Since the 1960s, a number of reports appearing in the literature have suggested the effectiveness of antidepressants in the relief of pain due to a wide variety of disorders.[18-24] Over the past several years, additional clinical studies have confirmed the usefulness of these drugs, at times independent of their antidepressant action. Clomipramine at doses of 10 or 20 mg given nightly to persons with chronic muscular and joint pains, when combined with conventional analgesic therapy, was effective in alterting pain threshold.[19-22] Another trial comparing the use of amitriptyline and fluphenazine (a phenothiazine derivative) found an improvement in perception of pain in diabetics with peripheral neuropathy within five days after initiation of amitriptyline.[20] These studies, however, were not well controlled.

Clinical double-blind, randomized studies have not provided consistent findings.[24] The administration of imipramine to 22 unselected patients with arthritis resulted in symptomatic improvement in only 60 percent, with less than one-third demonstrating improvement by muscular testing.[23] A multicenter double-blind clinical trial utilizing imipramine in combination with standard analgesic or antirheumatic therapy in arthritic patients found a statistically significant improvement in pain, stiffness, and grip strength more effective than with placebo.[19] However, a double-blind between-group comparison of imipramine and placebo in 59 patients with low back pain was not able to document a significant objective benefit over placebo, both groups showing significant improvement.[25]

A double-blind laboratory investigation of pain perception with doxepin given to healthy volunteers undergoing painful dental stimulation was not able to record significant changes in the detection threshold of pain.[26] However, a marked change in response bias against reporting stimuli as painful occurred soon after the subjects began taking either doxepin or placebo capsules. This effect was felt by the investigators to emphasize the importance of suggestion in modifying the response to pain.

More recently the use of antidepressants in a wide range of pain treatment has been found to be helpful.[27] A review of 40 placebo-controlled studies suggested that pain due to a variety of causes was able to respond to antidepressant therapy. These included headaches, facial pain, arthritic pain, and muscular pain. Individual differences existed with the different agents.[28] One study documented that the patient who received an antidepressant had less pain than almost 75 percent of the patients receiving placebos.[29] These analgesic effects, which were independent of a beneficial effect on mood, appear at relatively low doses and within a short time of starting therapy.[30,31,32]

Summary

In summary, more recent findings concerning primary analgesic activity of the tricyclic and some of the newly developed antidepressants suggest that although laboratory studies of their effectiveness maybe less than impressive, clinically, in certain types of pain, substantial relief can be obtained. Combination with conventional analgesic agents also is associated with a potentiation of analgesia. Although some of these responses may be due to relief of a reactive depression, the appearance of positive responses early in the course of treatment, at a relatively low dose of antidepressant, suggests that, as of yet, unidentified mechanisms may be operative. Today the use of these drugs is quite helpful in management of chronic pain even in their absence, especially in the presence of an overlying depression. This is discussed more fully in the chapters addressing pain management.

TOXICITY AND OVERDOSE

Tricyclic poisoning or overdose, although not as prevalent as that seen with other mood-altering drugs, is nonetheless not infrequent. Overdoses are of particular concern in children, who appear to be more susceptible to toxicity due to (1) lesser proportion of tricyclic binding to protein, (2) higher rates of hepatic biotransformation, and (3) a greater lean body mass in children compared to adults. This last factor is associated with relatively less drug being taken up by fatty tissues and more being available to reach the brain.[33-35]

Signs and Symptoms

In general, the toxic effects of the tricyclics are related to their anticholinergic and sedative properties. When administered in high doses, confusion, progressing to coma, may occur. Hyperpyrexia, hyperactivity including athetoid and choreiform movements, muscular rigidity, and increased intestinal activity can also be observed. In instances of tricyclic overdose, hypotension and tachycardia are frequently observed (Table 11.4). These findings may be accompanied by impaired cardiac conduction manifested by repolarization abnormalities, prolongation of the PR interval, widening of the QRS complex, bundle branch blocks, complete heart block, supraventricular and ventricular arrhythmias, as well as bradycardia and asystole.[36,37] Elevations of serum enzymes associated with myocardial damage and congestive heart failure have also been reported.

Treatment

The treatment of overdose is mainly supportive since tissue and protein binding do not allow for effective peritoneal or extracorporeal dialysis (Table 11.5). Diuretic agents are relatively ineffective due to a low renal excretory rate. If intervention occurs early and the patient is comatose, gastric lavage may be helpful. Administration of activated charcoal to diminish absorption is also useful. Activated charcoal, given within 30 minutes after a 75 mg dose of nortriptyline, can lower peak plasma levels by 60 percent. In vitro studies

TABLE 11.4. Cardiovascular Signs of Tricyclic Antidepressant Overdose

Arrhythmias
 Sinus tachycardia[a]
 Bradycardia
 Ventricular tachycardia and fibrillation
 Asystole
Conduction defects
 Repolarization abnormalities[a]
 Widening of QRS
 Heart block
Congestive heart failure
Hypotension[a]

[a]Most frequently observed

TABLE 11.5. Principles of Treating Tricyclic Antidepressant Overdose

Hasten elimination of agent[a]
 Emesis
 Activated charcoal
 Saline cathartics
Maintenance of satisfactory hemodynamic status
Prolonged cardiac monitoring
 Treatment of serious arrhythmias[b]
Pharmacologic therapy[c]
 Sodium bicarbonate
Physostigmine

[a] In an alert patient
[b] Type 1 antiarrhythmic agents contraindicated
[c] Only in cases that cannot be treated adequately by general supportive measures

have demonstrated a 10 gram packet of a commercial preparation containing 5 grams activated charcoal can absorb 3 grams of nortriptyline, a dose rarely exceeded in overdose reactions.[33,38-40]

It should be emphasized that the half-lives of the tricyclics are quite long, with plasma levels remaining elevated for several days. In instances of severe overdose (ingested dose greater than 1 gram), patients should be closely monitored in the intensive care unit for several days, even in the absence of initial cardiac findings.

Monitoring plasma TCA levels in treatment of tricyclic overdose is helpful and may correlate with both the severity and the duration of the QRS complex on ECG. Treatment of arrhythmias is necessary when symptoms develop. It should be emphasized that the prolonged half-life of amitriptyline mandates continuous cardiac monitoring for five to six days. The relationship of the tricyclics to the Type 1 antiarrhythmic drugs warrants prohibition of agents, such as quinidine and procainamide, to control arrhythmias. Similarly, beta blockers, noticeably propranolol (Inderal), potentially can cause tricyclic-induced contractility changes and should be avoided. Cardioversion and atrial pacing may also be of value in the presence of refractory arrhythmias or heart block. Digitalis may be used with caution in the absence of AV (atrio-ventricular) block when congestive heart failure exists. Sodium bicarbonate has been reported to be an effective therapeutic agent in the presence of oxidosis. The administration of sodium bicarbonate to children has been associated in a rapid conversion to regular rhythm.[34]

The use of physostigmine salicylate, a cholinesterase inhibitor, has been shown to be beneficial in reversal of the central nervous system effects of the tricyclics as well as having a salutary peripheral effect on the tachycardia in case of mild poisoning.[35,41,42,43] The recommended dose is 1 to 2 mg intravenously by slow infusion followed by another 2 mg in 15 to 20 minutes. The use of physostigmine, however, is not without hazard, as severe bradycardia, bronchospasms, and muscle weakness may be seen. Hypersalivation, which may also occur, can be quite dangerous in a comatose patient. Convulsions have been reported and in instances of severe poisoning, asystole can occur. Since most patients have only mild anticholinergic symptoms, treatment of cardiac complications with physostigmine should be considered only in those patients who cannot be adequately treated and carefully monitored.

DRUG INTERACTIONS

Since the tricyclics bind to plasma protein and affect the hepatic microsomal system, they can interact with a wide variety of drugs (Table 11.6).

Major Tranquilizers and Central Nervous System Depressants

Interference of metabolism of phenothiazines and tricyclic antidepressants, when both agents are used concomitantly, has also been reported as has the ability of phenothiazines to "competitively" diminish binding of tricyclics to plasma proteins, resulting in a greater likelihood of cardiac toxicity.[44,45]

TABLE 11.6. Drug Interactions of Tricyclic Antidepressants

Drug Increasing Plasma TCA Levels

    Aspirin, aminopyrine, cimetidine,
    fluoxetine, haloperidol, oral
    contraceptives, methylphenidate,
    phenylbutazone

Drugs Decreasing Plasma TCA Levels

    Barbiturates, charcoal, nicotine

Adverse Actions on Other Drugs

    Alcohol, barbiturates, and hypnotics
    Anticholinergics
    Clonidine
    Oral anticoagulants
    Guanethidine
    Levodopa
    Monoamine Oxidase Inhibitors
    Increased sedation
    Entrance anticholinergic effect
    Elevated blood pressure
    Increased bleeding
    Diminished antihypertension effect
    Delayed absorption
    Seizures, sweating, coma

Frequently, elderly patients presenting with a picture of complex depression will be treated with a combination of these two groups of drugs. In such cases, most especially in the presence of cardiac disease, serious consideration should be given toward an alternate therapeutic approach such as haloperidol. If a combination of phenothiazines and tricyclics is desired, careful, sequential electrocardiographic monitoring is mandatory.

Tricyclic therapy, in combination with administration of benzodiazepines, has also been advocated. Although hepatic metabolism of tricyclics can be stimulated with barbiturates and other sedatives, the effect of benzodiazepines on the microsomal system seems to be of minimal clinical importance. Synergistic interactions can occur between tricyclic antidepressants and drugs displaying anticholinergic effects, such as glutethimide (Doriden) and meperidine (Demerol). The combination with meperidine may result in a potentiation of the narcotic-induced respiratory depression.

Sympathetic and Sympathomimetic Agents

Numerous interactions have been reported to occur between the tricyclic antidepressants and cardiac medications. The actions of the tricyclics on noradrenergic neurons result in an interference with sympathomatic amines that predominantly act by being converted to NE in the neuron or stimulating release of NE from storage granules (Table 11.7). These drugs include ephedrine, metaraminol, mephentermine, and tyramine. Concomitant administration results in an inhibition of the pressor response caused by these drugs. Sympathomimetic drugs which have a predominantly direct action on the noradrenergic neuron have an enhanced pressor effect in the presence of tricyclics due to an increased concentration of NE at the receptor site. Clinically, this interaction may result in an augmented sympathetic effect in the presence of a tricyclic. Adverse symptoms have also been reported in patients maintained on tricyclics who receive local anesthetics containing epinephrine.

Antihypertensive Drugs

The use of antihypertensive agents in persons maintained on tricyclics must be accompanied by great caution.[46-48] Clonidine (Catapres) acts predominantly on the sympathetic cardiovascular medullary centers, decreasing the sympathetic neural activity of the heart, peripheral vasculature, and kidney, with resultant suppression of renin release. Clonidine, similar to methyldopa when utilized with a vasodilator and beta blocker combination, results in an additive therapeutic effect in persons with severe hypertension. The tricyclic antidepressants may inhibit clonidine's antihypertensive action through interaction in the central nervous system.

TABLE 11.7. Interactions Between Tricyclic Antidepressants and Sympathomimetic Drugs

Pressor Response Enhanced	Pressor Response Inhibited
Amphetamines	Ephedrine
Epinephrine	Metaraminol
Norepinephrine	Mephentermine
Phenylephrine	Tyramine

Guanidinium Derivatives

Guanidinium derivatives, such as guanethidine (Ismelin) and quanadrel sulfate (Hylorel), inhibit release of and progressively deplete NE by competing with it for reentry into the nerve terminal as well as causing a partial release of NE from the granule. The concomitant administration of tricyclic antidepressants can abolish guanethidine's antihypertensive effect secondary to the ability of imipramine and related drugs to block the active transport of guanethidine across axonal membranes.

Hypertension will, however, recur with an increased maintenance dose being required. Discontinuing of tricyclic therapy is associated with a gradual resumption of guanethidine effectiveness in approximately five days, although up to two weeks may be required. It should be emphasized that sudden discontinuation of doxepin may be associated with hypotensive reactions of considerable severity unless the dose of guanethidine is adjusted.

Reserpine

Reserpine and related rauwolfia alkaloids (Serpalan, Serpasil, Moderil, Rauwiloid) deplete catecholamines and 5-hydroxytryptamine by blocking uptake of both norepinephrine and dopamine in the granules. Since reserpine does not competitively enter the cell, its antihypertensive effect is not specifically antagonized by tricyclics. Since depression is not an unknown reaction to reserpine, however, combination with tricyclics would probably be unwise.

MAO Inhibitors

The monoamine oxidase (MAO) inhibitors have complex pharmacologic actions that may be related to enzyme inhibition of other enzymes in addition to MAO. Their basic effect is to increase concentration of dopamine and norepinephrine in the nerve endings through preventing their inactivation. Adverse effects with concomitant use of tricyclics have been well documented and may be quite severe.

Methyldopa

Methyldopa is one of the few autonomic antihypertensives that does not appear to interfere clinically with the tricyclic antidepressants. It is appropriate therapy, therefore, in patients taking tricyclics when hypotension cannot be controlled by a diuretic agent alone. However, hypertension and tachycardia have been observed with combined use of these agents.

Antiarrhythmic Agents

The similar action of some of the tricyclics to Type 1 antiarrhythmic drugs allows a potentiation of drug action with enhancement of toxicity when these agents are used concomitantly. Similarly, the concomitant use of any drug having a myocardial depressant effect might result in a synergistic myocardial depressant action.

Other Drug Interactions

Interference with microsomal metabolism of tricyclics can be seen with methylphenidate and progesterones. Concomitant administration of thyroid preparations may also enhance tricyclic toxicity. Selegiline (Eldepryl), an antiparkinson agent, when combined with use of tricyclics has been associated with high fevers, agitation, restlessness, reduced levels of consciousness, and rarely, fatalities.

Desipramine has also been shown to delay peak plasma levels of phenylbutazone when both drugs are administered concurrently.[49] This is believed to be due to an interaction at the level of the gastrointestinal tract preventing absorption of phenylbutazone. A potentiation of the alcohol-disulfiram reaction has also been reported in patients on amitriptyline.[50] These interactions, however, are based on sporadic reports, with more evidence being needed prior to assuming that concurrent use of these drugs with tricyclics should be prohibited.

NEWLY DEVELOPED ANTIDEPRESSANTS

The anticholinergic and adrenergic activities seen with tricyclics has stimulated investigators to develop new antidepressants devoid of undesirable side effects and potential cardiovascular toxicity. A number of these drugs are available; however, they should all be used only after one carefully reviews their indications, contraindications, and precautions.

TETRACYCLIC ANTIDEPRESSANTS

Maprotiline

Maprotiline (Ludiomil) is an antidepressant shown to be as effective as tricyclics when given in divided daily doses of 50 to 150 mg.[51,52] Its effect on the noradrenergic neuron is less than many of the tricyclics, and its use, therefore, is associated with a lower incidence of cardiovascular side effects. Yet it also is a weak blocker of the serotonin receptor. Its anticholinergic activity is considerably less than that seen with the tricyclics.

Trazodone (Desyrel)

Trazodone, a triazolopyridine derivative, exhibits antidepressant activity compatible to imipramine. Unlike the tricyclics, however, trazodone is devoid of noradrenergic activity, has minimal anticholinergic effects, and does not inhibit monoamine oxidase, antagonize reserpine, or potentiate L-dopa.[53]

In animals, the cardiovascular toxicity of trazodone is less than that observed with tricyclics. However, clinically, administration of trazodone to normal volunteers also receiving norepinephrine infusions was associated with a depression of blood pressure, suggesting a decreased sensitivity to norepinephrine. Clinical studies have also suggested that trazodone may be associated with rhythm abnormalities. The use of this drug in persons recovering from heart attacks or in those with existing severe cardiac disease is not recommended.

Preliminary findings suggest trazodone to be an effective antidepressant of special value in persons with underlying cardiac disease. The major side effect of this drug is sedation, which can best be minimized by administering the prescribed dose (50 to 800 mg per day) at bedtime.

INHIBITORS OF SEROTONIN UPTAKE

The inhibitors of serotonin uptake are the newest group of antidepressants. Associated with fewer undesirable effects than the tricyclics, they nonetheless do have side effects and interact with a number of other drugs. The most frequently used drugs of this group are listed in Table 11.8.

Fluoxetine

Fluoxetine (Prozac) is a bicyclic antidepressant with minimal anticholinergic and few sedative side effects. It is a potent inhibitor of 5-HT uptake with little effect on norepinephrine uptake or release. In a relatively short time it has become the most widely prescribed antidepressant in the United States with $1.2 billion in sales in 1993 and projections of $4 billion in sales by the year 2000.[54,55,56] In addition to its antidepressant action, it is believed to be effective in treating the pain associated with diabetic neuro-

TABLE 11.8. Drug Interactions with Serotonin Reuptake Inhibitors

Drug	Drug Interactions
Trazodone (Desyrel)	Alcohol Sedative Hypnotic Group Digoxin Monoamine Oxidase Inhibitor Phenytoin (Dilantin) Eldepryl Warfarin (Coumadin)
Fluoxetine (Prozac)	Diazepam (Valium) Eldepryl Haloperidol Lithium Monoamine Oxidase Inhibitor Tricyclic Antidepressants L Tryptophane
Sertraline (Zoloft)	Alcohol Diazepam (Valium) Eldepryl Lithium Tolbutamide Warfarin (Coumadin)
Paroxetine (Paxil)	Alcohol Cimetidine Eldepryl Monoamine Oxidase Inhibitor Digoxin Phenobarbital Phenytoin (Dilantin) L Tryptophane Warfarin (Coumadin)

pathy. Although it is an effective antidepressant, a moderate number of psychiatric symptoms have been reported. The most common side effects reported consist of nervousness, nausea, diarrhea, and sexual dysfunction. Clinically important drug interactions can occur with tricyclic antidepressant, monoamine oxidase inhibitor and neuroleptic drugs.

Nefazodone

Nefazadone (Serzone) is a phenylpiperazine related to trazodone and can inhibit norepinephrine and serotonin uptake. It is similar to imipramine in relieving depressive symptoms and exhibits less antihistaminic, anticholinergic, and sedative activity than the tricyclics and can interact with the benzodiazepines and the nonsedating antihistamines (Seldane, Hismanal) as well as monoamine oxidase inhibitors.

Sertraline

Sertraline (Zoloft) is a relatively new antidepressant that is a potent selective serotonin uptake inhibitor and is only comparable to amitryptline in treating depression. It is associated with minimum sedation. Side effects are minimal but most frequently involve the gastrointestinal tract.

Paroxetine (Paxil)

Paroxetine (Paxil) is chemically unrelated to other inhibitions of serotonin uptake which has been shown to be effective in treatment of depression. It is associated with a variety of side effects that were responsible for approximately 21 percent of patients discontinuing its use.

BUPROPION

Bupropion (Wellbutrin) is an antidepressant with a precise mechanism of action that remains to be clarified. It acts only weakly at noradrenergic and serotonergic receptors and does not inhibit monoamine oxidase. One of its most serious complications is induction of seizure activity, which may appear at doses as low as 450 mg per day. Although its clinical use has not been associated with abuse or dependency, its structural relationship to the phenylethylamines and its ability to produce mild amphetamine-like activity suggests it should be used cautiously. Drug interactions have been reported with carbamazepine, cimetidine, levodopa, monoamine oxidase inhibitors, phenobarbital, and phenytoin (Dilantin).

SUMMARY

Available evidence suggests that the use of antidepressants in the management of pain will be quite effective when a psychogenic component can be demonstrated. However, tricyclic antidepressants have not only been shown to potentiate morphine analgesia, but also have been reported to provide relief from pain in a wide variety of disorders. The potential interactions that may occur between antidepressants and a considerable number of other drugs often used in chronic pain states necessitates a careful individual evaluation prior to their use, especially in the elderly or in persons with cardiovascular disease.

REFERENCES

1. National Disease and Therapeutic Index. Listings from October 1973 to September 1974. Ambler, PA: IMA America, 1974.

2. Schildkraut JJ. Neuropharmacology of the affective disorders. *Annu Rev Pharmacol,* 1973, 13:427–454.

3. Cairncross KD. On the peripheral pharmacology of amitriptyline. *Arch Int Pharmacodyn,* 1965, 154:438–448.

4. Sigg EB, Osborne M, Korol B. Cardiovascular effects of imipramine. *J Pharmacol Exp Ther,* 1963, 141:237–243.

5. Borga O, Azarnoff DL, Forshell GP, Sjöqvist F. Plasma protein binding of tricyclic antidepressants in man. *Biochem Pharmacol,* 1969, 18:2135–2143.

6. Braithwaite RA, Goulding R, Theano G, Bailey J, Coppen A. Plasma concentration of amitriptyline and clinical response. *Lancet,* 1972, 1:1297–1300.

7. Coppen A, Ghose K, Montgomery S, Rama Rao VA, Bailey J, Christiansen J, Mikkleson PL, Van Praag HM, Van de Poel F, Minsker EJ, et al. Amtripyline plasma concentration and clinical effect. *Lancet,* 1972, 1:63–66.

8. Baldessarini RJ. Drugs and the treatment of psychiatric disorders. In: Gilman AG, Rall TW, Nies AS, Taylor P (eds.). *Goodman and Gilman's the pharmacological basis of therapeutics,* 8th ed. New York: Pergamon Press, 1990: 382–435.

9. Vohra J, Burrows GD, Soman G. Assessment of cardiovascular side effects of therapeutic doses of tricyclic antidepressant drugs. *Aust N Z J Med,* 1975, 5:7–11.

10. Freyschuss U, Sjöqvist F, Tuck D. Blockage of tyramine-induced pressure effects with tricyclic antidepressives. *Nord Med,* 1970, 84:1061–1062.

11. Thorstrand C, Lindblad LE. The effect of amitriptyline on forearm blood flow. *Scand J Clin Lab Invest,* 1976, 36:17–21.

12. Kantor SJ, Glassman AH, Bigger JR. The cardiac effects of therapeutic plasma concentrations of imipramine. Presented at American Psychiatric Association meeting, Toronto, May 1977.

13. Cardiovascular complications of tricyclic antidepressants. *N Z Med J,* 1971, 74:390–391.

14. Rawling D, Fozzard HA. Electrophysiological effects of imipramine on cardiac Purkinje fibers. *Am J Cardiol,* 1978: 41:387.

15. Giardina EGV, Bigger JT, Kantor SJ, Glassman AH, Perel JM. Electrocardiographic and antiarrhythmic effects of imipramine hydrochloride. *Clin Res,* 26:482A.

16. Gaultier M, Boissier JR, Gorceix A. The cardiotoxicity of imipramine in man. *Eur Soc Study Drug Tox,* 1976, 6:171–173.

17. Lee R, Spencer PS. Antidepressants and pain: A review of the pharmacological data supporting the use of certain tricyclics in chronic pain. *J Int Med Res,* 1977, 51:146–156.

18. Gringras M. A clinical trial of tofranil in rheumatic pain in general practice. *J Int Med Res,* 1976, 4 (Suppl. 2): 41–49.

19. Montgomery BJ. Psychotropic agents finding analgesic use. *JAMA,* 1978, 240:1225.

20. Hart FD. The use of psychotropic drugs in rheumatology. *J Int Med Res,* 1976, 4 (suppl. 2): 15–19.

21. Regalado RG. Anafranil in the management of long-term pain: A preliminary report. *J Int Med Res,* 1976, 4 (suppl. 2): 54–55.

22. Scott WA. The relief of pain with an antidepressant in arthritis. *Practitioner,* 1969, 202:802–807.

23. Kupers RK. Imipramine in the treatment of rheumatic patients. *Acta Rheumatol Scand,* 1962, 8:45–51.

24. Jenkins DG, Ebbutt AF, Evans CD. Tofranil in the treatment of low back pain. *J Int Med Res,* 1976, 4 (Suppl. 2): 28–40.

25. Chapman CR, Butler SH. Effects of doxepin on perception of laboratory induced pain in man. *Pain,* 1978, 5:253–262.

26. Max MB, Lynch SA, Muir J, Shoaf SE, Smoller B, Dubner R. Effects of desipramine, amitriptyline and fluoxetine on pain in diabetic neuropathy. *N Eng J Med,* 1992, 326:1250–1253.

27. Magni G. The use of antidepressants in the treatment of chronic pain: A review of the current evidence. *Drugs,* 1991, 42:730–748.

28. Onghena P, Van Houdenhove B. Antidepressant-induced analgesia in chronic nonmalignant pain: A meta-analysis of 39 placebo-controlled studies. *Pain,* 1992, 49:205–19.

29. Brown RS, Bottomlay WK. Utilization and mechanism of action of tricyclic antidepressants in the treatment of chronic facial pain: A review of the literature. *Anesth Prog,* 1990, 37:223–229.

30. Panerai AE, Bianchi M, Sacerdote P, Ripamonti C, Ventafridda V, DeConno F. Antidepressants in cancer pain. *J Palliat Care,* 1991, 7:42–44.

31. McQuay HJ, Carroll D, Glynn J. Low dose amitriptyline in treatment of chronic pain. *Anesthesia,* 1992, 47:646–652.

32. Smith RB, Rusbatch BJ. Amitriptyline and heart block. *Br Med J,* 1967, 3:311.

33. Thorstrand C. Clinical features in poisonings by tricyclic antidepressants with special reference to the ECG. *Acta Med Scand,* 1976, 199:337–344.

34. Crome P. Poisoning due to tricyclic overdose. *Med Toxicol,* 1986, 1:261.

35. Crocker J, Morton B. Tricyclic (antidepressant) drug toxicity. *Clin Toxicol,* 1969, 2:397–402.

36. Noble JJ, Matthews H. Acute poisoning by tricyclic antidepressant: Clinical features and management of 100 patients. *Clin Toxicol,* 1969, 2:403–421.

37. Crome P, Dawling S, Braithwaite RA, Masters, J, Walkey R. Effect of activated charcoal on absorption of nortriptyline. *Lancet,* 1977, 2:1203–1205.

38. Brown TC, Barker GA, Dunlop ME, Loughnan PM. The use of sodium bicarbonate in the treatment of tricyclic antidepressant-induced arrhythmias. *Anaesth Intensive Care,* 1973, 1:2.

39. Snyder BD, Blonde L, McWhirter WR. Reversal of amitriptyline intoxication by physostigmine. *JAMA,* 1974, 230:1433–1434.

40. Stewart GO. Convulsions after physostigmine (letter). *Anaesth Intensive Care,* 1980, 7:283.

41. Tobis J, Das BN. Cardiac complications in amitriptyline poisoning: Successful treatment with physostigmine. *JAMA,* 1976, 235:1474–1476.

42. Physostigmine for tricyclic antidepressant overdosage. *Med Lett Drugs Ther,* 1980, 22:55.

43. El Yousef MK, Manier DH. Tricyclic antidepressants and phenothiazines. *JAMA,* 1974, 229:1419.

44. Heiman EM. Cardiac toxicity with thioridazine-tricyclic antidepressant combination. *J Nerv Ment Dis,* 1977, 165:139–143.

45. Persson G, Siwers B. The risk of potentiating effect of local anaesthesia with adrenalin in patients treated with tricyclic antidepressants. *Sven Tandlak Tidskr,* 1975, 68:9–18.

46. Briant RH, Reid JL, Dollery CT. Interaction between clonidine and desipramine in man. *Br Med J,* 1973, 1:522–523.

47. Meyer JF, McAllister CK, Goldberg LI. Insidious and prolonged antagonism of guanethidine by amitriptyline. *JAMA,* 1970, 213:1487–1488.

48. Goldberg LI. Monoamine oxidase inhibitors: Adverse reactions and possible mechanisms. *JAMA,* 1964, 190:456–462.

49. Consolo S, Morselli PL, Zaccala M, Garattini S. Delayed absorption of phenylbutazone caused by desmethylimipramine in humans. *Eur J Pharmacol,* 1970, 10:239–242.

50. Pullar-Strecker H. Drug interactions in alcoholism treatment (letter). *Lancet,* 1969, 1:735.

51. Logue JN, Sachais BA, Feighner JP. Comparisons of maprotiline with imipramine in severe depression: A multicenter controlled trial. *J Clin Pharmacol,* 1979, 19:64–74.

52. Feighner JP. Pharmacology: New antidepressants. *Psychiatr Ann,* 1980, 10:388–394.

53. Larochelle P, Hamet P, Enjalbert M. Responses to tyramine and norepinephrine after imipramine and trazodone. *Clin Pharmacol Ther,* 1979, 26:24–30.

54. Gram LF. Fluoxetine. *N Eng J Med,* 1994, 1:1354–1361.

55. Freudenheim M. The drug makers are listening to Prozac: A host of similar antidepressants may soon join the fight in a $3 billion market. *The New York Times,* January 9, 1994.

56. Better than well. *The Economist,* April 6, 1996: 87–88.

Chapter 12

Marijuana

INTRODUCTION

Cannabis sativa, known to mankind since the early millenniums, is capable of abundant growth in both tropical and temperate climates. Since the inception of its cultivation in central Asia over 5,000 years ago, almost every human complaint has been treated with one form or another of this plant. Administration of cannabis preparations for the relief of pain was a recognized therapy until the end of the nineteenth century. Cannabis was felt to be particularly effective for headache, toothache, and menstrual cramps.[1] In fact, until the 1930s, preparations of cannabis were not only listed in the *Pharmacopeia* of the United States and the National Formulary but, in addition, could be found on shelves in pharmacies throughout the country. During the early 1900s, both the Eli Lilly and the Parke Davis Pharmaceutical Companies maintained farms where Cannabis americana, a potent strain of the plant, was grown. Increasing concern over the "evils" of this drug led to the passage of the Marijuana Tax Act in 1937, classifying marijuana as a narcotic and thereby effectively eliminating its legal distribution.[2] Today, although there are several synthetic forms of marijuana that exist, the use of this plant even for medical purposes remains controversial and prohibited.

PREPARATIONS

The strength or potency of marijuana is determined by its concentration of the psychoactive substance delta 9-tetrahydrocannabinol (Δ^9-THC). The fiber-type plant has a low Δ^9-THC content (usually less then 0.2 percent), whereas the type used for its psychoactive qualities has a Δ^9-THC content of between 1.4 to 5 percent.[3] Many local names have been assigned to cannabis products, depending on the portion of the plant consumed as well as the country of cultivation.

There are basically four major products that can be obtained from the cannabis plant. Hashish or charas, the resin extracted from the tops of the flowering plant, is considered to be much more potent than other preparations, containing 3 to 8 percent Δ^9-THC. It is usually mixed with tobacco prior to smoking. An extract of hashish oil can be produced with a Δ^9-THC content of 20 percent. Ganga refers to an extract of the smaller leaves. Preparations of dry leaves and flowering shoots have been termed *bang, kif, dugga,* and *machohna.*

Marijuana (grass) is the American term referring to the preparation made from all parts of the plant consumed to produce psychic changes. Most frequently, marijuana consists of the flowering tops, which, when crushed or chopped, can be smoked in cigarette form. An average marijuana cigarette weighs approximately 0.5 to 1 gram and contains 1 to 2 percent Δ^9-THC. However, there is a potent form of the plant (sinsemilla) whose Δ^9-THC may be as high as 15 percent.

PATTERNS OF USE

Marijuana is the most frequently used illicit drug. In 1971, the United States National Commission on Marijuana and Drug Abuse estimated 24 million Americans had used marijuana at some time.[4] In the 1980s approximately 60 percent of high school seniors had smoked marijuana at least once. During the early 1990s, the number of seniors and college students smoking marijuana decreased. A 1992 survey of high school and college students revealed an annual prevalence use of 22 to 28 percent, with the number of daily users decreasing markedly from 10.7 percent in 1970 to 2 percent in 1992. However, the 1994 survey found the marijuana use to have increased with 31 percent of high school seniors reporting using in the past year.

Although marijuana has long been proposed for a variety of medical conditions (Table 12.1), the appropriateness of its medical use has been revived recently with respect to its effectiveness as an analgesic and an antiemetic in persons with terminal disease (Table 12.1). The legality of authorizing marijuana use in selected groups of patients, however, remains in "turmoil." In fact, in 1994 after the U.S. Appeals Court upheld the position of the Drug Enforcement Agency not to reschedule marijuana, a small program under the auspices of the United States Public Health Service to supply marijuana medically to a small number of patients began to be phased out. To date, all attempts to carefully evaluate the medical use of marijuana have been prevented.

PHARMACOLOGY

Regardless of the components of the plant consumed, the active principles are the cannabinoids (Table 12.2), with Δ^9-THC primarily responsible for the psychic effects of the drug. Cannabinol (CBN) and cannabidiol (CBD), the two other major cannabinoids, are essentially inactive in humans.[7] In most instances, consumption of marijuana is by smoking. When used in this manner, a variable amount of Δ^9-THC is lost through exhaled air, the respiratory dead space, or elimination in the smoke. Pyrolysis (burning) also destroys some of the drug, although it is likely that volatilization in the smoke may occur prior to the actual burning of the tobacco. The efficacy of delivery of marijuana through smoking has been reported to range from 20 to 80 percent, with an average efficiency of 50 percent.[8]

Smoking a 500 mg marijuana cigarette containing approximately 5 to 20 mg Δ^9-THC results in absorption of 2.5 to 5 mg. Oral doses of Δ^9-THC are also effective, with the equivalent dosage needed reported to be two and one-half to three times higher. This is probably related to the destruction of marijuana in the gastrointestinal tract.

TABLE 12.1. Proposed Medical Uses of Marijuana

AIDS Wasting Syndrome
Analgesic
Anticonvulsant
Antidepressant
Antiemetic
Bronchodilator
Glaucoma
Sedative

TABLE 12.2. Constituents of Cannabis Isolated from Cannabis Sativa

Cannabinol (CBN)
Cannabidiol (CBD)
Cannabigerol (CBG)
Cannabicyclol
8-Tetrahydrocannabinol (Δ^8-THC)[a]
9-Tetrahydrocannabinol (Δ^9-THC)[a]

[a]Psychoactive substances

After smoking, Δ^9-THC, which is highly lipophilic, is absorbed rapidly by the mucous membranes, with pharmacological effects noted within minutes. Subjective effects persist for three to five hours. When ingested, a delay in appearance of plasma levels occurs with effects not being felt for at least 30 minutes.

Δ^9-THC is an avid binder of plasma proteins. Plasma concentrations reach peak values between 10 to 30 minutes, with an initial rapid fall reflecting a wide distribution to lipid-rich tissues.[9] Peak plasma levels following ingestion of Δ^9-THC do not occur for 30 to 120 minutes. Plasma levels may remain elevated for more than two hours although traces of TCH can be found in the plasma for up to several days. This finding probably reflects a gradual metabolism as well as the release of Δ^9-THC from tissues. The plasma half-life of Δ^9-THC and its metabolites is five to eight days.[10] Complete elimination after a single dose may take up to 30 days.

There had been little evidence to indicate that consumption of repeated small amounts of marijuana for several days or daily smoking for several weeks will produce permanent, clinically detectable accumulation in tissues. The availability of a more potent form of marijuana over the last few years, however, may result in tissue accumulation. Increased dosages at interval levels of less than eight to ten days will result in persistent accumulation of Δ^9-THC and its metabolites, and storage in lipid-rich tissues is considerable. The development of a steady state whereby the amount of the drug eliminated equals the amount absorbed can be reached after only four weeks of daily administration.[8]

Δ^9-THC is metabolized in the liver and excreted predominantly in the feces and the urine, with urinary metabolites able to be detected for weeks. Chronic marijuana smokers metabolize Δ^9-THC more rapidly than do nonsmokers.[11] This might explain the considerable amount of tolerance that has been observed clinically in regular users of cannabis products.

EFFECTS ON ORGAN SYSTEMS

The effects of marijuana on organ systems may be related not only to the active ingredients in cannabis but also to the manner in which the drug is taken. Smoking marijuana mixed with tobacco has all of the hazards associated with the effects of tobacco smoke on pulmonary and cardiovascular function. A great deal of investigation has accumulated concerning the pathophysiological effects of marijuana. The following section attempts to summarize these findings, emphasizing those appearing to be of particular clinical relevance.

Central Nervous System

The cerebral effects of marijuana administration have been well described.[12] Acute administration is associated with a variety of subjective experiences, which show a good deal of individual susceptibility. The most common feeling is euphoria accompanied by calm. When taken in isolation, a sedative effect may be experienced. However, when the drug is taken in a social setting, an opposite reaction—stimulation and increase in spontaneous activity—may occur. Short-term memory may be impaired, as may gait. With low doses, performance of relatively simple tasks may not reveal any difficulty in muscle coordination; however, complex tasks, such as driving ability and other related skills, may be accomplished only with difficulty. Sensory function is often reported as being enhanced; however, on objective evaluation, it is more often found to be unchanged or depressed. Auditory and visual acuity may be decreased. At times, although the smoker may not experience any signs or symptoms of impairment, objective testing reveals the opposite. One study of airline pilots found 10 of 19 to have substandard performance after smoking one marijuana cigarette, with impairment detected up to 24 hours later.[13]

In higher doses, marijuana can induce panic or anxiety reactions as well as feelings of paranoia and, at times, frank hallucinations. These adverse psychological effects of marijuana are more apt to appear in elderly patients or younger, inexperienced users. It should be emphasized that these reactions following "street use" of marijuana may be related to the presence of other hallucinogens rather than a specific effect of Δ^9-THC.

Electroencephalographic changes have been reported with both acute and chronic marijuana administration. These changes are mostly dose-related, consisting of alpha-wave slowing as well as slow-wave and spike activity in deep brain structures. Loss of REM sleep associated with an increase in total sleep time and an unaffected stage-four slow-wave sleep may occur. Cessation of marijuana use is accompanied by a rebound in REM sleep as well as in eye movements. Actual structural brain damage due to use of marijuana has not been demonstrated.[14]

Paralysis of the fourth cranial nerve has been reported with heavy use of marijuana.[15] However, these findings were noted in a drug treatment clinic where prevalence of polydrug use was considerable. A subsequent study of peripheral nerve function using electrostimulation did not reveal any evidence of conduction defects.[16]

Chronic marijuana users may develop a constellation of symptoms referred to as the antimotivational syndrome (Table 12.3). Whether these effects occur with intermittent use at low doses remains to be determined.

TABLE 12.3. Characteristics of the Antimotivational Syndrome

Apathy Dullness Fatigue Impaired judgment, concentration, memory Low frustration threshold Lack of concern with appearance or interpersonal relationships

Cardiovascular System

Marijuana can exert an effect on the cardiovascular system, primarily through the actions of Δ^9-THC. The magnitude of such an effect, however, is dependent on: (1) dose employed, (2) route of administration, (3) prestudy status of the subject with respect to the presence of chronic marijuana usage or cardiovascular disease, and (4) whether such effects are measured acutely or on a long-term basis (Table 12.4).

Studies of cardiac performance in normal subjects given intravenous infusions of Δ^9-THC at a rate equivalent to smoking one 5-mg Δ^9-THC marijuana cigarette reveal a significant increase in heart rate and left ventricular ejection time, with a shortened preejection period. There is no change in blood pressure, unless large doses are given, at which time orthostatic hypotension can occur.[17] Administration of propranolol can prevent the tachycardia, whereas the presence of alcohol will enhance the increase in heart rate.[18]

Electrocardiographic changes, in addition to tachycardia, have been reported with marijuana use. Sinus automaticity is enhanced and nonspecific ST segment and T-wave changes may occur. Premature ventricular contractions and bigeminal rhythms with syncope have also been observed.[19]

Marijuana's attributes as an antianxiety or euphoria-producing drug suggest the possibility of its use in coronary artery disease to alleviate the anxiety and tension frequently found in the anginal or postmyocardial infarction patient. Administration of marijuana to patients with angina, however, is associated with a significant decrease of up to 48 percent in mean exercise performance. Marijuana also increases the systolic pressure-heart rate product, resulting in a further increase in myocardial oxygen demand and the potential for causing angina.[20]

Congestion of the conjunctival blood vessels is one of the most consistent findings. The congestion persists longer than tachycardia, being apparent over 90 minutes after smoking. It is dose-related and considered to

TABLE 12.4. Hemodynamic Effects of Marijuana Administration

Dose	Heart-beat	Blood pressure	Orthostatic changes	Plasma volume	Myocardial contractility
Acute administration, small or moderate dose	↑	V	–	–	–
Chronic administration or administration of large, single dose	↓	↓	+	↑	NM
Coronary artery disease, acute administration	↑	↑	–	NM	↓

Note: ↑ = increase; ↓ = decrease; V = variable responses reported; – = no change; NM = not measured.
Reprinted with permission from Stimmel (1990).

be secondary to a direct effect of cannabis on the conjunctival vessels rather than an irritant effect of the cigarette smoke.

Respiratory System

Experimentally, discernible adverse pulmonary effects can be produced by chronic inhalation of marijuana in laboratory animals.[31] Analysis of the hydrocarbon fractions, or marijuana smoke condensates, has revealed that marijuana, due to active pyrolysis of its constituents, in fact contains higher amounts of carcinogenic hydrocarbons than pure tobacco smoke. The extent of the pulmonary lesions in animals is related to the duration of exposure as well as dose inhaled. However, changes were still present months after discontinuing inhalation.

Clinically, reports of the acute effects of marijuana smoking have been contradictory. Some investigators have noted statistically significant increases in bronchodilation as well as reversal of experimentally induced bronchospasm in adults with bronchial asthma.[21] Others have noted a failure of improvement of any parameters of pulmonary function in persons with reversible airway obstruction.[22]

Chronic marijuana smoking has long been associated with chronic cough, bronchitis, and obstructive pulmonary defects. Impairment in pulmonary function tests, manifested by decrease in vital capacity, functional expiratory volume, maximal mid-expiratory flow rate, and specific airway conductance, have also been noted in young smokers. These changes appeared between three to eight weeks after heavy marijuana smoking, persisting for at least one week after smoking ceased. Although a specific link with marijuana use and lung cancer has not been demonstrated, the practice of holding one's breath to obtain more of the drug allows for the potential to introduce more carcinogens into the blood stream than when smoking a cigarette. Depression of the respiratory response curve with either synthetic or natural marijuana has also been reported in a group of chronic users.[23]

Metabolic and Endocrine Effects

The effects of marijuana on reproductive function have come under scrutiny during the past several years.[24-28] Levels of plasma testosterone have been reported to be depressed in chronic marijuana smokers. Although conflicting findings exist, most recent studies confirm a decrease in sperm count in otherwise normal chronic users of marijuana. This oligospermia may be accompanied by an increase in abnormal sperm forms and a decrease in motility. Possible reasons for this depressant effect may be marijuana-induced inhibition of gonadotropins, FSH and LH associated with a subsequent reduction in testosterone, or a direct effect of marijuana on the germinal epithelium. Frequently, marijuana is consumed with other mood-altering drugs, such as alcohol, which also have been reported to effect spermatogenesis adversely. Gynecomastia in male marijuana users has been described, but not confirmed, hypothesized to be related to changes in serum prolactin levels.

Other Actions

Marijuana has also been reported to produce a variety of other effects.[29,30] These include weight gain, alteration of cell-mediated immunity, and diminished intraocular pressure, as well as inhibition of nausea and vomiting. The multiple effects of marijuana on the organ systems have resulted in its being postulated as being useful in a wide variety of clinical states (see Table 12.1). However, its effectiveness in virtually all of these conditions remains to be determined through carefully designed studies.

ANALGESIC ACTIVITY

One of the earliest uses of marijuana was for the relief of pain. Although its effectiveness as an analgesic was mainly anecdotal, a number of experimental studies have suggested that, under certain conditions, marijuana may indeed enhance or induce analgesia.[31,32] The underlying mechanisms for a possible analgesic effect of marijuana remain to be determined. It has been postulated that any analgesia induced by marijuana is primarily due to its hydroxymetabolites, and may depress the cells of the mid-brain and dorsal raphe nucleus.[33,34]

Smoking and Pain

The analgesic effects of marijuana in humans under experimental conditions have been studied by several investigators with often conflicting findings. The inhalation of marijuana smoke was accompanied by a decreased or an increased tolerance and heightened or unchanged pain. A study comparing the effects of intravenous administration of marijuana with that of diazepam and placebo found significant increases in detection thresholds without any evidence of analgesic effect on pain tolerance thresholds, suggesting its effect was primarily one of disruption of normal sensory signals, rather than elevation of pain tolerance.[35]

Clinical reports of the analgesic effectiveness of marijuana have been far less consistent. Paraplegics hospitalized in a VA hospital, with a history of marijuana use, reported the use of marijuana to be associated with a decrease in spasticity as well as in headache pain accompanied by an increase in pleasant sensations.[36] A double-blind study found pain tolerance to be greater in experienced marijuana smokers after marijuana administration. No effect on pain sensitivity was noted.[34] The administering Δ^9-THC to persons with angina did not confirm protection from experimentally induced chest pain.[20]

A study of the effects of 10 and 20 mg Δ^9-THC in patients with terminal cancer found that the higher dose was associated with impaired concentration and fuzzy thinking in 70 percent of persons.[37] However, an equal proportion did report being calmer. Dizziness, blurred vision, ataxia, and slurred speech were the dose-limiting effects. Although Δ^9-THC was shown to be a mild analgesic, the 20-mg dose was prohibitively sedating as well as intoxicating. The 10-mg dose rarely presented severe problems; however, sedation was also present and occasionally was associated with complaints of dizziness, blurred vision, and impaired thinking. These investigators concluded that the 10-mg dose of Δ^9-THC was effective in producing relaxation and appetite stimulation, which allowed for a reduction in the amount of both other analgesics and hypnotic drugs.

Similarly, in persons with acquired immune deficiency syndrome (AIDS), inhaled marijuana is proported to be an extremely helpful antiemetic agent, appetite stimulant, and analgesic. It is estimated that as many as 2,000 persons with AIDS in San Francisco are using street marijuana for these purposes.[38] Unfortunately, studies to determine its effectiveness have been opposed by the Drug Enforcement Agency and the National Institute of Drug Abuse. To date there has been no convincing evidence that marijuana has specific analgesic properties. It is, however, commonly accepted "on the street" that for many marijuana can be quite helpful in relieving pain in a variety of chronic painful conditions.[41,42]

Δ 9-THC Analogs

The dysphoric effects accompanying the use of Δ^9-THC for analgesia led to the development of analogs able to retain analgesic activity but devoid of other adverse effects. At least six analogs have been synthesized that have been demonstrated to be analgesic when tested in laboratory animals.[39,40,43] One of these, benzopyranopiperidine, has also been tested in the clinical setting and was double-blind crossover protocol, and was found to provide analgesia equal to codeine.[39] These results have remained to be confirmed.

Dronabinol

Dronabinol (Marinol) is the synthetically available form of marijuana approved for the treatment of nausea and vomiting associated with chemotherapy. Tolerance to its effects can develop, and instances of withdrawal have been reported. Unfortunately, many persons who find smoking marijuana to be effective in preventing chemotherapy-induced nausea do not find Marinol an effective alternative.

Hyperanalgesia

Reports have also appeared associating marijuana use with increased pain or hyperalgesia in patients with neoplastic disease. Bone pain experienced by these patients subsided on discontinuing smoking marijuana.

DEPENDENCE, TOLERANCE, AND WITHDRAWAL

Although psychological dependence to marijuana can readily develop, until recently there has been little if any associated physical dependence reported, even under conditions of extremely heavy use.[44] However, several reports have appeared describing physical symptoms after discontinuing marijuana use. These symptoms include irritability, restlessness, anorexia, nausea, vomiting, diarrhea, tremor, and sleep disturbances.[45] Most recently, experimental work with laboratory animals has suggested that high doses of marijuana can be associated with physical dependence.

TOXICITY

Adverse physical reactions to marijuana are relatively rare when the drug is smoked or consumed orally, with nausea and vomiting being most frequently reported after taking large doses. In the street setting, marijuana is rarely injected intravenously and physiologic overdose reactions are infrequent.

The major toxic reaction to a marijuana overdose is a marked change in mental state, which may range from mild anxiety to severe panic. Marked disturbance in thought patterns are not prominent in contrast to toxic reactions to major hallucinogens. The most accurate means of diagnosis is to obtain a history from either the patient or friends concerning the presence of marijuana ingestion. It is, however, extremely important to eliminate the possibility of ingestion of other mood-altering drugs. The most common form of treatment of marijuana toxicity in the absence of adverse physiological change is quiet reassurance. Marijuana overdose in persons with cardiac disease may be associated with precipitation of angina or hypertension. The presence of these symptoms requires appropriate therapy.

Intravenous injection is associated with considerable toxicity.[46] Toxic effects may be dependent on the dose injected as well as on the presence of allergic or idiosyncratic reactions to contaminants or other substances. Following injection, nausea, vomiting, and diarrhea are frequent. Hypotension, renal failure, and associated hematologic alterations, consisting of a leukemoid reaction, anemia, and thrombocytopenia, have also been reported.

The hypotension, which at times may be considerable, may be related to a hypovolemia secondary to copious diarrhea or may be the result of central nervous system effect of marijuana on the vasomotor receptor. The occurrence of renal failure is related to the preceding hypotension and is quite transient, responding quickly to fluid replacement.

Chronic regular use of marijuana may lead to antimotivational syndrome. This state is marked by a loss of social drive, passivity, and slowed mentation. The frequent recognition of this syndrome among younger chronic users has become of increasing concern.

DRUG INTERACTIONS

Since metabolism of marijuana occurs mainly through the hepastic microsomal enzyme system, interactions with other drugs also metabo-

lized through this pathway may occur (Table 12.5). Metabolism of
Δ^9-THC can be accelerated by pretreatment with phenobarbital and inhibited *in vitro* by acute administration of nortriptyline and desmethylimipramine, phenobarbital, amphetamine, and meprobamate.[47]

The clinical relevance of these reactions remains unknown. The combined use of marijuana and some tranquilizers, however, may result in adverse effects. The use of marijuana is frequently associated with consumption of other mood-altering drugs in 75 percent of users, with alcohol and stimulants being the most common.

Since marijuana acts on the autonomic nervous system, it is possible that combined use of similarly acting drugs might have added deleterious effects. The combined use of marijuana and dextroamphetamines can cause additive increases in heart rate and elevation of systolic blood pressure.[48] This was not associated with any interactive effect on psychomotor performance. Alcohol has also been shown to enhance Δ^9-THC-induced tachycardia, with synergistic effects also observed on impairment of psychomotor performance.[49] Administration of secobarbital and marijuana smoking can produce effects similar to that seen with alcohol with respect to both subjective responses and psychomotor impairment.[50]

TABLE 12.5. Interactions of Other Mood-Altering Drugs with Marijuana

Drug	Clinical Effects
Alcohol	Impaired psychomotor performance; enhancement of Δ^9-THC-induced tachycardia.
Amphetamines	Synergistic effect on heart rate and blood pressure.
Atropine	Synergistic effect on heart rate and blood pressure.
Barbiturates	Synergistic impairment of both subjective and psychomotor responses.
Diazepam	Enhancement of diazepam-induced CNS depression.
Ether	Prolongs ether anesthesia.
Naloxone	Attenuation of cannabis-induced analgesia; attenuation of naloxone-induced narcotic withdrawal.
Narcotics	Enhancement of narcotic-induced CNS depression.

The effect of marijuana on glucose metabolism may result in an impairment of glucose tolerance, as noted above. Although the clinical significance of this action remains unclear, marijuana use in diabetics may be associated with untoward effects.

Narcotic-marijuana interactions also occur. Intravenous administration of Δ^9-THC to healthy subjects pretreated with oxymorphone results in prominent central nervous system depression, marked by drowsiness and difficulty in arousal.[51] Similar effects occur when parenteral diazepam is administered after intravenous Δ^9-THC. Clinically important potentiation of narcotic effects with concomitant use of marijuana, however, has not been consistently demonstrated.

Atropine administered to patients on chronic Δ^9-THC can result in an increase in blood pressure.[52] Whether this interaction is central or peripheral has not been clearly defined. Concomitant use of parasympathetic blocking agents and Δ^9-THC may result in potentially dangerous drug interactions. Prolonged postoperative tachycardia in a series of patients who had smoked marijuana within 72 hours before undergoing outpatient general anesthesia with oral surgery has been reported.

SUMMARY

An analgesic response to marijuana has not been consistently demonstrated in the clinical setting. In addition, the undesirable side effects accompanying the use of this drug, especially in elderly or naive users, may make its use as an analgesic quite limited even if permitted. However, its antiemetic action, combined with its mood-elevating effects, has made its use quite attractive to some terminal cancer patients undergoing chemotherapy as well as in some persons with AIDS and severe muscle wasting. Unfortunately, existing government regulations preclude its medical use under these circumstances and controlled studies of its effectiveness have not been supported, despite surveys of oncologists that have revealed up to 44 percent recommend marijuana as an antiemetic and a slightly higher proportion indicate a willingness to prescribe this drug if legal. Although highly effective antiemetic agents are currently available, they are extremely expensive, and synthetic marijuana does not appear to be as effective an agent as in the natural drug.

At present there remains considerable controversy within the medical profession as to whether this drug has any clinical applicability.[54,55] This is due to most of the evidence concerning its effectiveness being anecdotal. Hopefully, with time, reason will prevail to allow execution of well-designed studies to determine marijuana's medical effectiveness.

REFERENCES

1. Gaoni Y, Mechoulam R. Isolation, structure, and partial synthesis of an active component of hashish. *J Am Chem Soc*, 1946, 86:1646–1647.

2. Cohen S. Marijuana: Does it have a possible therapeutic use? *JAMA*, 1978, 240:1761–1763.

3. Nahas G. Symposium on marijuana: Rheims, France 22-23, July 1978. *Bull Narc*, 1978, 30:23–32.

4. Shafer RP. *Marijuana, a signal of misunderstanding, Shafer report*. First report of the National Commission on Marijuana and Drug Abuse, March 1972. Washington, DC: US Government Printing Office, 1972.

5. National Institute on Drug Abuse. *Marijuana and health: Fourth annual report*. Rockville, MD: Department of Health, Education, and Welfare, 1974.

6. Johnston LD, O'Malley PM, Bachman JG. National survey results on drug use from monitoring the future study. 1975-1992. Rockville, MD: U.S. Dept. Health and Human Services; Public Health Service, National Institute Drug Abuse, 1993.

7. Hollister LE. Cannabidiol and cannabinol in man. *Experientia*, 1973, 29:825–826.

8. Hollister LE. Marijuana in man: Three years later. *Science*, 1971, 172:21 – 29.

9. Kreuz DS, Axelrod J. Delta 9-tetrahydrocannabinol: Localization in body fat. *Science*, 1973, 179:391–393.

10. Paton WDM. Pharmacology of marijuana. *Annu Rev Pharmacol*, 1975, 15:191–220.

11. Lemberger L, Tamarkin NR, Axelrod J, Kopin IJ. Delta-9-tetrahydrocannabinol: Metabolism and disposition in long-term marijuana smokers. *Science*, 1971, 173:72–74.

12. Borg J, Gerson S, Alpert M. Dose effects of smoked marijuana on human cognitive and motor functions. *Psychopharmacologia*, 1975, 42:211–218.

13. Yesavage JA, Leirer VO, Denari M, Hollister LE. Carry-over effects of marijuana intoxication on aircraft pilot performance: A preliminary report. *Am J Psychiatry*, 1985, 142:1325–1329.

14. Co BT, Goodwin DW, Gado M, Mikhael M, Hill SY. Absence of cerebral atrophy in chronic cannabis users: Evaluation by computerized transaxial tomography. *JAMA*, 1977, 237; 1229–1230.

15. Coleman JH, Tacker HL, Evans WE, Lemmi H, Britton EL. Neurological manifestations of chronic marijuana intoxication. Part I: Paresis of the fourth cranial nerve. *Dis Nerv Syst*, 1976, 37:29.

16. DiBenedetto M. Electrodiagnostic evidence of subclinical disease states in drug abusers. *Arch Phys Med Rehabil*, 1976, 57:62–66.

17. Benowitz NL, Jones RT. Cardiovascular effects of prolonged delta-9-tetrahydrocannabinol ingestion. *Clin Pharmacol Ther*, 1976, 18:287–297.

18. Kanakis C, Jr, Pouget JM, Rosen KM. The effects of delta-9-tetrahydrocannabinol (cannabis) on cardiac performance with and without beta blockade. *Circulation*, 1976, 53:703–707.

19. Miller RH, Dhingra RC, Kanakis C, Jr, Amat Y, Leon F. The electrophysiological effects of delta-9-tetrahydrocannabinol (cannabis) on cardiac conduction in man. *Am Heart J,* 1977, 94:740–747.

20. Aronow WS, Cassidy J. Effect of marijuana and placebo marijuana smoking on angina pectoris. *N Engl J Med,* 1974, 291:65–67.

21. Shapiro BJ, Tashkin DP. Effects of β-adrenergic blockage and muscarinic stimulation on cannabis bronchodilation. In: Braude MC, Szara S (eds.). *Pharmacology of marijuana.* New York: Raven Press, 1976: 277–286.

22. Abramson HA. Respiratory disorders and marijuana use (editorial). *J Asthma Res,* 1974, 11:97.

23. Tashkin DP, Shapiro BJ, Lee YE, Harper CE. Subacute effects of heavy marihuana smoking on pulmonary function in healthy men. *N Engl J Med,* 1976, 294:125–129.

24. Cushman P, Jr. Plasma testosterone levels in healthy male marijuana smokers. *Am J Drug Alcohol Abuse,* 1975, 1:269–275.

25. Kolodny RC, Lessin P, Toro G, Masters WH, Cohen S. Depression of plasma testosterone with acute marihuana administration. In: Braude MC, Szara S (eds.). *Pharmacology of marihjuana.* New York: Raven Press, 1976: 217–225.

26. Hembree WC, Nahas GG, Zeidenberg P, Dyrenfurth I. Marijuana effects upon the human testes. *Clin Res,* 1976, 24:272A.

27. Harmon JW, Aliapoulios MA. Marijuana-induced gynecomastia: Clinical and laboratory experience. *Surg Forum,* 1974, 25:423–425.

28. Lemberger L, Crabtree R, Rowe H, Clemens, J. Tetrahydrocannabinols and serum prolactin levels in man. *Life Sci,* 1975, 16:1339–1343.

29. Petersen BH, Graham J, Lemberger L, Dalton B. Studies of the immune response in chronic marijuana smokers. *Pharmacologist,* 1974, 16:259.

30. Dawson WW. Cannabis and eye function (editorial). *Invest Ophthalmol,* 1976, 15:243–245.

31. Kaymakcalan S, Turker RK, Turker MN. Analgesic effect of delta-9-tetrahydrocannabinol in the dog. *Psychopharmacologia,* 1974, 35:123–128.

32. Parker JM, Dubas TC. Automatic determination of the pain threshold to electroshock and the effects of 9-THC. *Int J Clin Pharmacol,* 1973, 7:75–81.

33. Hill SY, Schwin R, Goodwin DW, Powell BJ. Marihuana and pain. *J Pharmacol Exp Ther,* 1974, 188:415–418.

34. Milstein SL, MacCannell K, Karr G, Clark S. Marijuana-produced changes in pain tolerance: Experienced and non-experienced subjects. *Int Pharmacopsychiatry,* 1975, 10:177–182.

35. Raft D, Gregg J, Ghia J, Harris L. Effects of intravenous tetrahydrocannabinol on experimental and surgical pain: Psychological correlates of the analgesic response. *Clin Pharmacol Ther,* 1976, 21:26–33.

36. Dunn M, Davis R. The perceived effects of marijuana on spinal cord injured males. *Paraplegia,* 1975, 12:175.

37. Noyes R, Jr, Brunk SF, Avery DH, Canter A. Psychologic effects of oral delta 9-tetrahydrocannabinol in advanced cancer patients. *Compr Psychiatryy,* 1976, 17:641–646.

38. Grinspoon L, Bakalar JB, Doblin R. Marijuana, the AIDS wasting syndrome, and the U.S. Government. *N Eng J Med*, 1995, 333:670–671.

39. Harris LS. Cannabinoids as analgesics. In: Beers RF, Bassett EG (eds.). *Mechanisms of pain and analgesic compounds*. New York: Raven Press, 1979: 467–473.

40. Jochimsen PR, Lawton RL, Ver Steeg K, Noyes R, Jr. Effect of benzopyranoperidine, a delta-9-THC congener, on pain. *Clin Pharmacol Ther*, 1978, 24: 223–227.

41. Nieburg HA, Margolin F, Seligman BR. Tetrahydrocannabinol and chemotherapy (letter). *N Engl J Med*, 1976, 294:168.

42. Sallan SE, Zinberg NE, Frei E, III. Antiemetic effect of delta-9-tetrahydrocannabinol in patients receiving cancer chemotherapy. *N Engl J Med*, 1975, 293:795–797.

43. Wilson RS, May EL. 9-nor-delta 8-tetrahydrocannabinol, a cannabinoid of metabolic interest. *J Med Chem*, 1974, 17:475–476.

44. Low MD, Klonoff H, Marcus A. The neurophysiological basis of the marijuana experience. *Can Med Assoc J*, 1973, 108:157–165.

45. Jones RT, Benowitz N. The 30-day trip: Clinical studies of cannabis tolerance and dependence. In: Braude MC, Szara S (eds.). *Pharmacology of marihuana*, New York: Raven Press, 1976: 627-642.

46. Farber SJ, Huertas VE. Intravenously injected marihuana syndrome. *Arch Intern Med*, 1976, 136:337–339.

47. Siemens AJ, De Nie LC, Kalant H, Khanna JM. Effects of various psychoactive drugs on the metabolism of delta 9 tetrahydrocannabinol by rats in vivo and in vitro. *Eur J Pharmacol*, 1975, 31:136–147.

48. Evans MA, Martz R, Rodda BE, Lemberger L, Forney RB. Effects of marihuana-dextroamphetamine combination. *Clin Pharmacol Ther*, 1976, 20:350–358.

49. Macavoy MG, Marks DF. Divided attention performance of cannabis users and non-users following cannabis and alcohol. *Psychopharmacologia*, 1975, 44: 147–152.

50. Dalton WS, Martz R, Lemberger L, Rodda BE, Forney RB. Effects of marihuana combined with secobarbital. *Clin Pharmacol Ther*, 1975, 18:298–304.

51. Smith TC, Kulp, RA. Respiratory and cardiovascular effects of delta-9-tetrahydrocannabinol alone and in combination with oxymorphone, pentobarbital, and diazepam. In: Cohen S, Stillman RC (eds.). *The therapeutic potential of marijuana*. New York: Plenum Press, 1976:123–132.

52. Beaconsfield P. Some cardiovascular effects of cannabis. *Am Heart J*, 1974, 87:143–146.

53. Gregg JM, Campbell RL, Levin KJ, Ghia J, Elliott RA. Cardiovascular effects of cannabinol during oral surgery. *Anesth Anal*, 1976, 55:203–213.

54. Doblin R, Kleiman MAR. The medical use of marijuana: The case for clinical trials. *J of Addictive Diseases*, 1995, 14(1):5–11.

55. Schwartz RH, Voth EA. Marijuana as medicine: Making a silk purse out of a sow's ear. *J of Addictive Diseases*, 1995, 14(1):15–21.

SECTION III:
THE PRACTICAL MANAGEMENT OF PAIN

Chapter 13

General Principles
of Pain Management

INTRODUCTION

An assessment of a person in pain should not differ from the approach used in other medical disorders. A comprehensive history and physical examination are mandatory to determine both the presence of underlying disease as well as contributory factors that may be influencing symptoms. However, unlike other medical problems, there will be a considerable individual variation in the intensity of the pain regardless of etiology. In addition, often a precise cause will not be able to be clearly defined or, if defined, may not appear to be of sufficient magnitude to result in the intensity of pain experienced. Finally, especially in instances of chronic pain, a person may see a physician with definite perception of what is needed to obtain relief, which frequently may conflict with the physician's perception.

It is therefore imperative to remember the objectives that should exist when trying to relieve pain (Table 13.1); the primary objective always is to promote comfort to the greatest extent possible.[1] Toward this end, the general approach to pain management, be it acute or chronic, should be carefully examined (Table 13.2).

GUIDELINES FOR PAIN MANAGEMENT

Identifying the Source of Pain

It is obvious, but often forgotten, that in order to provide maximal pain relief, the source of the discomfort must be identified. All too often, persons in pain without an obvious source, are considered neurotic or, at the worst, hysterical. It is therefore essential that a careful effort be made

TABLE 13.1. Objectives in Management of Pain

Provide immediate relief from pain through elimination or reduction in incidence and severity
Educate as to what may be done to prevent or diminish future painful episodes
Develop individual guidelines to enhance functioning on a long-term basis

TABLE 13.2. Guideline to Approaching a Person in Pain

Identify source of pain
Assess severity of the pain
Identify existing modifying psychologic or environmental factors
Determine prior successful means of managing pain
Set appropriate goals and objectives
Decide whether drug therapy is warranted

to determine the origin of the pain. In general, organically based pain can be related to a variety of physiologic factors (Table 13.3). Most often the interplay among these factors must be addressed in order to obtain maximal relief.

Assessing Severity

A comprehensive description of the pain will aid in allowing an assessment as to its seriousness as well as the need for medical intervention. The mnemonic PQRST (Table 13.4) is most helpful in remembering the characteristics of pain to be explored.[2] Such an assessment should start with the perception of the pain, its characteristics, and the response to it. Although there are a variety of psychologic measurements that can be used to attempt to quantify the pain intensity, the results will nonetheless remain subjective. At times simply asking the person to rate the pain on a scale of 1 to 10 (with 10 being the most severe pain imaginable) can enable the physician to better understand the person's discomfort as well as establish a baseline to use as interventions occur. A somewhat more objective assessment however, is also possible through measurement of the actual

TABLE 13.3. Etiologic Factors in Selected Pain States

Mechanisms	Headache	Chest Pain	Abdominal Pain	Extremity Pain
Anxiety	+	+	+	+
Compression	Intracranial lesions Cervical rib Scalenus anticos syndrome	Mediastinal mass	Abdominal mass	Nerve outlet syndromes
Inflammation	Temporal ateritis, sinusitis	Aortitis, Herpes zoster, Myocarditis, Pleuritis, Costochondritis	Appendicitis Peritonitis	Arthritis Bursitis Myositis Osteomyelitis Tendonitis
Metabolic	Migraine states, pheochromocytoma	Thyrotoxicosis	Uremia, ketoacidosis, lead poisoning	Gout
Muscular	Cluster Ocular muscle	Spasm intercostal scalene, and pectral muscles	Abdominal wall pain	+
Neoplastic	+	+	+	+
Traumatic	Confusion Subdural or subarachnoid hemorrhage	Dissecting aneurysm, pneumothorax, esophaegeal rupture	Ruptured viscus	Ligamentous Synovial cyst rupture
Vascular	Angioma Aneurysm Basilar or vertebral arterythrombosis Hypertension	Myocardial Pulmonary	Embolus Sickle cell disease	Acute arterial occlusion, erthromeyalgia, thromboangiitis obliterans

physiologic responses to pain, such as heart rate and respiration. At the end of the assessment, a complete picture of the painful experience should be formed.

Recognizing Modifying Psychologic Factors

Particular attention should be placed on factors known to modulate the pain threshold (Table 13.5). Most important is the realization that a person's "understanding" the reason for pain can be a key to successful therapy. Pain is almost always associated with anxieties; a fear that a serious underlying disease exists and an inability to exert control over one's body to obtain relief are the most frequent. Providing an explanation as to why the pain is experienced can often be accompanied by a decrease in its intensity.

Similarly, concern with overmedication or fear of dependence or addiction may prevent a person from taking a narcotic analgesic appropriately to obtain relief. With chronic pain, this fear of addiction may lead one to become high on tranquilizers in a futile attempt to obtain relief instead of taking an appropriate analgesic that will enhance comfort and functioning.

TABLE 13.4. PQRST Characteristics of Pain

Palliative and provocative factors
Quality
Radiation
Severity
Temporal factors

TABLE 13.5. Factors Affecting Pain Threshold

Lowering Threshold	Elevating Threshold
Discomfort	Sleep
Insomnia	Sympathy
Fatigue	Understanding
Anxiety	Diversion
Fear or anger	Mood elevation
Depression	
Isolation	
Last painful experience	

Educating the patient and his or her family about the care and management of the pain is essential, yet is all too often neglected.

The presence or absence of the provocative and palliative modifiers of the pain describe both the psychological reaction to the discomfort, as well as possible precipitating causes. Although at times, identification of these factors may aid in the separation of primary psychogenic from organic disorders (Chapter 4), it should be reemphasized that all types of pain are variably influenced by stress and anxiety.

Pain precipitated by environmental stress or anxiety, which subsides slowly regardless of treatment employed, responds least well to analgesic agents. In such instances, supportive psychotherapy or even the use of psychotropic drugs may be quite helpful. Psychogenically induced pain, however, may frequently be associated with underlying organic disease. As an example, anxiety-induced angina or peptic ulcer pain are both accompanied by pathophysiological alterations that must be addressed with equal attention in order to relieve the pain. It is also important to emphasize that identifiable organic-based pain often facilitates development of psychological dysfunctioning. Indeed, the difficulty in distinguishing organic from psychogenic pain furthers the concept of a common pathophysiologic pathway.

Identifying Prior Successful Ways of Pain Relief

Listening to previous attempts on the part of a person to control the pain can be most helpful, not only in assessment but also in formulating treatment plans. It is in this area that physicians and other health care providers often fail by not believing a person's description of what provides relief, especially if the treatment is not in strict accordance with medical guidelines or common practice. Frequently, analgesia obtained when a drug is taken in an unusual manner may provide an insight into the origin of the pain or even allow a physician to realize that a "common pattern" of usage may not be consistent with a drug's pharmacologic actions. A frequent example of the latter instance can be seen daily in almost any hospital when meperidine (Demoral) is prescribed for acute pain. Frequently, an order is written for meperidine to be given at 50 to 75 mg doses every four hours, although virtually all persons with acute pain report the need for the drug at higher doses at two to three hour intervals. The patients' needs are in fact in accordance with the drug's pharmacologic actions, though not with its "common usage."

Setting Appropriate Goals

In evaluating pain as a symptom, a decision must be made as to whether the pain is of sufficient importance to warrant further medical evaluation or even therapy. Sporadic, transient pain is part of the daily activity of living, often initiated by sudden motion or anxiety. It is only when this pain becomes a prominent feature or begins to interfere with daily function that medical help is sought. Similarly, the presence of chronic debilitative disease such as arthritis may never allow one to be free from some discomfort. Help is sought only when the level of pain is such as to interfere with daily activities. A specific set of goals and objectives must be developed for each person in pain, consistent with the expectation of the individual, rather than that of the physician. These objectives should be openly discussed with the patient and, if appropriate, the family.

Determining Whether Drug Therapy Is Indicated

In many instances, pain may be relieved without the use of any medication (Table 13.6). Although it is much easier to take a "pill" for relief, depending on the cause of the discomfort, medication may not, in fact, be helpful or may even be contraindicated.

PRINCIPLES OF PHARMACOLOGIC THERAPY

Once it is decided that drug therapy is needed, there are certain principles that should be followed in order to assure maximal relief[3] (Table 13.7).

TABLE 13.6. Nonpharmacologic Methods for Pain Relief

Behavioral
Biofeedback
Imagery
Meditation
Relaxation
Physical
Active and passive exercise
Acupuncture
Application of heat or cold
Transcutaneous electrical nerve stimulation
Surgical nerve block or receptors

TABLE 13.7. Principles of Pharmacologic Treatment of Pain

Identify the source of pain and select a specific drug therapy.
Develop appropriate objectives.
Start with the weakest analgesic that can provide relief.
Individualize route of administration.
Give each drug an adequate trial.
Do not use analgesics on an as-needed (PRN) basis.[a]
Use equianalgesic doses when changing analgesics.
Be aware of side effects and treat prophylactically when possible.
Avoid excessive sedation.
Be aware of dependence and tolerance.
Use drug combinations carefully.
Confront personal biases.

[a]In acute pain states

Those principles that must be modified, depending on whether the pain is acute or chronic, will be discussed in Chapter 14.

Identify Source of Pain and Select a Specific Drug Therapy

A knowledge of the existing pathophysiology as well as the mechanism of a drug's action (Table 13.8) will facilitate selection of appropriate therapy. Pain caused predominantly by specific organ system pathology may often be best treated with analgesics only in the acute stages to provide immediate relief. The primary treatment of pain of infectious origin is antibiotics, initially combined with anti-inflammatory drugs. The sole use of analgesics is contraindicated because alleviation of symptoms may allow for progression of the underlying infection. Arthritic pain of metabolic origin, such as gout, responds quickly to the use of drugs affecting uric acid metabolism. Similarly, administration of analgesics for abdominal pain in the absence of an etiologic diagnosis may result in a masking of potentially catastrophic states, such as perforation. Ischemic cardiac pain or angina may be promptly relieved by vasodilators, beta blockers, or calcium channel blockers; however, effective analgesia with narcotic agents may occur only when relatively high doses are administered. Muscular pains may not require oral analgesia, but rather an injection of a local anesthetic to affect trigger-point activity after exercise. Pain secondary to neoplastic disease may be modified by radiation, chemotherapy, or hormonal treatment rather

TABLE 13.8. Mechanisms of Action of Drugs Used to Relieve Pain

Mechanism	Drugs
Interference with conduction of pain in peripheral pathways	Local anesthetics
Alteration of central nervous system perception of pain	Narcotics
Interference with release of substances mediating pain peripherally	Antipyretics
Relief of anxiety or depression	Sedatives, hypnotics, tranquilizers, antidepressants, marijuana
Alteration of consciousness	Anesthetics/hypnotics
Reversal of specific pathophysiology	
Infection	Antibiotics
Inflammation	Anti-inflammatory agents
Gout	Hypouricemic agents
Vasospasm	Vasodilators
Muscle spasm	Muscle relaxants
Vasodilation	Vasospastic agent

than long-term use of analgesic agents, although acute administration of analgesic is often warranted for immediate relief.

DEVELOP APPROPRIATE OBJECTIVES

Prior to prescribing an analgesic, it is essential to develop short-term as well as long-term objectives that can be clearly agreed upon by both patient and physician. Included in this must be an understanding by both physician and patient that if relief is not obtained, existing concerns will be readily discussed. This is especially important in the treatment of chronic pain, which, depending on the etiology, may either not be able to be completely controlled or may require considerable effort to achieve adequate analgesia.

Start with Weakest Analgesia That Can Provide Relief

Effective analgesia should be attempted with the weakest analgesic able to relieve the pain, associated with the least side effects. The World Health Organization has described the analgesic ladder, which uses progressively more potent drugs as the severity of the pain increases. Analgesics can

generally be divided into three groups: (1) the nonnarcotic (opioid) or peripherally active analgesics (acetaminophen, aspirin, the NSAIDs) and the antidepressants for neuropathy comprise the first step of treatment; (2) the centrally
acting analgesics (opioid and opioid antagonists) comprise the second step;
and (3) increased doses of more potent opioids (step 3) used as the pain
becomes more severe. In addition there are a number of nonrelated drugs that
may be of value in treating specific painful states.

Nonnarcotic (Nonopioid) Analgesics

These drugs are the most widely used analgesics for mild and even
moderate pain. In most instances, the use of aspirin 300 to 600 mg or
acetaminophen 300 to 600 mg orally every four hours will be sufficient.
Controlled studies have repeatedly demonstrated that the analgesia produced by aspirin is superior to that produced by placebo and equally effective as the usual doses of commonly used weak narcotic drugs. As discussed
in Chapter 5, a number of special aspirin preparations have appeared commercially in an attempt to promote better analgesia (Table 13.9). Although
the effectiveness of these preparations depends on the rapidity of the aspirin
absorption from the gastrointestinal tract, a poor correlation exists between
blood salicylate levels and analgesic effects. The use of enteric-coated aspirin is associated with a minimal degree of gastric irritation as compared to
other preparations.[4-7] The difficulty with using these drugs as the severity of
the pain increases is that they all exhibit a "ceiling effect" to analgesia, and
the risk of toxic effects increases with increased doses. However, it is
important to remember, with respect to the NSAIDs, that failure of one drug
to obtain relief does not mean another NSAID will not be effective.

Narcotic (Opioid) Analgesics

The opioids (Chapters 6 and 7), both the pure agonists and the mixed
agonist-antagonist, all have the potential to cause dependency and tolerance with chronic use, as well as withdrawal when stopped abruptly. The
intensity of these reactions depends on both dose and duration of use. The
narcotic antagonist-agonists are believed to present less of a problem with
dependence than the pure agonists. However, objective evidence of this is
not overwhelming. The opioid agonists may be used either orally or intramuscularly, depending on the clinical setting. The specific drug selected
should be readily absorbed from the gastrointestinal tract and associated
with minimum side effects. Codeine, the most widely used narcotic analgesic for mild to moderate pain, is accepted as a standard for comparison

TABLE 13.9. Summary of Commonly Used Aspirin Preparations*

	Claims	Observations
Plain aspirin	Rapid effective analgesia	Role of absorption determined by dissolution rate. No studies indicating one brand superior over others.
Buffered tablets	Variably diminish gastric acidity	Equal degree of gastric irritation as plain aspirin.
	Increase in rate of absorption	No evidence of more rapid analgesia.
Buffered solutions	Diminish gastric acidity	Less gastric irritation due to increased buffer.
	Increase in rate of absorption	More rapidly absorbed; high sodium content; alkinization of urine results in increase in urine salicylate and lower plasma levels.
Enteric-coated time release	Less gastric irritation	Less gastric irritation due to dissolution mainly in small bowel.
	Prolonged analgesia	Absorption delayed by prolongation of analgesia questionable.

*See also Chapter 5

286

for drugs in this category. Although effective in relieving pain, codeine is quite capable of producing all of the adverse effects seen with other more potent opioids. The incidence of serious side effects, however, is rather low and, when combined with its low cost, codeine is the narcotic agent of choice in treatment of mild to moderate acute pain.

Moderate to severe pain will usually require the use of more potent analgesics, either parenteral if the pain is acute, or orally in chronic pain. It is important to emphasize that one should be aware of equianalgesic doses of both opioid and nonopioid analgesics to allow for a smooth transition once a decision has been made to administer another analgesic drug (Tables 13.10 and 13.11).

Individualize Route of Administration

The route of administration should suit the patient's needs (see Table 13.10), which depend on the pain intensity. The commonly used routes are oral, rectal, transdermal, or parenteral.

Parenteral use will provide rapid, effective analgesia but will also be accompanied by a more rapid development of tolerance. Parenteral analgesics may be given by the intramuscular, intravenous, or intrathecal routes. Intramuscular injection results in a relatively slow onset with highly variable plasma levels that may result in therapeutic levels only one-third of the time with the patient being either under- or overdosed in the interim.

Intravenous injections provide rapid analgesia but also can result in "peak and valley" levels of the drug in the bloodstream. A continuous intravenous infusion can regulate this, but it requires intensive nursing supervision to monitor the infusion rate. On the other hand, patient-controlled analgesia, as described later in this chapter, allows for improved pain control with less nursing care, lower effective dose with better analgesics, and less respiratory problems.

Intrathecal analgesics, the placement of a catheter within the membrane of the spinal cord, can provide steady analgesia with less systemic side effects. However, it is often associated with a spinal headache. In addition it may be cumbersome for the person to move about without anxiety.

Most recently an implantable pump with an inextinguishable power supply has been approved by the Food and Drug Administration to continuously administer intrathecally a preservative-free form of morphine. This is felt to be quite advantageous for those in severe pain who no longer respond to conventional analgesics. Other such pumps are also on the market. Their effectiveness in relieving pain on a long-term basis remains to be determined as the use of these devices increases.

TABLE 13.10. Commonly Used Routes of Administration of Analgesic Modification

ROUTE	ADVANTAGES	DISADVANTAGES
Oral	Useful for mild and moderate pain Widely available Administered at home by patient	Side effects may limit dose Ceiling effect with nonnarcotic analgesics
Rectal	Easy to administer if person unable to take by mouth Continuous administration without infusion Administered at home by patient	May not be accepted Side effects Slow onset of action Possible risk of infection if immunocompromised
Transdermal (Fentanyl)	Long duration of action with single patch Useful in severe pain in home setting Continues administration without needles	Absorption may be variable Side effects not as easy to reverse Slow onset action Difficult to modify dose rapidly Local skin irritation May require short active drug for breakthrough pain
Intramuscular/Subcutaneous Injection	More rapid onset than oral route	Slow onset compared to intravenous route Variable plasma levels
Subcutaneous Infusion	Pain relief if intravenous access not possible Can be used at home	Only limited volume can be administered Irritation at infusion on site Requires infusion pump and skilled nursing support

ROUTE	ADVANTAGES	DISADVANTAGES
Intravenous Infusion	Rapid pain relief No limitation on volume Permits dose titration by patient	Requires infusion pump and skilled nursing support Local infection and infiltration may occur
Epidural/Intrathecal Infusion	Local anesthetics can be added	Increased rate of tolerance Local infections Skilled physicians and nurses needed Spinal headache may occur Urinary retention possible Infusion pump needed Limits patient mobility

Adapted from *Clinical practice guidelines: Management of cancer pain*, 1994 (9); U.S. Department of Health and Human Services, Washington, DC: pp. 42, 43.

TABLE 13.11. Equianalgesic Doses of Mild to Moderate Analgesics

	Trade Name	Oral dose (mg)	Frequency of Administration (hours)
Acetaminophen		650-975	4-6
Aspirin		650-975	4-6
Codeine		32	4-6
Diflunisal*	Dolobid	250-500	12
Etodolac	Lodine	200-400	6-8
Fenoprofen	Nalfon	200	4-6
Ibuprofen	Motrin	400-600	6
Ketoprofen	Orudis	25-75	6-8
Magnesium Salicylate		650	4
Meclofenamate	Meclomen	50-100	4-6
Meperidine		300	2-3
Naproxen*	Naprosyn	250	6-8
Naproxen sodium*	Anaprox	275	6-8
Pentazocine	Talwin	150	3-4
Propoxyphene		65	4
Salsalate	Disalcid	500	4
Sodium salicylate		325-650	3-4
Trisilate		1,000-1,500	12

*Loading dose required

290

Oral administration, although accompanied by a slower onset of action, will result in a longer duration of analgesia and has additional advantages: it allows a person the psychological reassurance of not needing to take a drug frequently in order to be pain-free, and also allows a continuation of daily activities unencumbered by the need for injections. Similarly, rectal administration in a person unable to take analgesics by mouth allows for self-administration at home without the need for skilled nursing care. Transdermal administration also provides a person with the ability to self-administer medications without focusing on the need to take a drug at fixed time intervals. Each of these routes has its advantages and drawbacks with respect to both acceptability as well as consistency of analgesia (see Table 13.10).

If a change in route of administration is to be made, it is essential to utilize equianalgesic doses in order to provide a smooth transition. Administration of an inadequate dose will result in withdrawal reactions accompanied by a reappearance of pain and anxiety. Administration of a larger dose may result in excessive sedation or even respiratory depression.

Determine Frequency of Analgesic Administration

Analgesic medications should be prescribed regularly "around the clock" in the presence of acute pain or exacerbations of chronic pain. The intervals between administration should be sufficiently short to avoid drastic changes in pain levels. Both laboratory and clinical studies have shown that anxiety will cause an increased need for narcotics, thus setting up a vicious cycle for pain relief (Chapter 3). Sufficient plasma levels must be present at all times to provide effective analgesia. In treating chronic pain, the narcotic requirement over a 24-hour period should be calculated and a long-acting narcotic administered. "Breakthrough" analgesia with a short-acting narcotic should be available if needed.

It is unfortunate, but nonetheless true, that physicians more often than not prescribe narcotics at sufficiently infrequent intervals to allow for the appearance of anxiety and anticipatory pain. Inadequate pain control, ranging from moderate to severe and distressing pain, has been reported in as many as 73 percent of patients in pain.[8-11] At times, even if the interval between narcotic dosage is appropriate, the prescription is written for the drug to be given on an "as needed" (PRN) basis. Although PRN medication in acute pain is, in fact, contraindicated, many physicians still feel that this prescription will result in a better control of narcotic dosage, as well as a lesser likelihood of developing tolerance and dependence. This is incorrect.

When medication is ordered PRN, it requires a person to (1) ask for an analgesic, (2) have this request filtered through the nursing staff, and (3) wait in considerable pain for variable intervals prior to each injection, with many patients counting the minutes until they are permitted to receive their next injection.

In addition to providing adequate analgesia, administration of analgesics at regular intervals will also reduce anticipatory anxiety and decrease the total amount of analgesics required. Of equal importance, a person will develop a feeling of comfort and reassurance with his or her physician.

Individual physician resistance to regular administration of analgesics can be easily overcome by use of patient-controlled analgesia (Chapter 14). As noted previously, studies comparing the effectiveness of patient-controlled intravenous analgesia with traditional methods have suggested that this technique is associated with a lesser dosage, fewer complications, and more rapid and prolonged analgesia. Patients using this technique can appear to achieve pain relief without becoming high or developing undesirable side effects[12-14] (Chapter 14). In addition, the actual length of stay may be reduced by 20 to 30 percent.

Patient-controlled analgesia, however, does require the patient to focus on the pain in order to adjust both the narcotic dose and frequency of administration. For this reason, appropriate physician prescription of an analgesic in sufficient doses at frequent intervals is still preferred by many. A compromise solution is for orders to be written with several possible doses. The person would then be asked at each interval if additional pain relief is needed to warrant the larger dose. This allows for both patient control of symptom relief, as well as appropriate flexibility in dosage due to fluctuation in pain intensity.

Give Each Drug an Adequate Trial

When a specific drug is chosen, it must be given an adequate trial before considering it ineffective and switching to another agent. Use of the more potent NSAIDs may often result in relief of moderate pain without the need for the narcotic analgesics. Several of these drugs (Dolobid, Postel, Anaprox, and Toradol) require a loading dose in order to provide the most effective pain relief. Ketorolac (Toradol), the only injectable NSAID, has been shown to be effective in moderate to severe pain, producing analgesia comparable to morphine 12 mg or meperidine (Demerol) 100 mg when given intramuscularly. Its duration of action (six hours) is also considerably longer than Demerol.

Although combining different NSAIDs does not provide any additional analgesia, individual differences do exist between the ability to obtain pain relief from a specific agent. If one NSAID is not effective, another can be tried. In the presence of severe, noninflammatory pain, however, narcotic analgesics remain the most effective agents.

A decision concerning a specific analgesic should also take into consideration the cost of the drug prescribed. The cost of analgesics may vary greatly and may be of specific importance when prescribing large quantities of analgesics for patients in chronic pain.[8]

Use Equianalgesic Doses When Changing Analgesics

Once a decision has been made concerning the severity of the pain and whether an oral or an injectable analgesic is preferred, there is rarely a need to change narcotic analgesics unless the analgesic dose is such that (1) on a volume basis, the administration of a more potent agonist will result in the injection of a smaller volume or the ingestion of a lesser number of pills; (2) individual sensitivity exists to a particular drug; or (3) coexisting renal or hepatic diseases are present. The most frequent reason given for changing narcotics, that of ineffective analgesia, is rarely valid. Most often, a therapeutic failure is due to inadequate dosage or inappropriate frequency of administration. It should also be emphasized that changing drugs does not lessen the risk of addiction if the drugs used are all within the same pharmacologic group.

If a decision is made to change analgesics, initial equianalgesic doses must be given (Table 13.12).[11,12] When converting to another opioid, the easiest method is to calculate the total dose taken over 24 hours and then initially administer two-thirds of that dose, utilizing the appropriate frequency and equivalent dose of the new drug.

There are, however, differences between the narcotic analgesics that must be recognized. Since methadone is a long-acting analgesic, its initial use will be accompanied by slowly rising plasma levels that may result in excessive sedation during the first day of therapy. The dose, therefore, may need to be adjusted, especially when used in the elderly. The use of the narcotic agonist-antagonists should not begin if the person has been taking a pure narcotic analgesic for relief until this drug has been eliminated from the system. Prescribing an agonist-antagonist while levels of a narcotic analgesic exists in the body can precipitate withdrawal.

Be Aware of Side Effects

The use of analgesics, similar to other drugs, is associated with side effects. These are discussed fully in the sections describing the different groups of drugs. In order to better evaluate the potential for developing a

TABLE 13.12. Equianalgesic Doses of Commonly Used Potent Analgesics[a]

Trade name	Dose (mg) i.m.	Freq (hr)	Dose (mg) p.o.	Freq (hr)
Morphine	10	3-4	30	3-4
Buprenorphine (Temagesic)	0.4	6-8	NA	
Butorphanol (Stadol)	2-3	3-4	NA	
Codeine	75	3-4	130	2-4
Diacetylmorphine (Heroin)	5	NA	NA	
Fentanyl[c]	0.1	2	NA	
Hydromorphone (Dilaudid)	1.5		8	
Ketorolac[c]	30	6		
Levorphanol	2	6-8	4	6-8
Meperidine (Demerol)	75-100	3	300	2-3
Methadone	10	6-8	20	6-8
Oxymorphone (Numorphan)	1	3-4	NA	
Oxycodone[b]	NA		30	3-4
Nalbuphine (Nubain)	10	3-4	NA	
Hydrocodone (Lorcet, Lortab, Vicodan)	NA		30	3-4
Pentazocine (Talwin)	NA		30	4-6

[a]See also Chapters 5,6,7.
[b]Oral forms commonly available containing 4.5 mg oxycodone HCl, 0.38 mg oxycodone terephthalate, and 325 mg aspirin (Percodan, Percobarb) or 500 mg acetaminophen (Percocet 5, Tylox).
[c]Available now in patch form for one-month lasting analgesia.
NA = Not available

side effect from a specific analgesic, it is helpful to understand the terms pharmacokinetics and pharmacodynamics.

Pharmacokinetics describes what the body does to a drug to effect its absorption, distribution, and metabolism. Although the pharmacokinetics of a drug are well defined before appearing on the market, individual variability can result in considerable differences. Most adverse drug reactions are related to the variability in elimination of the drug from the body. This is of most concern in persons with liver or kidney disease since most drugs are either excreted in the urine or metabolized in the liver.

Pharmacodynamics describes what the drug does to the body through its action on the tissues or at specific receptors. In control of pain, often drugs with different mechanisms of action are used simultaneously in order to heighten analgesia while diminishing the adverse effects that might occur if a single drug was used at a higher dose. A prime example is the use of aspirin or acetaminophen with narcotics such as codeine or oxycodone. Use of agents that have identical mechanisms of action, however, may cause adverse effects. The use of narcotics and drugs in the sedative group, which both result in central nervous system depression, is an example.

Concerning the narcotics (opioids), it is important to emphasize that the frequency of serious side effects is in reality quite low when compared to the frequency of inadequate analgesia usually accompanying their use. Respiratory depression, the most serious narcotic side effect, rarely develops with appropriate prescribing practices. Tolerance to the analgesic effects of narcotics necessitating increased doses is accompanied by tolerance to respiratory depression, making overdose unlikely.

Avoid Excessive Sedation

When opioid analgesics are needed, the patient should be watched closely to make certain that excessive sedation is avoided. It is important to emphasize that when opioids are prescribed appropriately for chronic pain, although drowsiness may initially occur at times accompanied by mental clouding, these symptoms usually subside within several days. In fact, once pain is relieved and the person becomes tolerant to the sedative effects of the drug, cognitive and psychomotor function is little impaired.[14,15]

The use of sedatives and hypnotics, such as barbiturates, nonbarbiturate hypnotics, or benzodiazepines as discussed earlier, may result in respiratory depression or excessive sedation and at times even delirium. Although these drugs can be used concomitantly with narcotic agents when appropriately monitored, the indication for their use should never be to enhance analgesia.

Be Aware of Dependence and Tolerance

The most common rationale accompanying the physician prescription of inadequate analgesia or a person's refusal to take a narcotic analgesic for relief is the fear of addiction on the part of both physician and patient. One should always be aware of the potential to develop dependence with subsequent tolerance to the analgesic effects of narcotics. However, if satisfactory analgesia cannot be obtained with the use of nonnarcotic analgesics, a fear of dependence should not be a contraindication to administering a narcotic. As discussed earlier (Chapter 3), the appropriate administration of narcotics to provide analgesia is rarely in and of itself associated with addiction.[16,17] Dependence that will develop with medically supervised chronic use is important only due to the development of tolerance to the analgesic effect. For this reason, the dose of narcotic should be increased or decreased as needed, corresponding to alterations in levels of pain intensity. Withdrawal from narcotics once the source of pain has been removed can be easily accomplished.

Dependence or addiction to narcotics, however, is a real risk when these drugs are prescribed in the absence of any cause of pain. In such situations, often the drug is taken for the high that can be obtained by varying the dose and the frequency of administration. For this reason, these drugs should never be prescribed in a cavalier manner. Yet, when an indication exists in the presence of either acute or chronic pain, they should be used appropriately with the primary object being relief of pain.

Use Drug Combinations Carefully

Combinations of drugs should be administered only when additional specific effects are desired.[16,17,18] The rational behind their use is to: (1) provide more effective analgesia while diminishing the incidence of side effects; (2) address existing anxiety concerning the pain; and (3) diminish the risk of narcotic dependence. Although analgesic combinations are often effective, at other times the rational for their use is less than clear.

Over- the-Counter Analgesics

Analgesic combinations of aspirin, acetaminophen, or other NSAIDs are exceedingly common in prescription as well as over-the-counter medications. It is generally believed that caffeine, in combination with aspirin, is particularly useful in the presence of central nervous system depression. The evidence of any increased effectiveness of these combinations, however, remains to be proven.[19] In addition, the amount of caffeine is usually less than one would obtain through drinking a cup of coffee. The use of caffeine combined with aspirin or acetaminophen for analgesia is believed to be helpful only when over 60 mg of caffeine is taken.

Aspirin-, Acetaminophen-Opioid Combinations

Aspirin in combination with pentobarbital, promazine, or propoxyphene has not been reported to be more effective than aspirin alone. Combinations of aspirin or acetaminophen with codeine, oxycodone, and pentazocine can result in an enhanced analgesic effect and, at times, allow a lower narcotic dose to be prescribed. None of these combinations offer any major advantage with respect to time required to achieve analgesia or duration of analgesia. A slight but definitive sedative effect is also noted with respect to aspirin in combination with propoxyphene, codeine, pentazocine, and oxycodone. The use of aspirin or acetaminophen combinations, when taken chronically, may also be accompanied by opioid dependence. Furthermore, if used inappropriately, such combination in high dosage will produce euphoria and addiction indistinguishable from that occurring with use of only a narcotic agent. Chronic use of aspirin combinations also creates the risk of gastrointestinal side effects when aspirin is used as a single agent, especially when high doses are needed to relieve pain.

Other Combinations Used to Promote Analgesia

Combinations of analgesics with other psychotropic agents may be indicated, depending on the specific circumstances (Table 13.13). The use of tricyclic antidepressants has been found to be an effective adjunct in therapy for persons who suffer from depression as a response to pain. In addition, as described in Chapter 6 the use of tricyclics or fluphenazine, a phenothiazine derivative in combination with a narcotic, can result in more effective analgesia. When administered alone, these drugs may diminish certain types of pain without the need for analgesics (Chapters 10 and 11).

In the treatment of acute pain, combinations of amphetamine and morphine have also resulted in potentiation of analgesia associated with the need for a lower dose of morphine as well as a diminution in central nervous system depression (Chapter 6). The use of hydroxyzine in combination with narcotics in treating acute pain has also been reported to reduce required morphine without any adverse increase in sedative effects (Chapter 10). When used in epidural analgia with morphine, clondine has been observed to increase the duration of morphine action by almost twofold.

TABLE 13.13. Psychoactive Agents Used in Treatment of Pain

Amphetamines
Carbamazepine
Butyrophenones
Haloperidol
Hydroxyzine
Phenothiazines
Chlorpromazine
Fluphenazine
Phenytoin[a]
Tricyclic antidepressants

[a]Primarily for pain associated with tic douloureux

Baclofen (Lioresal), a GABA Beta agonist, has recently been shown to considerably enhance morphine analgesia postoperatively. However, due to the frequent adverse reactions associated with its use, more clinical trials are needed.[20]

Combinations of analgesics with the benzodiazepines (Valium, Librium) frequently occur in the hospital setting under the premise that more effective pain relief can be obtained with a lower dose of narcotic analgesic. This is incorrect. The result of such combinations is most often increased sedation with persistent pain. As a result, the patient is often confused, yet, still in pain. Since these drugs can also centrally depress respiration when used with narcotics associated with an independent risk of dependence, their use should be avoided. A patient in pain who does not obtain relief with a narcotic analgesic should have the dose or the frequency of administration increased rather than be given a benzodiazine.

The concurrent administration of anti-inflammatory drugs with analgesics devoid of specific anti-inflammatory properties may be associated with a marked decrease in arthritic pain. In such conditions, however, the use of aspirin or a NSAID as sole medication will often result in appropriate relief. Combinations of anti-inflammatory agents and analgesics, therefore, should be reserved for individuals either unable to tolerate aspirin or NSAIDs or to obtain satisfactory analgesia despite appropriate use of these agents.

Confront Personal Biases

One of the most prominent factors responsible for inadequate pain relief is bias toward the use of analgesics, especially those in the narcotic group. On the part of the physician treating acute pain, an unreasonable fear of addiction often prevents appropriate analgesic prescription. In treating chronic pain, very often the frustration expressed by a person whose pain is unable to be relieved is perceived by the physician as manipulative in order to obtain mood-altering drugs. This is especially true if the origin of the pain cannot be precisely defined or if the intensity of the pain or the associated disturbance in function is greater than the physician thinks reasonable. In such circumstances, it is essential that the physician be nonjudgmental and carefully and appropriately assess the pain so that relief can be provided.

The bias of one in pain can also prevent adequate analgesia. The fear of addiction to narcotics often allows the pain to become much more intense than is necessary before medication is requested. This results in considerable anxiety and the need for a greater amount of medication to provide relief. Often a person who fears addiction will insist on taking tranquilizers rather than an opioid even though the former, in reality, is associated with an equal, if not greater risk of dependency and will not relieve the pain. Persons with chronic pain will often insist on taking a short-acting rather than a long-acting opioid such as methadone. This is due to their fear that taking methadone will label them "addicts" since methadone is also used in maintenance therapy for heroin addiction.

Finally, persons with chronic pain syndromes have often experienced such frustration in negotiating the health care system without obtaining relief that they are predisposed to believe that physicians will never take their complaints seriously, especially when their analgesic requirements are greater than usual due to the development of tolerance. In such instances, adequate patient-physician relationships are unable to develop, and often the amount of narcotic needed to provide relief is overstated in an attempt to obtain appropriate medication. All of these biases must be addressed by both physician and patient in order to afford relief.

The Use of Placebos

The use of placebos in the treatment of pain is often accompanied by greater risks than benefits and may seriously affect the patient-physician relationship.[21,22,23] Placebos cannot be utilized to assess the prominence of psychological components of pain as up to 30 to 40 percent of persons with of organic pain may obtain relief with placebos. Correspondingly, when administered in a laboratory setting, narcotics may not be accompanied by an analgesic response even though, when given clinically, consistent analgesia is seen (Chapter 4).

Unfortunately, all too frequently physicians are unaware of the effectiveness of placebos in treating organic pain. Physicians most often prescribe placebos not to relieve suffering but to prove that the pain is without organic basis. Placebos are given to patients who are disliked or are suspected of exaggerating their symptoms. There is little evidence to suggest that pain relieved by placebo is not real. In fact, evidence suggests just the opposite. Malingerers and narcotic addicts are often less likely to report relief with placebos.

One survey of the use of placebos in a teaching hospital found that placebo misuse not only resulted from a lack of knowledge but also from a feeling of frustration in attempting to provide analgesia.[20] Placebos were given to patients in situations where extreme physician-patient or staff-patient conflicts had developed. The use of placebos under such conditions can only worsen the physician-patient relationship and exacerbate the symptoms.

SUMMARY

Relief of pain can best be obtained if a thoughtful approach is carried out by both the physician and the person in pain. This is not difficult. Even if complete relief is not possible, which may be the case for some chronic pain, an understanding of the cause of the pain, as well as what can be done by both physician and patient to minimize it, will allow the patient to better tolerate the discomfort and to continue his or her daily activities.

REFERENCES

1. U.S. Agency for Health Care Policy and Research. *Acute pain management: Operative or medical procedures and trauma*. Rockville, MD. U.S. Department of Health and Human Services; 1992, 14.

2. Twycross RG. Pain and analgesics. *Curr Med Res Opin,* 1978, 5:497–505.

3. Stimmel B. Pain, analgesia, and addiction: An approach to the pharmacologic management of pain. *Clin J of Pain*, 1985, 1:14–22.

4. Halpern LM. Analgesic drugs in the management of pain. *Arch Surg,* 1977, 112:861–869.

5. Cronk GA. Laboratory and clinical studies with buffered and nonbuffered acetylsalicylic acid. *N Engl J Med,* 1958, 258:219–221.

6. Blythe RH, Grass GM, MacDonnell DR. The formulation and evaluation of enteric coated aspirin tablets. *Am J Pharm,* 1959, 131:206–216.

7. Lanza FL, Royer GL, Jr, Nelson RS. Endoscopic evaluation of the effects of aspirin, buffered aspirin, and enteric-coated aspirin on gastric and duodenal mucosa. *N Engl J Med*, 1980, 303: 136–138.

8. Marks RM, Sachar EJ. Undertreatment of medical inpatients with narcotic analgesics. *Ann Intern Med,* 1973, 78:173–181.

9. Charap AD. The knowledge, attitudes and experience of medical personnel treating pain in the terminally ill. *Mt Sinai J Med,* 1978, 45:561–580.

10. Oden RV. Acute postoperative pain: Incidence, severity, and the etiology of inadequate treatment. *Anesthesiol Clin of North Am,* 1989, 7:1–15.

11. Donovan M, Dillon P, McGuire L. Incidence and characteristics of pain in a sample of medical surgical patients. *Pain,* 1987, 30:69–78.

12. McIntosh DG, Rayburn WF. Patient controlled analgesia in obstetrics and gynecology. *Obstet Gynecol,* 1991, 78:1129–1135.

13. Camp JF. Patient-controlled analgesia. *Family Physician,* 1991, 44:2145–2150.

14. Hanks GW. Morphine sans Morpheus. *Lancet,* 1995, 346:652–653.

15. Vainio A, Ollila J, Matikainen E, Rosenberg P, Kalso E. Driving ability in cancer patients receiving longterm morphine analgesia. *Lancet,* 1995, 346:667–670.

16. Angell M. The quality of mercy (editorial). *N Engl J Med,* 1992, 306:98–99.

17. Porter J, Jick H. Addiction rare in patients treated with narcotics. *N Eng J Med,* 1987, 302:123.

18. Beaver WT. Combination analgesics. *Am J Med,* 1984, 77:38–53.

19. Moertel CG, Ahmann DL, Taylor WF, Schwartzn N. Relief of pain by oral medications: A controlled evaluation of analgesic combinations. *JAMA,* 1974, 229:55–59.

20. Gordon NC, Gear RW, Heller PH, Paul S, Miaskowski C, Levine JD. Enhancement of morphine analgesia by the GABA B agonist baclofen. *Neuroscience,* 1995, 69:345–349.

21. Goodwin JS, Goodwin JM, Vogel AV. Knowledge and use of placebos by house officers and nurses. *Ann Intern Med,* 1979, 91:106–110.

22. Moertel CG, Taylor WF, Roth A, Tyce FA. Who responds to sugar pills? *Mayo Clin Proc,* 1976, 51:96–100.

23. Shapiro AK, Struening EL, Barten H, Shapiro E. Correlates of placebo reaction in an outpatient population. *Psychol Med,* 1975, 5:389–396.

Chapter 14

Management of Acute and Chronic Pain

INTRODUCTION

The principles to be followed in the management of pain are the same, regardless of whether the pain is acute or chronic (Chapter 13). There are, however, specific pragmatic differences between these two states (Table 14.1). Acute pain is associated with a specific injury to the body (nociceptive) that is usually easily identifiable, frequently expected (postoperative pain), and usually limited in time and location. Chronic pain, while often caused by tissue injury, may also be due to an injury to the central nervous system that disturbs the normal transmission of sensations (deafferentation pain) or may have a psychogenic component manifested by considerable pain without an obvious cause. The chronicity of the pain, regardless of cause, also produces psychologic disturbances that must be addressed if successful pain relief is to occur.

ACUTE PAIN

Acute pain often serves a useful physiologic purpose, signaling the presence of a potentially serious disturbance in homeostasis. If resulting from external forces, the pain focuses attention on the injured part and, by limiting motion, prevents further tissue damage. Although psychological factors are rarely primary in acute pain, as discussed in Chapter 4, the immediate response to severe injury may be pain-free if survival or "winning" rather than treatment is the immediate cause of concern. Once these feelings have subsided, pain may start to be experienced. In this setting, the autonomic response to pain is similar to that of anxiety states directing attention to treatment of the pain, as well as the accompanying anxiety to obtain effective relief.

Persistence of acute pain, however, does not only result in increasing discomfort but is also associated with the onset of a number of deleterious

TABLE 14.1. Comparison of Acute and Chronic Pain States

	Acute pain	**Chronic pain**
Relief of pain	+	+
Sedation	May be desirable	Avoid
Duration of analgesia	Until acute event subsides (hours to days)	As long as possible
Administration	At regular intervals	At regular intervals
Route	Parenteral may be preferred	Oral
Dose	Usually standard	Individually determined
Other medications	Not often required	Commonly required
Dependence and tolerance	Unusual	Common
Psychological component	Usually not prominent	May be major determinant of response

physiologic responses. As an example, chest pain (angina) in persons with coronary artery disease serves as a warning signal that the patient is engaging in a level of activity exceeding the capability of the arterial system to deliver sufficient oxygen to the heart muscle. Persistent angina indicates a continuing inadequate blood supply to the heart and can result in a heart attack, or myocardial infarction. Pain associated with a heart attack intensifies the physiologic response to pain with further deleterious effects.

Most episodes of mild or moderate acute pain resulting from nonintentional injury can be adequately treated with acetaminophen, aspirin, or one of the analgesic nonsteroidal anti-inflammatory drugs. Not infrequently, one of these agents combined with a mild narcotic can also provide adequate relief. Relief of severe acute pain, including postoperative pain, however, will usually require a narcotic drug. The choice of specific analgesics is discussed in Chapter 13. The following sections discuss the severe acute pain most often encountered after surgery.

Postoperative Pain

In the postoperative setting, pain is an expected response. It has been estimated that over 23 million operations are performed annually. Unfortunately, many are accompanied by pain that is not adequately treated.[1,2] The management of postoperative pain should, in fact, begin prior to the surgery during the time a history is taken by either the surgeon or the anesthesiologist. This history should include information concerning the patient's previous experience with pain (Table 14.2). It is most important to learn to what had been helpful in the past to relieve pain or whether the person is currently taking an analgesic that may result in a tolerance to the usual dose of a narcotic.

In addition to receiving information from the patient, the physician should also provide information as to what is to be expected when anesthesia wears off. The need for a person to be forthright about the intensity of the pain experienced, rather than adopting a stoical approach should be emphasized. If the analgesic is not effective or is being given too infrequently, this should also be brought to the physician's attention. If a person expresses concern over loss of control in obtaining effective pain relief, the possibility of patient-controlled analgesia (PCA) should be fully discussed and offered as an option, if appropriate.

Equally important to reassuring a person that the pain will be adequately controlled is the need to fully explain the surgery and the postsurgical environment. This is critical for those patients who will go directly from the operating room to the intensive care unit. These "high tech" units with their numerous monitors and alarms and the many tubes or lines that may be inserted into a person's body all serve to increase anxiety and lower the pain threshold. By knowing what to expect, anxiety will be diminished and pain easier to manage.

In relieving postoperative pain, a patient should be monitored constantly to be certain adequate analgesia is being obtained. Since considerable individual variation exists as to the dose that is required to obtain pain relief, the prescribed dose should be targeted to relieve pain without pro-

TABLE 14.2. Factors To Be Addressed in Preoperative Assessment of Pain Relief After Surgery[1]

Prior painful episodes and the person's response
Presence of concurrent medical conditions that might affect postoperative analgesic regimen
Most methods effective in obtaining pain relief
Attitudes toward use of narcotics or tranquilizing agents
Past history of chronic pain syndromes or current analgesic use that may result in tolerance to usual analgesic doses
Current expectations of postoperative pain

ducing excessive central nervous system depression. For the first 24 to 48 hours, the narcotic should be administered on a regularly scheduled basis; then, both frequency and dose should be adjusted to continue pain relief. It is important to remember that if a person is alert and in pain, the current dose of narcotic is insufficient, regardless of actual dose administered. Since the first sign of an excess of narcotic analgesia is sedation, an alert responsible person in pain is insufficiently medicated.

Inadequate analgesia may also be associated with adverse systemic effects. Increased pain may affect deep breathing and cough with the potential for atelectasis, pooling of secretions, and respiratory infections. Persistent abdominal pain may prolong the normal recovery period. Severe muscular discomfort associated with restricted movements may promote vascular stasis with subsequent slowing of blood flow, increasing clot formation. Once the source of acute pain has been clearly identified, therefore, it is quite important to provide adequate rapid analgesia.

Management of Severe Acute Pain

Clinically, the narcotic that is generally preferred for moderate to severe acute pain is meperidine (Demerol). The reasons for this are unclear but may relate to the misconceptions that synthetic narcotics are safer than morphine and that meperidine can prevent smooth muscle spasms, which reportedly occur with other narcotics. These beliefs persist despite the fact that when meperidine's analgesic effect is examined, little advantage with respect to toxicity, dependence, or addiction liability among narcotics is found. In addition, when given intramuscularly, meperidine is quite irritating and has a short duration of action. Finally, in postoperative patients who became delirious, the use of meperidine was found to significantly increase the risk of developing delirium.

It is unfortunate that the preference of physicians for meperidine is generally unrelated to their knowledge of its pharmacological actions. The customary meperidine prescription is usually 50 to 75 mg every four hours as needed (PRN) even though 100 to 150 mg is well within the therapeutic range for treatment of severe pain and is comparable to 10 mg of morphine. This results in inadequate analgesia and increased patient anxiety. The latter is most often handled by prescribing diazepam (Valium) 5 to 10 mg every eight hours and the addition of the phenothiazine phenergan to enhance analgesia. In such situations, pain remains unrelieved and the patient becomes sedated and at times confused.

The use of meperidine is also accompanied by the accumulation of a toxic metabolite normeperidine, which can cause increased irritability, confusion, and ultimately convulsions. Since normeperidine has a relatively long half-life of 15 to 20 hours and is excreted through the kidney, younger persons with impaired renal function as well as the elderly are particularly susceptible to these toxic effects. Meperidine is an effective analgesic but only when used appropriately. Its use in acute pain is most appropriate for short periods in healthy young people. Although all of the narcotic agonists or those with mixed agonist-antagonist characteristics can be effective if the dose is adjusted appropriately, if one disregards individual susceptibility, morphine provides the most effective analgesia with the least side effects for the least cost. In certain groups of persons, such as those with cardiac disease, the use of some of the narcotic antagonist-agonists analgesics is contraindicated due to their negative effects on cardiac muscle (Chapter 7).

Ketorolac, an injectable NSAID, has also been reported to provide effective relief without the need to use narcotic analgesics. Intramuscular Ketorolac is felt to be nonirritating to tissues and as effective as 12 mg of morphine but longer-acting.

In some cases, combinations of a narcotic with amphetamine or hydroxyzine may be helpful (Chapter 6). Some studies have also reported the effectiveness of indomethacin and NSAIDs in lowering the dose of narcotic analgesics needed.[3] These findings, if confirmed, may be helpful in cases of ambulatory surgery (when a person is discharged the same day). Other drugs may be used as adjunctive or even primary medications, depending on the etiology of the pain.

Patient-Controlled Analgesia (PCA)

Perhaps as a response to dissatisfaction by both physician and patients with providing effective analgesia, over the past several years PCA has become an increasingly acceptable and highly effective method of relieving postoperative pain.[1,4,5,6] With this technique, the patient is allowed to self-administer intravenous doses of narcotics as needed with limits of frequency and dose being set on the dispensing unit through "lock out" times. An example of PCA would be the ability to self-administer morphine at 1 mg per hour with a lock out time of eight to ten minutes. Even if the administration is too frequent, the resulting sedation usually prevents a person from "overdosing."

Numerous studies have not only demonstrated the effectiveness of PCA but, in addition, have documented the total narcotic analgesics requirement to be lower, the incidence of side effects less, and the hospital stay actually shortened by 20 to 30 percent.[4,5,6] As with any technique, monitoring is important and tolerance will develop with time.

Epidural or Intrathecal Analgesia

Frequently, postoperative analgesia may be obtained in an intensive care setting by infusing opioids through the membranes of the spinal cord in persons with abdominal or lower extremity pain. This technique is associated with a lower dose of opioid, a longer duration of action, and no risk of sedation. At times, infrequent side effects may occur, ranging from confusion, urinary infection, shock to respiration, and depression. As a result, this technique is best reserved for critically ill patients in specialized care centers.[1,7]

Analgesia Due to Locally Applied Opioids

Although the effects of opioids on the central nervous system are well known, evidence has recently been presented demonstrating the ability of narcotic agents to produce analgesia by local administration to peripheral nerve terminals. Morphine in systemically ineffective doses applied to intramarticular surfaces during knee surgery has resulted in significant reduction of pain similar in magnitude to commonly used local anesthetics.[8]

Summary

Acute pain of mild to moderate intensity can often be relieved by aspirin, acetaminophen, or the NSAIDs, alone or in combination with a narcotic agent (Chapter 13). If the pain is moderate to severe, an oral or injectable narcotic will usually be required to provide relief.

Once the cause of the pain has subsided, the narcotic, if administered for a relatively short time, may be abruptly discontinued without any major untoward effects. It should be noted, however, that administration of a narcotic around-the-clock for even several days can be associated with the production of a mild degree of dependence and a mild withdrawal reaction consisting of nervousness and irritability, usually clinically undetected. This is well tolerated by the patients and should not stand in the way of prescribing appropriate analgesia.

CHRONIC PAIN

Chronic pain, unlike acute pain, which may serve as a useful warning signal to impending physiologic damage, has minimal useful biologic function. In fact, its presence serves to severely restrict one's productive activities and frequently is also associated with considerable sociological and psychological disturbances. There are a variety of conditions responsible for the common presentation of nonmalignant pain. These include pain of central origin, headache, temporal mandibular pain (TMJ), trigeminal neuralgia, chronic muscle pain syndromes, low back pain, and arthritis.[9] It has been estimated that 14 percent of people suffer limitation of activity due to chronic pain, with 9 percent experiencing major limitations in their activities.

Regardless of the origin of the pain, however, it is apparent that relief is more often than not incomplete. This is not only due to inadequate prescribing patterns of physicians but also to persons' perceptions of the risks of taking analgesic medications. A national pain survey by Louis Harris and Associates found that 60 percent of persons in chronic moderate pain were reluctant to take analgesics for relief despite the pain being so debilitating that one-third were unable to engage in their normal activities for at least one out of every three days of the year. Even when treated, 50 percent continued to have pain while on analgesics.

CONDITIONS ASSOCIATED WITH CHRONIC PAIN

In the sections that follow, the incidence of pain in a variety of selected conditions will be discussed, followed by general principles of diagnosis and therapy. The chapter will end with a discussion of specific therapy for particularly vexing chronic pain states. Pain due to malignant diseases is of particular importance and will be discussed in Chapter 17.

Central Pain

The various causes of central pain syndrome (CPS) have been already discussed (Chapter 1), the most common being stroke although spinal cord injury, multiple sclerosis, and Parkinson's disease can all be associated with CPS. It has been estimated that as many as 100,000 persons in North America may be suffering from CPS and, unfortunately, many remain inadequately treated due to the lack of objective findings, resulting in physicians often being quite skeptical as to the degree of pain described.[10] In addition, due to the characteristics of CPS (Table 14.3), a person's understanding of the cause of the pain is often lacking. Since CPS also does not always respond well to narcotic analgesics, the mainstay of most chronic pain states, the anxiety accompanying CPS is also considerable, often contributing to persisting distress.

TABLE 14.3. Characteristics of Central Pain Syndrome

History of trauma to, or disorder of, the central nervous system.

Symptoms of pain usually appear distant in time to primary injury or disease.

Pain may vary greatly in intensity, but is poorly located, unremitting, or caused by stimuli not usually painful.

Physical examination cannot usually identify origin of pain.

Psychologic factors can markedly influence pain.

Headache

Headache is such a prevalent symptom that it almost defies demographic analysis. It has been estimated that at least 80 percent of the population suffer from headaches annually, with 20 percent seeking a physician's advice primarily due to this symptom. Severe disabling headaches may exist in up to 20 percent of men and 32 percent of women, resulting in a total cost to society of up to 10 billion dollars.[11]

Face and Jaw Pain

Pain in the jaw presenting with a constellation of symptoms labeled as temporomandibular disorders (TMD), temporal mandibular joint-myofascial pain dysfunction syndrome (MPDS), and craniomandibular dysfunction (CMD). These conditions afflict a large number of people. They are often associated with few physical findings, but nonetheless, accompanied by considerable disability, and pain that may be experienced whenever one speaks or eats. Facial pain due to disturbances of the fifth cranial nerve (Trigeminal neuralgia, tic douloureux) is an extremely painful paroxysmal condition that can cause persistent pain for weeks at a time. Although the cause of the pain may be related to pressure being placed on the nerve root, most often a specific physical cause cannot be identified.[12,25]

Muscle Pain Syndromes

There are several conditions associated with chronic muscle pain (myalgias) and fatigue (Table 14.4). Together they cause considerable numbers of people great pain and are often accompanied by depression and frustration. Frequently family life, interpersonal relationships, and social productivity are impaired. Those with these conditions are particularly frustrated in their attempts to obtain relief, as many health care providers are either unaware of the reasons for the pain or do not recognize these states as real clinical entities, attributing symptoms primarily to anxiety and depression.

Fibromyalgia and Myofacial Pain

Fibromyalgia (FS) is characterized by a generalized aching or muscular pain, tingling sensations (paresthesia), fatigue, and nonrestorative sleep, associated with specific identifiable trigger points in the involved muscles that may affect 2 to 6 percent of the population and other disorders including tension headaches, chronic fatigue syndrome, and temporomandibular joint syndrome.[12-17] Often this symptom complex is accompanied by bowel disturbances. The expression of the myofascial pain (MFP) syndrome is quite similar to fibromyalgia except it is more localized to several muscle groups. A variety of factors have been implicated as contributing to the pathophysiology of these disorders (Table 14.5). The identification of actual trigger points (Table 14.6) not only is helpful in providing local relief but firmly establishes the diagnosis. Although some feel that the presence of trigger points leads to a diagnosis of MFP rather than fibromyalgia when the pain is often diffuse and the relationship with trigger points

TABLE 14.4. Syndromes Associated with Chronic Muscle Pain

Chronic Fatigue Syndrome
Eosinophilia Myalgia Syndrome
Fibromyalgia
Myofascial Pain Syndrome
Lyme Disease

TABLE 14.5. Contributory Factors in Fibromyalgia

Dysfunction of Neurotransmitters
Abnormal Pituitary Hypothalamic Adrenal Axis
Serotonin Deficiency
Dysfunction of Immune System
Disturbed Central Pain System
Tissue Trauma

TABLE 14.6. Characteristics of Trigger Points Causing Muscle Pain

Deep localized tenderness in defined muscle groups
Presence of a defined tight muscle band
Eliciting a twitch response in affected muscle
Presence of referred pain similar to that experienced when stimulated

is less than clear, considerable overlap exists between these two conditions.

Chronic Fatigue Syndrome

Similar generalized symptoms when preceded by a viral infection are considered to be part of the clinical complex termed chronic fatigue syndrome (CFS). At times persons with this entity have been found to have high titers to Epstein Barr virus (EBV), as well as immunologic abnormalities. However, since EBV infections are extremely common, with many completely asymptomatic persons having elevated titers, its relationship to the CFS remains unclear.[18,19]

Eosinophilic Myalgia Syndrome

The eosinophilia myalgia syndrome, a condition associated with consuming contaminated preparations of tryptophan, is accompanied by diffuse myalgias, psychologic dysfunction, and markedly elevated eosinophil counts.

Joint Pains

Arthritis is another prevalent condition, believed to afflict 26 million persons. Of this group, it is estimated that 6 million have symptoms of sufficient intensity to markedly interfere with daily function. This disability is predominantly due to pain rather than actual mechanical limitations in joint mobility. Estimates in societal costs due to chronic arthritic pain exceed 13 billion dollars annually.

Low Back Pain

Low back pain is one of the most common causes of discomfort in the United States, affecting virtually everyone at some time during their life.

In persons under 45 years of age, it is the most common cause of disability. Although 90 percent of persons with acute low back pain will recover spontaneously within a month, the remainder will continue to have symptoms. A stratified sample of 1,135 persons between the ages of 18 and 64 found 18 percent to report the presence of low back pain, with 62 percent having pain of sufficient intensity to warrant radiologic evaluation and 4 percent having had surgery.[21] An estimated 2 to 5 percent of all adults will be partially or totally disabled due to back pain, with 15 percent incapacitated for up to six months at an annual cost to society of up to $50 billion.[9,20,22] Litigation frequently accompanies and perhaps intensifies complaints. One study of over 200 people with chronic pain involved in litigation revealed 63 percent to have primarily an emotional rather than an organic component.[23]

Summary

Chronic pain, regardless of etiology, is of considerable societal as well as individual concern because it affects nearly one-third of the American population, disabling over 50 million people at an annual loss of 700 million work days and 60 billion dollars.[18] It should be emphasized that in many instances, it is not the underlying pathology that produces the disability but rather the recurrent pain and its accompanying depression. It is, therefore, incumbent upon both physicians and patients to be aware of the multiple factors responsible for producing chronic pain as well as appropriate principles of management.

DIAGNOSIS

The approach to the patient in chronic pain is at times quite complex and not infrequently tests the physician's capacity to deal with this problem in a holistic manner. The initial evaluation must emphasize principles discussed earlier (Chapter 13) and address a number of objectives (Table 14.7). First, an accurate diagnosis as to the origin of the pain must be provided. This necessitates a careful medical history to make certain that appropriate measures have been undertaken to identify an organic basis. If organicity has not been able to be established, it is essential to convince oneself that nothing further can be done to identify a specific cause. The importance of this cannot be overstated. As a person with chronic pain moves from physician to physician in an attempt to obtain relief, the actual diagnostic tests done to identify the cause of the pain frequently become blurred. Successive physicians take at face value the patient's feeling that there is

TABLE 14.7. Objectives in the Evaluation of Chronic Pain

Establish an accurate diagnosis of the origin of the pain.
Identify existing iatrogenic factors.
Obtain a comprehensive and psychosocial assessment.
Obtain a complete description of the characteristics of the pain identifying all factors exacerbating or alleviating the pain intensity.

no identifiable cause and often relegate the symptoms to a psychogenic origin. In addition, even in the face of a known cause, a pain intensity greater than expected may indicate the presence of a concomitant, yet unrecognized problem.

However, it must also be mentioned that the presence of an abnormal finding on an extremely sensitive diagnostic test does not necessarily identify the cause of the pain. Magnetic resonance studies (MRIs) can frequently detect subtle abnormalities that exist in many people who have no discomfort. The physician must therefore carefully evaluate and interpret the significance of any abnormal results.

Psychosocial Assessment

Persons with nonmalignant chronic pain severely tax the physician's time and resources. Frequently they are considered "undesirable" patients. The most common physician responses are referrals to a psychiatrist, to a pain "specialist," or prescription of the requested medications. At times, if the patient appears satisfied, medication renewal occurs routinely. As a result, almost invariably the physician's response becomes problematic and may result in unnecessary diagnostic or therapeutic procedures that may cause further pain, and exacerbation of psychological disabilities. A complete psychiatric and psychosocial assessment is, therefore, mandatory (Table 14.8). This assessment should include the effects that the pain has had on family interrelationships as well as the extent of the secondary gain that the pain and disability have on everyday function.

At times this assessment may provide information suggesting that the experience of pain is more contrived than real or, at best, has a considerable psychologic overlay. Information elicited suggesting this includes obvious exaggeration of symptoms, willingness to undergo repetitive invasive procedures to document pain in spite of previous negative findings on similar examinations, refusal to allow a discussion of pain with immediate family members, continued self-manipulation known to exac-

TABLE 14.8. Psychosocial Evaluation of Chronic Pain

Encourage detailed, open discussion of pain experience.
Review typical day with respect to appearance of pain and limitation of activities.
Define effect of pain on employment history and current income, including disability income.
Assess family interrelationships, including the specific impact of the painful disorder.
Determine types of medication currently taken as well as specific reasons for any effects of each individual drug.

erbate pain, history of poor compliance with suggested treatment regimens, and resistance to a formal psychiatric evaluation.

Description of Pain Experience

It is most important to obtain a comprehensive description of the pain experience. The symptoms attributed to pain are often in reality due more to anxiety or, if narcotic dependence is present, to the onset of withdrawal. Consideration of factors precipitating or altering the intensity of the pain is also of value. By eliminating adverse environmental conditions, changing the frequency of analgesic administration, or improving the interactions between the patient and family members, the intensity of the pain can be diminished.

Classification

Persons with chronic pain can generally be categorized into one of several groups (Table 14.9).[26] The first consists of people who have no identifiable premorbid psychological dysfunction and an apparent organic cause of the pain. Chronic nonmalignant pain is extremely common, seen

TABLE 14.9. Categorization of Chronic Pain States

Physical cause with a normal premorbid personality
Physical cause present—previous personality disorder
No observable physical cause—identifiable previous personality disorder
Conscious malingering without any organic basis

in up to one-third of all cases. Although primary treatment is directed at the cause of the pain, related psychological symptoms, if present, should also be addressed. In the second group, a physical cause may or may not be present; however, some difficulty in psychological function can be identified prior to initiation of the painful event, and anxiety and depression are prominent. This includes individuals with cognitive impairments, often reflected as chronic pain syndrome in the elderly, the presence of situational stresses such as those seen in industrial-related injuries, chronic unremitting headaches, and readily identifiable personality disorders. In the third group, an obvious personality disorder exists in the absence of any identifiable cause of pain. These patients, presenting the greatest therapeutic challenge, have been termed polysymptomatic and are often seen among the "intractable" patients attending pain clinics.[26]

Finally, there are the true "malingerers," individuals who complain of chronic pain and present with symptoms associated with an identifiable disease state, but have no pathology. In some instances, these symptoms are used to obtain mood-altering drugs. In others, the need to identify with painful serious conditions represents a severe psychologic state, termed the Munchausen Syndrome. It is essential that prior to categorizing a person with chronic pain as a malingerer, a careful thoughtful evaluation is performed.

MANAGEMENT

Integrative Responses

The prevalence of chronic pain in numerous disorders of varying etiologies does not allow for a single explanation. Regardless of the neuroanatomical or physiological hypothesis, it must be emphasized that psychological factors also play an overwhelming role, and, as noted in Chapter 4, cannot be clearly separated from the "organic." As chronicity develops, the primary autonomic response to acute pain becomes less prominent, and signs and symptoms, such as sleep disturbances, irritability, and depression, appear. Alternatively, these reflexes may become hyperactive and serve as a further source of discomfort and anxiety. Finally, the environment in which the pain is experienced and the quality of existing interpersonal interactions further modify the pain response. All of these factors must be considered in addressing the management of chronic pain.

Available Nonpharmacologic Therapies

Currently available modalities for the management of chronic pain may be broadly classified as pharmacologic, anesthetic, surgical, physical, and psychological. The nonpharmacologic treatments may be divided into non-invasive and invasive (Table 14.10). Each of these techniques may be effective with specific disorders or in individuals with different disorders. Although the following discussion will focus on the pharmacological approach, it must be emphasized that in many instances the administration of analgesics or other mood-altering drugs may not be successful in patients with an exaggerated response to pain or with pain having no demonstrable organic cause. Not only will a psychotherapeutic approach be the most effective, but the prescription of analgesics will frequently give rise to dependence and addiction without any measurable effect on relief of pain. Similarly, many instances of chronic muscular pain cannot only be treated with exercise and relaxation techniques, but regular use of these modalities can often prevent recurrence and promote an overall feeling of well-being. Finally, educational approaches to help a person better understand his or her disease, as well as participate in therapeutic decisions, have also been shown to be effective in reducing pain.

Pain Clinics

Many persons with chronic pain can be treated effectively only by the multidisciplinary holistic approach available in pain clinics.[27-29] Clinics specializing in the treatment of pain provide a vast array of services that cut across disciplines. All current methods of treating pain are usually available. The staff, through their interest and availability, are knowledgeable in the pathophysiology of intractable pain as well as comfortable in dealing with patients' demands, which are considerable. Surprisingly, many patients en-

TABLE 14.10. Approaches to Treatment of Pain

Noninvasive	Invasive
Behavior modification	Acupuncture
Biofeedback	Ablative procedures
Heat	Cordotomy
Biogenics	Cingulotomy
Exercise	Sympathectomy
Hypnosis	Tractotomy
Ice massage	Laser Therapy
Pharmacologic	Central nervous system
Psychotherapy	stimulation of thalamic areas
Transcutaneous nerve	Percutaneous nerve
stimulation (TENS)	stimulation
Relaxation	
Stress Management	

tering a clinic may not be taking an analgesic or may be on these drugs despite their ineffectiveness in providing relief. Frequently, treatment may be directed toward interruption of pain pathways through nerve blocks or drugs other than analgesics. Studies have suggested that people able to participate in pain clinic regimens have a significant increase in functioning, including a return to work, as well as a decreased use of analgesics, especially those that are dependency-producing.[29]

Nonetheless, the majority of persons in chronic pain never visit a pain clinic. Even those who ultimately receive a referral have usually been unsuccessfully treated by their physicians and may often experience a considerable waiting time prior to a first appointment. Relapse following initial successful treatment may be high, and persons will frequently reject the concept of a "clinic" environment, regardless of how helpful it might be.[33] It is therefore essential that the available pharmacologic options available be known to both physicians and patients. The following discussion concerning the pharmacological approach to chronic pain is, therefore, directed toward the primary care physician, as well as his or her patients.

Analgesic Therapy

Although the basic tenet in treating chronic pain is to use the weakest analgesic effective in providing relief (Chapter 13), most persons seeking a physician's care have already run the gamut of over-the-counter and prescription drugs. With respect to oral analgesics, it should be repeated that there is little evidence to indicate that any of the weaker narcotics, such as codeine, propoxyphene, meperidine, and the narcotic antagonist-agonist pentazocine, when given in equianalgesic oral doses, are much more effective than 650 mg of aspirin or acetaminophen. It is quite possible, however, that the inability to obtain relief with oral medications is related more to the way in which the drug is administered rather than the presence of refractory pain. A careful history concerning prior analgesic use, including dose and frequency of administration, is quite important, therefore, especially with respect to the interval between the appearance of pain and analgesic ingestion. At times, merely adjusting the medication schedule to take the analgesic prior rather than subsequent to the onset of pain may be effective.

As previously discussed, depending on etiology, the pain may not respond at all to analgesics but to drugs whose actions focused on the actual pathologic disturbance. At times, the actions of analgesics may be enhanced or diminished depending on the cause of pain. An example is the effectiveness of narcotics in inflammatory pain. For various reasons sensitivity to narcotics in the presence of inflammation is enhanced whereas in the presence of neuropathic pain, morphine analgesic is diminished.

A person whose pain medication has progressed from oral analgesics to parenteral narcotics without obtaining appropriate relief has usually seen several physicians and is often quite resistant to seeing another. The main objective is often to convince the physician to prescribe the narcotic exactly as requested. Narcotic dependency is invariably present and the drug is often taken for euphoric as well as analgesic effects. In such a setting, it is extremely important for the physician to be nonjudgmental and to carefully define with the patient the goals and objectives to be followed.

When a person is using a narcotic appropriately, the feeling should be conveyed that dependency is a necessary accompaniment of narcotic use and not in and of itself to be avoided if that is the only way to relieve the pain. At the same time, appropriate information concerning the detrimental effects of taking narcotics specifically to get high as well as the risks associated with long-term uncontrolled parenteral use should be discussed. If a determination is made that a narcotic is needed, a drug that can be taken in oral form is quite preferable.

Choice of Analgesic

As previously emphasized, depending on the nature and severity of the pain if a nonopioid analgesic such as a NSAID is able to provide effective relief, its use is preferable. If an opioid analgesic is required, however, a drug should be chosen that has a long duration of action. Unlike the NSAIDs, the opioids have no ceiling on their effectiveness—increasing the dose is accompanied by increasing analgesia.

The physiological basis for the use of a long-acting oral opioid rather than injections of short-acting opioids has long been well described.[31,32] Injections of a potent short-acting opioid will result in an extremely high blood level for a relatively short period. This phenomenon results in production of a pharmacologic withdrawal in brain cells sensitizing those cells to the next narcotic dose. It may be that these effects facilitate the development of the addictive behavior so frequently seen in persons having chronic pain with a defined cause. Analgesic treatment in chronic pain should therefore be focused on the use of long-acting oral or transdermal preparations, rather than injections to provide relief (Table 14.11).

Several sustained-release preparations of morphine sulfate are available for use in chronic pain. Sustained-release morphine (MS Contin, Oramorph SR) has been shown to provide effective analgesia for moderate to severe pain without undue side effects.[32,33] Fentanyl, an extremely potent short-acting narcotic has been made available in a patch (transdermal)

TABLE 14.11. Long-Acting Analgesics Used in Treatment of Chronic Pain

Drug	Trade Name	Duration of Action (hours)
Morphine Sulphate	Ms. Contin Oramorph SR Roxanol SR	8-12
Fentanyl Transdermal	Duragesic	48-72
Methadone	Dolophine	6-8

form to provide analgesia for chronic pain states.[34] The patch, which can be easily applied, may have a duration of action of up to 72 hours. Since an increase in serum fentanyl concentrations can occur over the first 24 hours of wearing the patch, several days should pass before a decision is made to increase the dose, and a full week may be needed for an equilibrium to occur once a dose is altered. This is an effective form of analgesia when a functional GI track is not present or when nausea and vomiting exists. However, the actual dose delivered may be difficult to control at times and local allergic reactions to the patch may limit its usefulness.

Methadone was one of the first drugs used to treat chronic pain. As described in Chapter 6, when given orally, methadone does not produce rapid peak levels in the blood or brain. Its slow release from tissue reservoirs into the bloodstream permits a fairly stable narcotic level with even analgesia. Changes in concentration are quite slow with an average plasma half-life of 24 hours. Even with increasing doses, peak blood levels are not reached until two to four hours after the dose is ingested. Other oral narcotics either are not as well absorbed from the gastrointestinal tract or are insufficiently bound to tissues to allow for a slow release to the bloodstream as the blood level of the narcotic falls. With repeated administration of a fixed methadone dose, tolerance will develop to its analgesic activity in the manner similar to that seen with other narcotics. In such instances dose adjustments must be made at appropriate intervals. It should also be remembered that the accumulation of methadone in the tissues with repeated doses can predispose to toxicity, especially in the elderly. For this reason, when initiating methadone therapy, careful monitoring for the first 72 hours is needed.

Changing from Injections to Oral Medications

Although all narcotics can be interchanged freely, provided equianalgesic doses are used, almost invariably a fear will be expressed concerning the ability of oral medication to provide satisfactory analgesia. The fear of inadequate analgesia with oral analgesics may be so prominent that even though a patient may be suffering from sterile abscesses due to recurrent parenteral narcotic use and may have a limited body surface area for further injections, great resistance is encountered in attempting to discontinue injections. This fear is not entirely unfounded as most patients have been treated inappropriately with oral narcotics, utilizing drugs that are either poorly absorbed or given at insufficient intervals to provide satisfactory analgesia.

If oral analgesics are to be initiated in persons chronically dependent on parenteral narcotics, the use of methadone is preferred. Switching analgesia from parenteral narcotic use to oral methadone is a relatively simple process. The total amount of parenteral narcotic administered in a 24-hour period is converted to an oral methadone dosage, which is then administered every six to eight hours. The patient should be told that it may take a day or more for a blood level of methadone sufficient to provide analgesia to be reached. In order to relieve anxiety during the first several days, orders should be written for an injection of narcotic if pain occurs.

Since individual tolerance with respect to analgesic efforts of methadone may vary, a person should be carefully monitored during the first 48 hours to make certain that the dose administered will not cause respiratory depression. The interactions of methadone with drugs in the alcohol-barbiturates-sedative group, notably diazepam, make it mandatory that concurrent use of diazepam be separated by at least two hours from the methadone dose. If satisfactory analgesia is unable to be maintained with the initial methadone dose, the dose may be adjusted upward at the rate of 20 mg per day until a plateau level is reached.

As an alternative to methadone, sustained-release morphine or transdermal fentanyl may be used. Since transdermal fentanyl (Duragesic) has a duration of action of up to 72 hours, care must be taken not to initially "overshoot the mark" to avoid sedation or actual overdose. In general, a fentanyl providing 100 micrograms of fentanyl an hour is equivalent to 10 mg of morphine by intramuscular injection every four hours. To convert a person to transdermal fentanyl, one calculates the previous 24-hour analgesic requirement successful in relieving pain. This is then converted to an equianalgesic oral morphine dose, and then the appropriate patch strength of fentanyl is selected. Once stabilization on oral or transdermal medications has occurred and there is no longer a need for an injection every three to four hours to obtain relief, a more complete evaluation considering psychological needs can occur. The person is now able to carry out daily activities without focusing on medication schedules.

ADJUNCTIVE MEDICATIONS IN SPECIFIC BRAIN STATES

Adjunctive medications, usually comprising different classes of psychotropic drugs, may not only be of great value in enhancing analgesia but, depending on the type of pain, may also be of primary value in providing relief (Table 14.12).

Central Pain Syndrome

Central pain can be both superficial and deep, most often described as a constant or intermittent — but regular —burning sensation. Although central pain syndromes often respond poorly to narcotic analgesics, the use of drugs that block adrenergic, serotonergic, and dopaminergic neurons have shown to be effective, especially in treatment of neuropathic pain. The use of tricyclic antidepressants, notably amitriptyline and nortriptyline, has been associated with relief of post-stroke pain, independent of the antidepressant properties.[10,35] Baclofen, a drug that inhibits transmission of gamma ammobutyric acid (GABA) has been found helpful in relieving sensory symptoms seen in CPS.[10] Clonidine, available as a transdermal patch, has also been shown to be helpful in relieving the pain of causalgia.[36] Calcitonin has also been suggested as helpful in relief of phantom limb pain.[37] Whether these agents will prove to be effective over time remains to be determined.

Headache

Headaches are most often treated adequately with one of the nonnarcotic analgesics, which include aspirin and acetaminophen alone or in combination with other drugs as well as the nonsteroidal anti-inflammation drugs (NSAIDs). Absorption of these drugs may be increased with the use of metoclopramide (Reglan), which can also decrease the nausea that may often accompany severe headache pain, especially for migraine attacks. However, for those suffering with the severe unremitting pain that is associated with several types of headaches, a wide variety of medications are available that address the specific pathophysiology present (Table 14.13). It is therefore essential that cause and type of headache be precisely identified. In addition, treating the pain without determining the etiology of a headache can be quite hazardous, especially if the headache is related to an underlying systemic

TABLE 14.12. Adjunctive Medications Useful in Selected Pain States

Bone pain due to osteoporosis or Paget's disease calcitonin

Central pain states

    Antidepressants: amitryptiline, nortriptyline
    Andrenergic agents: clonidine, B blockers
    Anticonvulsants: carbamazine
    Phenothiazines
    Haloperidol

Muscle spasm

    Benzodiazepines
    Orphenadrine citrate
    Meprobamate
    Haloperidol (spasmatic torticollis)
    Baclofen (spasm of demyelinating disease)
    Dantrolene (spasm of demyelinating disease)

Peripheral nerve (neuropathic pain)

    Capsaicin
    Clonidine
    Guanethidine
    Antidepressants: amitriptyline, desipramine, doxepine, fluoxetine, paxil
    Phenothiazines
    Haloperidol
    Anticonvulsants: carbamazepine, diphenylhydantoin,
        sodium valproate, clonazepam
    Oral local anesthetics: flecainide, mexiletine, tocainide
    Topical anesthetics: eutectic mixture of local anesthetics (EMLA-cream),
        Lidocaine gel

Trigeminal neuralgia

    Baclofen
    Carbamazepine
    Clonazepam
    Diphenylhydantoin
    Sodium valproate

[a]The use of many of these drugs is associated with frequent complications and side effects. The reader should consult an appropriate desk reference prior to prescribing these agents.

disorder such as hypertension, tumor, or aneurysm, not only leads to escalating doses of narcotic analgesics and antidepressants but also may have disastrous consequences.

Most recently sumatriptan (Imitrex), a serotonin antagonist that promotes constriction of cerebral blood vessels, has been found to be effective for the treatment of acute migraines and is being used as a replacement for both the ergot alkaloids and the narcotic analgesics in persons

TABLE 14.13. Classification of Primary Headache Syndrome

Classification	Nonanalgesics considered effective
Cluster headaches	Chlorpromazine, lithium, prednisone, methysergide (Sansert)[a], sumatriptan
Inflammatory	Antibiotics
Psychogenic	Antidepressants
Tension headaches[b]	Midrin[c], mild sedatives, diazepam[d], tricyclic antidepressants, propranolol, Periactin (cyproheptadine)
Vascular headaches	Ergotamine tartrate, dihydroergotamine (migraine variants), Midrin[c], propranolol, methysergide (Sansert)[a], MAO inhibitors, tricyclic antidepressants, clonidine, Periactin

[a]Can cause serious adverse effects; should be avoided if possible.
[b]Most tension headaches can be relieved by use of mild nonnarcotic analgesics alone or in combination with caffeine, or with a short-acting sedative or tranquilizer. Other medications are used in refractory severe cases.
[c]Isometheptene mucate, dichloral phenazone, acetaminophen.
[d]Use may be associated with dependency.

without a history of heart disease. Sumatriptan is available as an injection, an oral preparation, and in several countries as a nasal spray.

Preventing headaches, especially migraines, is often difficult. A variety of drugs have been advocated as being effective, with beta blockers such as propranolol and timolol being most frequently used. Other drugs that have been prescribed in an attempt to prevent attacks of migraine include calcium channel blockers, antidepressants, methysergide (Sansert), NSAIDs, and the anticonvulsant valproate.

Neuropathic Pain

Neuropathic pain may be initiated centrally or in the peripheral nervous system. Pain in the peripheral nervous system due to local trauma or systemic disease such as diabetes has been treated effectively by a variety of medications. These include the tricyclic antidepressants, as well as anticonvulsants such as carbamazepine and phenytoin.[10] Oral antiarrhythmic agents such as mexiletine, tocanamide, and flecainide have also been found to be helpful alternatives.[38] Transdermal, epidural, and intrathecal clonidine have also provided relief in neuropathic as well as cancer pain. Recently, capsaicin (Drysol), a substance derived from solanaceae plants, has been shown to deplete the neurotransmitter substance P found in sensory neurons. Topical application of capsaicin has been demonstrated to be effective in relieving neuropathic, as well as arthritic pains.[39,40] Topical application of anesthetic creams or gels under pressure dressings are effective in treating neuropathic pain. Newer antidepressants, such as venlafaxine (Effexor) and nefazodone (Serzone), and the anticonvulsants, gabapentin (Phenurone) and lamotrigine (Lamictal), have also been used. However, the effectiveness of these agents based on large scale trials remains to be determined.

Muscle Disorders

Treatment of the focal and generalized myalgias has remained far from satisfactory. Muscle relaxants, drugs affecting neurotransmitter function, antidepressants, abolition of specific trigger points with local anesthetics, and dietary supplements with amino acids (especially tryptophane) have all been used with varying results. Much more is needed to be learned about the actual pathophysiology of the conditions in an attempt to provide more consistently effective therapy.

Low Back Pain

The ubiquity of low back pain, be it due to an actual herniated disc, primarily muscle spasm, or arthritic changes, has resulted in a variety of medications being prescribed in an attempt to relieve pain and discomfort, as well as a number of surgical interventions (Table 14.14). The difficulties in providing consistent relief are related to the lack of clarity in defining the origin of the pain. As many as 90 percent of persons with low back pain do not have a definite diagnosis. There persists a poor correlation between symptoms, objective findings, and diagnostic studies. Psychological and sociological factors such as the possibility of compensation also serve to deter a precise surgical intervention when therapy is not consistently effective nor uniformly applied. As an example, the rates of surgery for low back pain differ by eightfold between the United States and England.[41]

In assessing a person with low back pain, the first step is to eliminate the presence of serious causes such as a vertebral fracture, a nerve compromise, through tumor, infection, or ruptured intervertebral discs. In the absence of such conditions, nonprescription analgesics often provide the best relief. Although muscle relaxants are often prescribed, there is little evidence that they are more effective than acetaminophen, aspirin, or the nonsteroidal anti-inflammatory drugs. The use of relaxants or more potent analgesics such as narcotics, although at times helpful, often may be associated with drowsiness and sedation.

Procedures that appear effective when evaluated in a controlled, blinded fashion often are found to offer no better relief than placebo. Even the most commonly accepted treatment of acute low back pain—prolonged bed rest—has now been shown to be less than helpful, with continuing normal activities, within the limits of pain control associated

TABLE 14.14. Current Therapies for Low Back Pain

General
Bed Rest
Traction
Exercises
Transcutaneous Electrical Nerve Stimulation
Pharmacologic
Muscle Relaxants
Cortisone Insertions into Facet Joints
Analgesics
Antidepressants
Anti-inflammatory Agents
Surgical
Removal of Herniated Discs
Fusion of Vertebrae

with more rapid recovery than either bed rest or specific exercise to mobilize the back muscles.[42,43] At present, the accepted therapy is limited bed rest with early exercise, accompanied by the use of the nonsteroidal antiinflammation drugs and when helpful, muscle relaxants. However as noted earlier in this chapter, most persons with low back pain improve regardless of therapy administered or type of health care providers seen.

It should also be remembered that low back pain is cyclic, almost regardless of therapy provided. A recent study of over 1,500 persons with low back pain who saw a variety of healthcare providers, including primary care physicians, orthopedic surgeons, chiropractors, and primary care physicians in health maintenance organizations, found the outcome to be the same regardless of the type of professional providing the care. Despite the marked differences in both evaluation and management, only 5 percent of persons had not reported functional recovery within six months.[24]

Trigeminal Neuralgia (Tic Douloureux)

Trigeminal neuralgia is an extremely painful condition, manifested as facial pain over the branches of the trigeminal nerve. The exact etiology of the pain has not been precisely identified but is felt to be related to vascular compression of the nerve root. The pain may cease spontaneously only to return in decreasing pain-free intervals. Treatment with carbamazine is often effective in up to 75 percent of cases. Other drugs include phenytoin, baclofen, and the newer anticonvulsants, gabapentin, and lamotrigine. Microvascular decompression of the trigeminal nerve has also recently been shown to provide persistent relief when pharmacologic therapy fails.[44,45]

PSYCHOLOGICAL SUPPORT

Psychological support is always a useful adjunct to pharmacologic therapy and, in certain instances, may ultimately allow for a marked reduction in analgesic medication even in the presence of a demonstrable organic lesion. The psychological devastation that accompanies unrelieved chronic pain cannot be overemphasized. The pain becomes a focus of the entire day's activities to the exclusion of other needs or relationships. At times the expression of chronic pain may, in fact, be considered a stress-related disorder that interferes not only with a person's ability to work, but with family and societal interactions as well. These findings reinforce the estrangement and isolation that may accompany persistent pain, thus emphasizing the need to address psychological as well as pharmacological

TABLE 14.15. Assessing the Effectiveness of Therapy in Chronic Pain

---

Objective improvement in functioning
Maintaining level of functioning
Slowing rate of physical deterioration
Decrease in pain perception
Improved mood and well-being
Obtaining satisfactory relief with oral rather than injectable drugs
Decrease in, or discontinuing of, narcotic agents

---

needs. In some instances, depending on the cause of the pain, psychological support may be the primary form of therapy (Chapter 18).

MEASURING EFFECTIVENESS OF THERAPY

The effectiveness of therapy in alleviating chronic pain may be measured by a number of parameters (Table 14.15). The most successful outcome is obviously the restoration of function without any residual deficits. Unfortunately, in persons with chronic pain, regardless of existing organic impairment, attaining this goal is usually quite difficult. A second, more reasonable objective would be supportive, maintaining existing functions with minimal further loss. In individuals with progressive destructive disorders or neoplastic diseases, the main objective would be palliative, attempting to prevent or slow the progression of symptoms realizing that little can be done to improve the underlying pathology.

In the face of irremediable deficits, improving the patient's mood and sense of well-being becomes a primary goal. Often allowing the patient to express feelings freely will enable a better adjustment as well as strengthen the physician-patient bond. This is especially true with respect to patients with neoplastic disease who all too frequently are given rather short shrift by physicians, nurses, and even friends and family (Chapter 16).

A final parameter of success is the ability to: (1) markedly decrease the frequency of taking analgesics, and (2) obtain analgesia with oral rather than parenteral drugs or with nonnarcotic rather than narcotic agents. This goal is best achieved once the psychosocial factors have been addressed and the patient is able to obtain a better understanding of his or her reaction to the underlying problem.

UNRELIEVED PAIN

Unfortunately, more often than not, regardless of origin, chronic pain is not adequately relieved. This is usually due to inappropriate behavior by both patients and physicians. Often patients minimize their symptoms due to a need to be stoic, as in an attempt to please the health care providers, or due to a perception that pain naturally accompanies the underlying disorder. At times, the secondary gain inherent in persistent suffering may also play a role. Frequently, compliance is the problem, with a person not taking the analgesic as suggested. This, in turn, with respect to narcotic drugs, may be related to a fear of becoming an addict. When the behavior of the patient is the major deterrent to achieving relief, often a frank discussion with the physician addressing existing concerns and fears will allow for the pain to be adequately treated.

It is more often the behavior of the physician, rather than the behavior of the person in pain, that causes persistent suffering. Physicians consistently prescribe inadequate doses of narcotic analgesics at too infrequent intervals, regardless of the actual cause of the pain. This problem is discussed in detail in Chapter 15.

SUMMARY

Having outlined a variety of parameters that can be used to evaluate the effectiveness of therapy for chronic pain, as well as specific agents used in therapy, it is discouraging to note that there are few large studies addressing this issue. Comparisons of invasive and noninvasive treatments are few, and cost-effective therapies are rarely discussed. Much more evaluation of effective measures to relieve pain is needed.

It must be emphasized, however, that whatever the method of therapy agreed on by the physician and patient, satisfactory long-term analgesia is not easily achieved. Indeed, analgesics are rarely effective in treating chronic pain due to a benign nonrecurrent disorder. Continuing patience is required, as is the development of a strong physician-patient relationship to build a bridge of mutual trust and respect that will withstand the inevitable frustration. Equally important is allowing a person to assume responsibility for participating in the decision making process.

REFERENCES

1. U.S. Agency for Health Care Policy and Research. *Acute pain management: Operative or medical procedures and trauma.* Rockville, MD: U.S. Dept. Health and Human Services, 1992.

2. Marks RM, Sachar EJ. Undertreatment of medical inpatients with narcotic analgesics. *Ann Intern Med,* 1973, 78:173–181.

3. Postoperative pain relief and nonopioid analgesics (editorial). *Lancet,* 1991, 337:524–526.

4. White PF. Use of patient-controlled analgesia for management of acute pain. *JAMA,* 1988, 259:243–247.

5. Camp JF. Patient-controlled analgesia. *Fam Physician,* 1991, 44:2145–2150.

6. McIntosh DG, Rayburn WF. Patient-controlled analgesia in obstetrics and gynecology. *Obstet Gynecol,* 1991, 78:1129–1135.

7. Bayless JM, Stanley TH, Have BO. Pain in the ICU: Using analgesics effectively. *J Critical Illness,* January, 1986: 19–27.

8. Stein C. The control of pain in peripheral tissue by opioids. *New Eng J Med,* 1995, 332:1685–1690.

9. Katzwa. Approach to the management of nonmalignant pain. *Am J Med,* 1996, 101 (Supp 1A): 54S–63S.

10. Gonzales GR. Central pain: Diagnosis and treatment strategies. *Neurol,* 1995, (Supp 9): S11–S16.

11. Rasmussen BK, Olesen J. Symptomatic and nonsymptomatic headaches in a general population. *Neurol,* 1992, 42:1657.

12. Sweet WH. The treatment of trigeminal neuralgia. *New Eng J Med,* 1986, 315:174–177.

13. Yunus MB. Toward a model of pathophysiology of fibromyalgia. Aberrant central pain mechanisms with peripheral modulation (editorial). *J Rheumatol,* 1992, 19:846–850.

14. Yunus MB. Research in Fibromyalgia and myofascial pain syndrome: Current status, problems, and future directions. *J of Musculoskel Pain,* 1993, 1:23 – 41.

15. Mense S. Peripheral mechanisms of muscle nociception and local muscle pain. *J of Musculoskel Pain,* 1993, 1:133–170.

16. Smythe H. Links between fibromyalgia and myofascial pain syndromes (editorial). *J Rheumatol,* 1992, 19:842–843.

17. Wolfe F, Simons DG, Friction J, Bennett RM, Goldenberg DL, Gerwin R, Hathaway D, McCain GA, Russell IJ, Sanders HO, Skootsky SA. The fibromyalgia and myofascial pain syndrome: A preliminary study of tender points and trigger points in persons with fibromyalgia, myofascial pain syndrome, and no disease. *J Rheumatol,* 1992, 19:944–951.

18. Holmes GP, Kaplan JE, Gantz NM, Komaroff AL, Schonberger LB, Straus SE, Jones JF, Dubois RE, Cunningham-Rundles C, Pahwa S, et al. Chronic fatigue syndrome: A working case definition. *Ann Intern Med,* 1988, 108:387–389.

19. Whelton CI, Salit I, Moldofsky H. Sleep, Epstein-Barr virus infection, musculoskeletal pain, and depressive symptoms in the chronic fatigue syndrome. *J Rheumatol,* 1992, 19:939–943.

20. Frymoyer JW, Cats-Baril WL. An overview of the incidence and cost of low back pain. *Orthop Clin North Am,* 1991, 22:263–271.

21. Loeser JD. Low back pain. In: Bonica JJ (ed.). *Pain.* New York: Raven Press, 1980:363–377.

22. Lister BJ. Dilemmas in the treatment of chronic pain. *Am J Med*, 1966, 101 (Supp 1A): 2S–5S.

23. Deyo RA. Fads in the treatment of low back pain. *N Engl J Med*, 1991, 325:1039–1140.

24. Carey TS, Garett J, Jackman A, McLaughlin C, Freyer J, Smuker DR, the North Carolina Back Pain Project. The outcomes and costs of care for acute low back pain among patients seen by primary care practitioners, chiropractors, and orthopedic surgeons. *N Eng J Med*, 1995, 333:913–917.

25. Gangarosa LP, Mahan PE, Ciarlone AE. Pharmacologic management of temporomandibular joint disorders and chronic head and neck pain. *Cranio*, 1991, 9:328–338.

26. Merskey H. The role of the psychiatrist in the investigation and treatment of pain. In: Bonica JJ (ed.). *Pain*. New York: Raven Press, 1980:249–260.

27. Aronoff G. *Pain centers: A revolution in health care*. New York: Raven Press, 1990.

28. Wilson RR, Aronoff GM. The therapeutic community in the treatment of chronic pain (editorial). *J Chron Dis*, 1979, 32:477–481.

29. Deardorff WW, Rubin HS, Scott DW. Comprehensive multidisciplinary treatment of chronic pain: A follow-up study of treated and nontreated groups. *Pain*, 1991, 45:35–43.

30. Turk DC, Rudy TE. Neglected topics in the treatment of chronic pain patients. *Pain*, 1991, 44:5–28.

31. Dole VP. Addictive behavior. *Sci Am*, 1980, 243:138–140,142,144.

32. Zenz M, Strumpf M, Tryba M. Long-term oral opioid therapy in patients with chronic nonmalignant pain. *J Pain Symptom Manage*, 1992, 7:69–77.

33. Deschamps M, Band PR, Hislop TG, Russthoven J, Iscoe N, Warr D. The evaluation of analgesic effects in cancer patients as exemplified by a double-blind crossover study of immediate-release versus controlled-release morphine. *J Pain Symptom Manage*, 1992, 7:384–392.

34. Portenoy RK, Southam MA, Gupta SK, Lapin J, Layman M, Inturrisi CE, Foley KM. Transdermal fentanyl for cancer path: Repeated dose pharmacokinetics. *Anesthesiol*, 1993, 78:36–43.

35. Sandford PR, Lindblom LB, Haddox JD. Amitriptyline and carbamazepine in the treatment of dysesthetic pain in spinal cord injury. *Arch Phys Med Rehab*, 1992, 73:300–301.

36. Davis KD, Treede RD, Raja SN, Meyer RA, Campell JN. Topical application of clonidine relieves hyperalgesia in patients with sympathetically maintained pain. *Pain*, 1991, 47:309–317.

37. Jaeger H, Maier C. Calcitonin in phantom limb pain: A double-blind study. *Pain*, 1992, 48:21–27.

38. Chabal C, Jacobson L, Mariano A, Chaney E, Britell CW. The use of oral mexiletine for the treatment of pain after peripheral nerve injury. *Anesthesiol*, 1992, 76:513–517.

39. Tandau R, Lewis GA, Krusinski PB, Badger GB, Fries TJ. Topical capsaicin in painful diabetic neuropathy controlled study with long-term follow-up. *Diabetes Care,* 1992, 15:8–14.

40. Deal CL, Schnitzer TJ, Lipstein E, Seibold JR, Stevens RM, Levy MD, Albet D, Renold F. Treatment of arthritis with topical capsaicin: A double-blind trial. *Clin Ther,* 1991, 13:383–395.

41. Investigation of failed low back surgery (editorial). *Lancet,* 1989; 939–940.

42. Deyo RA, Diehl AK, Rosenthal M. How many days of bed rest for acute low back pain? A randomized clinical trial. *N Engl J Med,* 1986, 315:1064–1070.

43. Malmivaara A, Häkkinen U, Aro T, Heinrichs M-L, Koskenniemi L, Kuosma E, Lappi S, Paloheimo R, Servo C, Vaaranen V, Hernberg S. The treatment of acute low back pain—bed rest, exercises, or ordinary activity? *N Engl J Med*, 1995, 332:351–355.

44. Fields HL. Treatment of trigeminal neuralgia. *N Engl J Med*, 1996, 334:1125–1126.

45. Barker II FG, Jannetta PJ, Bissonette DJ, Larkins MV, Jho HD. The long-term outcome of microvascular decompression for trigeminal neuralgia. *N Engl J Med*, 1996, 334:1077–1083.

Chapter 15

Unrelieved Pain:
The Role of the Physician

INTRODUCTION

As discussed earlier (Chapter 13), studies concerning the ability of persons in pain to receive adequate relief consistently demonstrate inappropriate physician prescribing patterns resulting in needless pain and discomfort. For many people, daily functioning is severely impaired as well as their interpersonal relationships with family and friends. There are a variety of reasons why physicians may not prescribe sufficient analgesic medications (Table 15.1). Each must be addressed if the physician's ability to relieve pain is to be maximized.

FEDERAL AND STATE REGULATIONS: FEAR OF SANCTIONS

The role of the physician in initiating drug dependence (iatrogenic dependence) is of concern not only to physicians and patients but also to legislative bodies.[1,2,3] Since the beginning of the twentieth century, federal legislation has been directed toward monitoring physician prescription of dependency-producing drugs without seriously restricting access to appropriate therapies. Currently, the control of dependency-producing drugs falls under the Controlled Substances Act, with responsibility for enforcement residing with the Drug Enforcement Administration (DEA). Many states, however, have also introduced their own regulations.

The Controlled Substances Act

Under the Controlled Substances Act of 1972, drugs with the ability to produce physical or psychological dependence, associated with the poten-

TABLE 15.1. Reasons for Inadequate Prescription of Analgesics

Inhibitory influences of federal and state regulations and disciplinary boards
Lack of suitable knowledge base
Fear of producing dependency and addiction
Cultural and societal barriers to use of narcotics
Adherence to customary prescribing behaviors
Unconscious bias toward different groups

tial for misuse or abuse, are classified into one of five categories. Each category represents gradations of the relative hazards and effectiveness of these agents ranging from Schedule I substances, which have high abuse potential and no acceptable medical use, to Schedule V substances, which have little abuse potential and can be purchased without a prescription (Table 15.2). It is important to emphasize, however, that any of the drugs that alter moods have the potential for abuse. Even some of those substances of Schedule V such as codeine, when taken inappropriately in high doses, can cause euphoria and dependence.

The Psychotropic Substances Act

This legislation enacted in 1978 resulted in an amendment to the Controlled Substances Act and stated that the legitimate and useful prescription of these drugs for medical purposes should not be restricted. It also provided for the Secretary of Health and Human Services, in consultation with the medical and scientific communities, to determine what constituted the ethical practice of medicine with respect to prescriptions of these substances.

The Uniform Controlled Substances Act (UCSA)

This act, initially written in 1970 and revised in 1990, forms the basis for the different states' controlled substances legislation. The revised UCSA recognizes the importance of the medical use of controlled substances, distinguishes patients from addicts, emphasizes the importance of patient confidentiality, permits the use of chronic narcotic analgesic therapy for intolerable pain, and establishes a program to detect drug diversions.

TABLE 15.2. Examples of Substances Classified Under the Controlled Substances Act*

	SCHEDULE I	SCHEDULE II	SCHEDULE III	SCHEDULE IV	SCHEDULE V
Stimulants	N-methylamphetamine	Amphetamines, methamphetamines, cocaine, phenmetrazine, methylphenidate	Benzphetamine, phentermine HCl, mazindol, phendimetrazine	Diethylpropion, mazindol, fenfluramine	
Barbiturates and nonbarbiturates, hypnotics and sedatives	Methaqualone	Amobarbital, pentobarbital, secobarbital Glutethimide Combinations: Tuinal	Methylprylon chlorhexadol, aprobarbital, butabarbital, thiopental	Barbital, phenobarbital, mephobarbital methohexital methylphenobarbital, chloral betaine, chloral hydrate, fethchloruynol, ethinamate, meprobamate, paraldehyde, enzodiazepines zolpidem	
Hallucinogens	Marijuana, lysergic acid diamide, tetra-hydrocannabinols, peyote, mescaline, psilocybin, phencyclidine	Dronabinol			
Narcotics	Heroin, Ketobemidone, Levomoramide racemoramide, benzylmorphine, dihydromorphnione, morphine-methylsulfonate nicocodine, nicomorphine	Opium, morphine codeine, hydromorphone, methadone, pantopon, meperidine, oxycodone, anileridine, levorphanol, oxymorphone, sufentanil, fentanyl, alfentanil	Paregoric opioids with limited quantities of morphine or codeine derivatives	Propoxyphene	Exempt narcotics
Narcotic Antagonists				Pentazocine	Buprenorphine

*Classification of specific drugs may change on periodic reassessments.
aNarcotic preparations with nonnarcotic active medical ingredients.

MONITORING SYSTEMS

A variety of monitoring systems exist at both federal and state levels to detect inappropriate sales and use of mood-altering substances. They include:

The Automation of Reports and Consolidated Orders Systems (ARCOS)

ARCOS operated by the Drug Enforcement Agency requires all manufacturers and distributors to report transfers of controlled substances.

Prescription Abuse Data System (PADS)

PADS, established by the American Medical Association, attempts to identify problems with drug prescriptions within a state as well as to develop a way of dealing with specific problems.

The Medicaid Control System (MADAS)

MADAS allows monitoring of all medicaid prescriptions of controlled substances that are paid for by Medicaid.

Multiple Copy Prescription Programs (MCPPs)

MCPPs, in existence in several states, require prescriptions for certain mood-altering drugs to be completed in either triplicate or duplicate with one copy going to the pharmacy and one to the state. If a triplicate form exists, the physician is usually required to keep a copy. Regulators feel that this system prevents forgeries, inhibits physicians from excessive prescribing, inhibits subsequent alteration of the original prescription, and is able to substantiate allegations of excessive prescribing against specific physicians. Many physicians, however, feel that such systems violate patient confidentiality, as well as inhibit physicians from appropriately prescribing these drugs for fear of harassment by state investigation units. In fact, surveys have shown that the response to such scrutiny is often an alteration in prescribing practices. Whether this improves or adversely affects patient care remains controversial.

In fact, both federal and state regulations pertaining to the prescription of these drugs are so detailed and yet so vague that they often discourage physicians from prescribing these substances.[1,2,3] Physicians remained concerned that prescription of Schedule II substances for prolonged periods, even when clearly indicated, will subject them to disciplinary action. This is enhanced by the confusion that often exists between addiction and physical dependence. Many state boards require physicians to have tried all alternative means of treatment prior to placing a person on chronic narcotic therapy, with some states requiring psychiatric consultations for chronic narcotic therapy, under the premise that a need for long-term narcotic analgesics suggests a coexisting disorder. This is especially true for chronic nonmalignant pain. Since these boards often consist of physicians with inadequate knowledge bases, a physician may be called to task for prescribing what in reality is appropriate. One survey of state disciplinary boards revealed that only 75 percent of its members felt that prescribing opiates for an extended time to treat cancer pain was appropriate. When opiates were prescribed for more than several months for chronic nonmalignant pain, only 12 percent thought the practice was legal and acceptable. Since most disciplinary boards act on the basis of "customary practice" of the community's physicians and most physicians characteristically underutilize narcotics, a physician who provides appropriate analgesia may well be exposed to sanctions. This is especially true in treating severe pain, which often requires a much greater than "usual" amount of opiate for relief. Several surveys have demonstrated a reluctance of many physicians, even oncologists, to prescribe opiates in appropriate doses due to their concerns with existing regulations.[2,3]

Protection from misuse or abuse of analgesic agents really cannot be legislated but must be accompanied by an understanding of the indications and risks associated with these drugs by physicians, the public, and the regulatory agencies. Competing public interests, mainly the prevention of diversion of legal drugs to illicit use and eliminating prescribing for profit, must be balanced with relief from pain and suffering, which should be the primary concern. All too often the regulatory agencies are more concerned with their policies rather than their effect on the medical community.

INADEQUATE PHYSICIAN KNOWLEDGE BASE

The appropriate use of analgesics and other mood-altering drugs is a subject that unfortunately receives too little attention in medical school and residency training. As a physician moves further away from basic pharmacology — where most of the information concerning drug action is taught — an increasing unfamiliarity with the specific actions of analgesics and other mood-altering agents develops. Drugs may be used more frequently than necessary due to the reliance placed on the publicity given to newer agents, often accompanied by patients' requests for "nonaddictive" substances.

At times, this may result in overprescription of mild narcotic analgesics or excessive use of tranquilizers, rather than a narcotic analgesic. Even today, most physicians consider propoxyphene (Darvon) a nonnarcotic effective mild analgesia. This is despite the fact that propoxyphene is an ester of methadone and in sufficient doses, can cause dependence, tolerance, overdose, and addictive behavior indistinguishable from more potent narcotics.[4-7] Codeine and oxycodone (Percocet), commonly prescribed analgesics, are also capable of producing dependence or addiction. One survey found codeine to be the most frequent drug of abuse in patients without a demonstrable cause of pain.[8] In many instances, those who take codeine are not even aware it is a narcotic.

The narcotic agonist-antagonists are prescribed freely by many physicians without concern of addiction. Yet pentazocine (Talwin), available as an analgesic since 1967, at one time was an attractive alternative to heroin.[9,10] Buprenorphine (Buprenex), now being marketed in a noninjectable form, remains uncontrolled despite addicts reporting its effects similar to heroin in clinical trials and its recognition as one of the leading drugs of abuse in New Zealand.[11]

On the other hand, the use of the benzodiazepines or antidepressants is considerable despite the ability of the former to produce dependence and the latter to cause euphoria when taken inappropriately.[12-14] Surveys have documented the prescription of (1) antidepressants to 27 percent of an alcoholic population although only 7 percent were felt to be depressed;[12] (2) psychotropic drugs to 58 percent of women admitted to a metropolitan correction center although only 23 percent were felt to need these medications;[13] and (3) a disproportional number of these drugs by family practitioners and internists compared to frequency of office visits.

FEAR OF ADDICTION

Fear of producing addiction to narcotics is foremost in the minds of most physicians when asked to provide medication for pain relief. This fear often interferes with their ability to provide adequate analgesia. One study demonstrated that those physicians who thought the probability of addiction was high after prescribing meperidine for ten days to a patient in pain were more likely to give lower initial doses, as well as to be less likely to respond to the need for increased medication with recurrent pain even if pain was due to terminal malignancy.[15]

A second study of 100 patients with malignant pain found 60 percent to be prescribed doses of meperidine of 50 mg or less, with 11 percent having to wait for five or more hours before another dose with all prescriptions written for PRN administration.[16]

In fact, the risk of initiating an addiction when narcotics are prescribed appropriately for relief of pain is quite small. Although historical references attribute physicians as initiating dependence on opiates, a survey reviewing addiction among a population of black heroin addicts found less than 2 percent to attribute their addictions to prescription of a narcotic for medical reasons.[17] Perhaps the largest the largest survey of iatrogenic narcotic dependence was done as part of the Boston Collaborative Drug Surveillance Program.[18] This program monitors all drug exposures in several hospitals, with information being extracted from clinical records and by interviews with patients and physicians. Of over 11,000 hospitalized medical patients who had narcotics administered during their hospital stay, only four were reported to have become addicted. A more recent analysis of publications pertaining to drug or alcohol dependence in chronic-pain patients found less than one-tenth of these publications used acceptable criteria for drug misuse or even gave percentages of dependence problems.[19]

Available data, therefore, suggest that when narcotics are utilized appropriately for acute pain in a hospitalized setting, the actual incidence of medically induced narcotic dependency is negligible. Even in chronic-pain populations, there is little evidence that drug abuse or addiction is common. Nonetheless, this misapprehension remains among many physicians and unfortunately, narcotic analgesics continue to be underprescribed. It has been suggested that the reason for this is the metaphysical use of narcotics, endowing them with mystical fearful powers that cause physician opiophobia.[3,16] This is clearly a fear that must be overcome.

ADHERENCE TO CUSTOMARY PRESCRIBING PRACTICES

Physicians' prescribing behavior has been described as consisting of an intermix of three components or modalities: instrumental, command, and customary.[20] *Instrumental* allows for a critical assessment of the specific condition, the properties of the drugs to be used, and their effectiveness. *Command* is the modality pursued when one acts to avoid any penalties associated with noncompliance. *Customary*, or traditional, behavior reflects actions approved by the community peer group. The prescription of narcotic analgesics most commonly follows the command and customary modalities. Physicians who prescribe inappropriate doses of meperidine or mixed narcotics and benzodiazepines do so not from ignorance, but from following what has been the customary practice of using opioids as conservatively as possible, and then only as a last resort. A recent study of physicians treating patients with metastatic cancer pain highlighted such customary practices.[21] When asked which medications they would prescribe for moderate to severe cancer pain, 38 percent did not choose an opioid first with 14 percent stating they would not choose such a drug even after palliative radiotherapy had failed.

UNCONSCIOUS BIAS

It is unfortunate but true that some of us react to a person's complaint based not on the specific complaint, as much as on the characteristics of the person complaining. It has been shown that physicians' attitudes toward alcoholic or drug-dependent persons may interfere with their diagnosis and treatment.[22] Another study assessing the use of analgesics in an emergency room found Hispanic patients with bone fractures to be twice as likely as non-Hispanic white patients to receive no pain medication.[23]

Similarly, persons in chronic pain who have seen many physicians without relief are, at times, thought by physicians to be less than honest concerning their symptoms. They are perceived as coming in for a visit only to request medication to allow them to get high. African-American patients have also been reported more likely to receive less than adequate analgesics. One study found patients attending cancer pain treatment clinics less likely to receive adequate analgesics when those clinics were treating primarily minority groups.[24] Patients with acute painful states, such as sickle cell disease, who may have developed a tolerance for narcotics and are in need of an increased dose, are often considered to be exaggerating their pain. Women and the elderly with metastatic cancer also were more likely to obtain less adequate analgesia than others. At times inadequate analgesics are prescribed because the patient appears less ill than the physician would expect if severe pain was present. One survey reported that 76 percent of physicians admit an inability to accurately assess pain, which suggests that many physicians only recognize pain when a person truly appears to be suffering or when function is severely impaired.[21]

CULTURAL AND SOCIAL BARRIERS

Finally, since people's beliefs are formed by the society in which they live, often when a physician wishes to prescribe appropriately to relieve pain, the patient refuses to take this drug, also displaying opiophobia. This is frequently seen when one tries to prescribe methadone to a person in chronic pain who is not receiving relief from his or her current medication regimen. Often the person is on impressive amounts of short-acting narcotic analgesics, as well as dependency-producing amounts of benzodiaze-pines and other sleeping pills. Although the person remains somewhat groggy, the pain persists and prevents functioning. Yet, methadone is refused because the person feels this will incur the label of "junkie" due to the use of methadone in maintenance therapy for heroin dependency. The same person, however, will have little concern about taking large doses of Demerol or Dilaudid. It is difficult to overcome these biases, yet it is essential to do so in order to maximize the chances of providing effective pain relief.

OVERPRESCRIPTION OF ANALGESICS

At times, inappropriate excessive prescriptions of analgesics occur. A physician may be aware of an individual's physical dependency but, because of compassion for the patient's efforts to obtain this drug, may rationalize its prescription in order to decrease the person's anxiety or concern. Persons dependent upon various prescription drugs often are able to manipulate a physician into prescribing medication for imagined ailments without the phy-sician realizing that these medications will only further a physical dependen-cy. In such cases, a person may visit many physicians, requesting only a small number of pills, returning in a sequential yet "spaced" pattern to prevent arousing suspicion of drug abuse.

Physicians who themselves have become physically dependent on pre-scription drugs may, in an attempt to rationalize their own dependence, prescribe these drugs in increasing dosage. Finally, a small but finite number of physicians uncaring of the hazards associated with misuse and abuse of such drugs may prescribe them solely for profit. Although these physicians represent an extremely small proportion of practitioners, none-theless, in certain instances, they may be responsible for the appearance of large numbers of drugs on the street.

THE DRUG-DEPENDENT PHYSICIAN

The epitome of iatrogenic drug dependence is the drug-dependent phy-sician. The psychological milieu in which many physicians function is quite conducive to drug abuse. Long working hours, stresses inherent in dealing with acutely ill patients, and the difficulty encountered in accept-ing personal limitations, accompanied by the unique availability of mood-altering drugs, predispose physicians toward the use of these agents to facilitate coping with prevailing life stresses.

It is quite difficult to determine the degree of physician drug dependence with any accuracy. The easy availability of psychotropic drugs allows long periods of use prior to detection. A 1966 survey of medical students' amphetamine use revealed 35 percent to have taken amphetamines at least once.[25] A 20-year follow-up of a physician cohort found them to have taken more sedatives, stimulants, and tranquilizers than other college graduates.[26,27] Other studies have confirmed the particular vulnerability of physicians to drug dependence, with physicians considered to be almost twice as likely to misuse mood-altering drugs when compared to others in comparable socioeconomic groups, and 30 to 100 times greater than the general population.[28,29,30,31,32,33] Conflicting findings, however, have been reported with dependence problems among physicians believed not to be significantly higher than other professional groups.[29]

Once a dependency problem is detected, however, the physician is often hesitant to seek help. Hesitancy of other physicians to report a colleague also delays treatment and reinforces continued drug-taking behavior.[25,30,31,32] Treatment of dependent physicians is often quite difficult. Similar to nonphysicians, they are manipulative and show a considerable facility in vacillation, rationalization, and prevarication that interferes greatly with the treatment process. Therapeutic success is usually related to underlying psychologic disturbance rather than to the drug abused or intensity of dependency. At present, increasing attention is being focused on the impaired physician. Most states have instituted impaired-physician programs and medical centers have established committees to identify, treat, and most important, prevent the impaired physician from providing inappropriate care.

SUMMARY

Existing evidence suggests that iatrogenic drug dependence is a real phenomenon but one that occurs infrequently when dependency-producing drugs are prescribed in an appropriate manner. Consistent narcotic use in chronic pain of known etiology that is unable to be relieved by other means, while associated with physical dependence, may nonetheless allow an individual to function in a productive manner. The potential for the development of iatrogenic dependence to barbiturates or other drugs used inappropriately to promote or enhance analgesics is much greater. Since physicians are often less inhibited in prescribing these medications, the indication for their use are frequently interpreted rather liberally. The many factors involved in inappropriate prescription of analgesics are all able to be identified, and when this is done, effective pain relief can occur.

REFERENCES

1. Hill CS, Jr. The negative influence of licensing and disciplinary boards and drug enforcement agencies on pain treatment with opioid analgesics. *J Pharmaceut Care in Pain and Symptom Control*, 1993, 1:43–61.

2. Joranson DE. Regulation influence on pain management: Real or imagined? *J Pharmaceut Care in Pain and Symptom Control*, 1993, 1:113–118.

3. Stimmel B. Underprescription/overprescription: Narcotic as metaphor. *Bull NY Acad of Med*, 1985, 61:742–752.

4. Miller RR. Propoxyphene: A review. *Am J Hosp Pharm*, 1977, 34:413–423.

5. National Institute on Drug Abuse. *Phase report*, Drug Abuse Warning Network, Project DAWN: U.S. Department of Justice, U.S. Department of Health, Education, and Welfare, July-Sept 1977.

6. New warning on propoxyphene. *FDA Drug Bulletin*, 1979, 9:22–23.

7. Smith RJ. Federal government faces painful decision on Darvon. *Science*, 1979, 203:857–858.

8. Maruta T, Swanson DW, Finlayson RE. Drug abuse and dependency in patients with chronic pain. *Mayo Clin Proc*, 1979, 54:241–244.

9. Bailey WJ. Nonmedical use of pentazocine (letter). *JAMA*, 1979, 242:2392.

10. Inciardi JA, Chambers CD. Patterns of pentazocine abuse and addiction. *NY State J Med*, 1971, 71:1727–1733.

11. Lavelle TL, Hammersley R, Forsyth A, Bain D. The use of buprenorphine and temazepam by drug injectors. *J Addictive Diseases*, 1991, 10(3):5–14.

12. Glatt MM. Alcoholism (letter). *Lancet*, 1983, 2:735.

13. Shaw A. Women inmates are being overtranquilized. *The Journal*. Toronto, October 10, 1983.

14. Chambers CD, White OZ, Linquest JH. Physicians' attitudes and prescribing behavior. A focus on minor tranquilizers. National Meeting on Prescribing. New York: City College of the City University of New York, 1981.

15. Marks RM, Sachar EJ. Undertreatment of medical inpatients with narcotic analgesics. *Ann Intern Med*, 1973, 78:173–181.

16. Morgan JP, Plect DL. Opiophobia in the United States. *The undertreatment of severe pain in society and medication: Conflicting signals for prescribing of patients*. Lexington, MA: Lexington Books, 1983, 313–326.

17. Chambers CD, Moffett AD. Negro opiate addiction. In: Ball JC, Chambers CD (eds.). *The epidemiology of opiate addiction in the United States*. Springfield, IL: Charles C Thomas, 1970:288–300.

18. Porter J, Jick H. Addiction rare in inpatients treated with narcotics (letter). *N Engl J Med*, 1980, 302:123.

19. Fishbain DA, Rosomoff HL, Rosomoff RS. Drug abuse, dependence, and addiction in chronic pain patients. *Clin J Pain*, 1992, 8:77–85.

20. Termin P. *Taking your medicine: Drug regulations in the United States*. Cambridge, MA: Harvard University Press, 1980:12–17.

21. Cleeland CS, Gonin R, Hatfield AK, Edmonson JH, Blum RH, Stewart JA, Pandya KJ. Pain and its treatment in outpatients with metastatic cancer. *New Engl J Med*, 1994, 330:592–596.

22. Chappel JN, Schnoll SH. Physician attitudes: Effect on the treatment of chemically dependent patients. *JAMA,* 1977, 237:2318–2319.

23. Todd KH, Samaroo N, Hoffman JR. Ethnicity as a risk factor for inadequate emergency department analgesia. *JAMA,* 1993, 269:1537–1539.

24. Blendon RJ, Aiken LH, Freeman HE, Corey CR. Access to medical care for black and white Americans: A matter of continuing concern. *JAMA,* 1989, 261:278–281.

25. Smith SN, Blachly PH. Amphetamine usage by medical students. *J Med Educ,* 1966, 41:167–270.

26. Vaillant GE, Brighton JR, McArthur C. Physicians' use of mood-altering drugs: A 20-year follow-up report. *N Engl J Med,* 1970, 282:365–370.

27. Vaillant GE, Sobowale NC, McArthur C. Some psychological vulnerabilities of physicians. *N Engl J Med,* 1972, 287:372–375.

28. Johnson RP, Connelly JC. Addicted physicians: A closer look. *JAMA,* 1981, 245:253–258.

29. Winick C. Physician narcotic addicts. *Soc Prob,* 1961, 9:174–186.

30. McAuliffe WE, Rohman M, Wechsler H. Alcohol, substance use, and other risk-factors of impairment in a sample of physicians-in-training. *Advances in Alcohol and Substance Abuse,* 1984, 4(2):67–87.

31. Bissell L, Jones RW. The alcoholic physician: A survey. *Am J Psychiatry,* 1976, 133:1142–1146.

32. Vincent MO, Robinson EA, Latt I. Physicians as patients. *Can Med Assoc J,* 1969, 100:403–412.

33. Green RC, Jr, Carroll GJ, Buxton WD. Drug addiction among physicians: The Virginia experience. *JAMA,* 1976, 236:1372–1375.

SECTION IV:
MANAGEMENT OF PAIN
IN SPECIAL POPULATIONS

Chapter 16

Pain Relief in Children and the Elderly

INTRODUCTION

In the preceding chapters the pharmacological actions of analgesics and other drugs used to facilitate analgesia have been described, as have the basic approaches to be used by the physician confronted with a patient in pain. Although the information presented is applicable regardless of the etiology of the pain, there are certain groups who may be particularly sensitive to drug effects or who, by virtue of an underlying medical or psychologic disorder, may be particularly recalcitrant to therapy.

Each practicing physician frequently comes in contact with these individuals. Recognition that such individuals require some additional thought before prescribing an analgesic may prevent untoward drug reactions, provide more satisfactory analgesia, and, most important, facilitate the development of a stronger physician-patient bond. This chapter will focus on special aspects of management of pain in the young and the elderly.

CHILDREN

Although the treatment of pain in adults is far from optimal, evidence from a wide variety of sources suggests that relieving pain in children is even less adequate for reasons that are less than valid (Tables 16.1, 16.2). However, the consequences of allowing children to remain in pain are considerable and often either minimized or derided by many health care providers.

Ability of Newborns to Experience and Remember Pain

On the basis of early and inadequate studies, it was believed that the biology of the newborn did not include actual pain perception. As a result,

TABLE 16.1. Analgesic Use in Children

Frequently analgesics not prescribed for painful procedures
Prescribed analgesics often not administered
PRN orders rarely carried out
When possible, least potent analgesic administered regardless of intensity of pain
For similar procedures, children less likely to receive analgesics than adults

TABLE 16.2. Rationalizations for Inadequate Prescribing of Analgesics to Children

Newborns not capable of perceiving pain
Children will not remember painful experiences
Pain in children cannot be accurately measured
Response to potent analgesics will cause serious side effects
Use may promote addiction in the future
Children may exaggerate degree of pain
Children are more susceptible to respiratory depression than adults

analgesics even during surgical procedures were frequently not provided.[1,2,3,4] This has been shown to be incorrect. Pain pathways are well developed by the eighth month of gestation, and studies of newborns have demonstrated that they do respond to painful stimuli. Children most certainly experience pain which, similar to adults, is accompanied by considerable stress and anxiety. Unlike adults, however, children are less able to express their dissatisfaction with the absence of relief for their pain or even indicate their desire for pain medication. Early adverse experience of pain may affect the child or later the adult's response to pain. The difficulties that persist in providing effective treatment can be illustrated by a survey of anesthesiologists in England. Although the majority of those surveyed believed neonates experienced pain, few provided analgesics for postoperative pain.

Evidence suggests not only that newborns experience pain, but also that they have the capacity to remember painful experiences.[5] Studies of circumcision have found that such changes may affect the responses of newborns to their environment, including the parent/infant bond, as well as later psychological sequela.

Measurement of Pain in Children

It has often been said that children are not accurate reporters of pain due to the secondary gain that occurs when pain is expressed. There is no reason to believe, however, that children would be any less accurate in expressing their discomfort than adults. In fact, when children are allowed to self-administer narcotic analgesics such as the use of patient-controlled analgesics for sickle-cell crises, they have been found to be quite responsible.

It is also not difficult, as described below, to measure the degree of pain a child might be experiencing. However, as with adults, if the child appears to be in more pain than the physician considers appropriate, the response should be weighted toward taking the child's word and relieving the pain.

The Use of Opioids and Their Side Effects

It is commonly believed that children may experience more serious or frequent adverse effects from opioids and, equally important, have a greater risk of developing an addiction in later life. Both of these beliefs are incorrect.[6] Although newborns may be somewhat more susceptible to respiratory depression that adults, children are not. With either population, one should prescribe narcotics appropriately to avoid respiratory depression. If respiratory depression does occur, adequate monitoring will detect this quickly and immediate reversal of the depression can occur with narcotic antagonists.

There is similarly no evidence that appropriate use of opioids in children promotes addiction during adulthood. Of all the parameters associated with addictive behaviors, appropriate treatment of pain in children has not appeared as a risk factor. This fear of addiction is actually more prevalent in physicians than in patients and is responsible at times for rather strange behavior. This is best exemplified by physicians treating newborns who are undergoing narcotic withdrawal due to their mother's dependency on opioids, with pharobarbital rather than tincture of opium. Although studies have shown that opium or paregoric (a mild narcotic) are the best drugs to use, phenobarbital is most commonly preferred so as not to "perpetuate a narcotic addiction." Yet phenobarbital itself is dependency-producing and is clearly not the drug of choice. This fear of addiction is also the primary reason why, although guidelines exist for pain management in children (similar to guidelines for adults), they are not more closely adhered to when treating children.

Pain Management

It is therefore quite important to optimally manage painful states in children. One must not only assess the potential for an event to produce pain, but must attempt to diminish as much as possible the intensity of the pain that the child may experience. In order to accomplish this, the guidelines promulgated by the Agency for Health Care Policy and Research should be carefully followed (Table 16.3). Assessing the presence of and intensity of pain is especially important. Frequently, children who are in pain or who are anxious will not be able to express their feelings clearly.

The monitoring of objective parameters, such as pulse, blood pressure, and respiration, often helpful in adults to indicate pain, is of much less value in children due to the ever-present anxiety that affects these parameters in a similar manner. As a result, suggestive responses, such as facial expression, continual restlessness, and extreme limitation in movement of a body part may be indications of continuing pain. Reassurance, maintaining physical contact, such as holding the child's hand, and the presence of the parents or a cherished object may assist in relieving the anxiety and allowing a better assessment of the pain. If a child is able to verbalize the presence of pain, the intensity should be assessed, as should the suitability of patient-controlled

TABLE 16.3. Guidelines for Management of Pain in Hospitalized Children

• Treat anticipated procedure-related pain prophylactically
• Provide unhurried adequate explanation of procedure to child and family
• Introduce child to all physicians and other personnel who will be providing care before procedure
• Be attentive to environmental stimuli and carefully explain environment to child
• Do not delay expected time of procedure
• Provide preprocedure medication whenever appropriate
• Allow parents to be with the child whenever he/she is awake, regardless of location of the child
• Do not administer drugs in a painful manner   —Intramuscular and rectal administrations should be avoided
• Use both pharmacologic and nonpharmacologic means to relieve pain
• Develop an accurate means of assessing presence and intensity of pain
• Consider appropriateness of patient-controlled analgesic

Source: Adapted from Reference 3.

analgesia (PCA). PCA has been used effectively in children as young as age ten.

Choosing an Analgesic

The choice of an analgesic to relieve pain in a child should be made in accordance with the general principles previously discussed (Chapter 13). However, with respect to children, certain differences exist in their responses to specific analgesics. Aspirin, although an extremely effective analgesic, should not be used in children due to its association with Reye's syndrome. It may also have a proportionally greater effect on gastric secretion and platelet aggregation than in adults. Other NSAIDs are effective in treating pain, especially in the presence of inflammation, and have been approved for pediatric use. Acetaminophen is also an effective analgesic for mild pain and can enhance the analgesic actions of narcotic analgesics.

In selecting a narcotic analgesic, it is important to remember that newborns and very young children may be slightly more susceptible to the respiratory depressant effects than adults, due to altered metabolic pathways and slower rates of excretion. Doses must therefore be adjusted accordingly. Narcotics can be given by intravenous, oral, transmucosal, or transdermal routes. The use of meperidine in children should be carefully considered as renal function is normally diminished during the first days after birth. Normeperidine, the active metabolite of meperidine, is a potent convulsant and, when used in children with immature renal function, may be associated with toxic effects. Similarly, the mixture of meperidine, promethazine (Phenergan), and, at times, chlorpromazine (Thorazine) often used in adults should not be given to children due to a high incidence of adverse effects. Fentanyl, an extremely potent analgesic, is cleared rapidly in the newborn, suggesting that an increased dose in neonates may be required. However, fentanyl's long half-life can be associated with accumulation in the tissue with a potential for respiratory depression.

Summary

There is no reason why a child's pain is not taken as seriously as pain experienced by an adult. Guidelines exist to assist physicians less knowledgeable in pain management to provide appropriate relief. Such guidelines should not only be widely disseminated to physicians who care for children but, in appropriate form, to parents whose children are to have surgical procedures and who suffer with chronic painful conditions.

THE ELDERLY

Management of pain in the elderly may present both diagnostic and therapeutic challenges. The aging process is believed to be accompanied by an elevation in pain threshold secondary to degeneration of neurons in the dorsal columns, resulting in a diminished sensory awareness.[7] However, studies in the elderly have not clearly demonstrated a change in pain sensation. Clinically, sensory complaints in the elderly are quite common, even in the absence of objective findings.[8] The presence of pain in nursing home residents has been estimated to be between 45 and 80 percent, with the prevalence of analgesic use only 40 to 50 percent.[8] This is no surprise, as more than 80 percent of the elderly suffer from arthritis and its complications. Yet, little attention has been focused upon pain and its management in the elderly. It has been observed that of the more than 4,000 papers on pain published annually, less than 1 percent describe pain in the elderly.[9]

Determining the Cause of the Pain

Pain that may be of relatively minor significance in a younger person may, in the elderly, signal serious disease.[10,11] Headaches unrelieved by simple analgesics may be the first sign of transient ischemic attacks, temporal arteritis, cervical osteoarthritis, subdural hematomas, or subarachnoid bleeding. Chest pain, which may be mild, nonetheless may represent a broad spectrum of disorders, such as an acute myocardial infarction, arthritis of the spine, herpes zoster infection, or even referred pain from abdominal crises. Abdominal pain due to visceral disease may also present differently. In acute inflammatory states, the expected elevation of white blood cells may be blunted. Localization of pain might be quite difficult. Back pain, a frequent symptom, although most often secondary to degenerative vertebral changes, may also be due to more serious etiologies such as Paget disease, metastatic cancer, or osteomyelitis. Neuropathic pain syndromes due to diabetes, peripheral vascular disease, or herpes zoster infections are not infrequent.

In addition, depression, common among the elderly, may also considerably modify pain perception. At times, chronic pain may be a manifestation of another functional impairment that is perceived as pain. Most often this can occur in the presence of cerebral deficits associated with difficulty in short-term memory or in carrying out perceptual motor functions. Attributing these problems to the presence of pain allows the individual to rationalize an inability to participate in activities. In contrast, unrelieved and unrecognized pain may result in depression and inability to function. It is, therefore, quite important to assess pain symptoms in the elderly carefully in order to identify the cause, as well as develop an appropriate management plan.

Pharmacokinetics of Aging

Although the general principles outlined for treatment of pain (Chapter 13) should be followed in the elderly, the pharmacological approach must be modified due to the effects of aging on the pharmacokinetics of different drugs as well as the tendency for the elderly to be on multiple medications (Table 16.4).

Absorption of drugs from the gastrointestinal tract is altered with aging. These changes may be due to a number of factors, including decreased gastric acidity, absorptive surface, and blood flow to abdominal organs, increased incidence of duodenal diverticula, and prolongation of gastric emptying time.[12] Physiologic changes occurring as part of the aging process can influence drug distribution once absorption has been completed. These alterations include decreases in intracellular fluid, serum albumen, and body weight as well as an increase in the proportion of fatty tissue to lean muscle mass.[13] Age-related changes in the volume of distribution of a drug will have a variable effect depending on the degree of the drug's lipid solubility. Those drugs with a high lipid solubility will have an increased volume of distribution and correspondingly diminished blood levels. Highly ionizable drugs, however, will exhibit a decreased volume of distribution and increased blood levels. In the presence of age-related decreases in serum albumen, drugs highly bound to plasma proteins will have an increased plasma concentration of unbound drugs, which may be associated with a greater potential for toxicity.

A number of age-related physiologic changes promote alterations in biotransformation and ultimately the excretion of drugs.[14] Liver size and activity of the hepatic microsomal enzyme system diminish with age. An associated age-related decrease in renal function may also affect drug excretion. Investigators have demonstrated that an approximately 50 percent decrease in renal function or renal blood flow may enhance plasma half-life and the potential for drug toxicity.[15] Clinically, however, toxicity may not occur if the prolongation in half-life and decrease in biotransformation can be offset by the presence of an increased volume of distribution resulting in an unchanged plasma clearance.

Adverse Effects of Analgesic and Other Mood-Altering Drugs

The elderly are susceptible to all of the side effects generally described with the use of mood-altering drugs used to provide or facilitate analgesia.

TABLE 16.4. Physiologic and Pharmacokinetic Changes Associated with Aging

Physiologic changes	Pharmacokinetic effects
Cardiovascular	
Decrease in cardiac output Decrease in arterial flow Alteration of circulation to organ systems	Redistribution of blood flow from liver and kidneys, resulting in prolonged plasma half-life and diminished biotransformation[a]
Gastrointestinal	
Decrease in gastric acidity Prolonged gastric emptying Decrease in absorptive surface Decrease in liver size and in activity of hepatic microsomal system Increase in incidence of duodenal diverticula	Alteration of ionization and solubility Decrease in drug absorption Decrease in rate of biotransformation[a] Increase in plasma half-life[a] Increases the potential for malabsorption
Metabolic	
Decrease in intracellular fluid Decrease in body weight Decrease in serum albumen Increase in serum globulin Increase in proportion of fatty tissue to muscle mass	Increased effects with standard dosage[a] Increase in free to bound drug ratio[a] Increase in storage of lipid soluble drugs[a] Increase in plasma half-life[a] Increase in volume of distribution[a]
Neuronal	
Increase in rate of neuron loss	Increased susceptibility to hypoxia[a] Increased sensitivity to central depressants[a] Potential for confusion about drug regimen
Renal	
Decrease in renal clearance	Increased plasma half-life[a]

[a]Enhances potential for drug toxicity.

These have been reviewed in previous chapters and will not be discussed here. Certain drug effects, however, may occur with a greater frequency in the elderly, enhancing the possibility of toxic reactions (Table 16.5). This enhanced susceptibility may be due either to the altered physiology of aging or the presence of specific disease states commonly encountered in the elderly.

TABLE 16.5. Selected Age-Related Adverse Effects of Analgesic and Other Mood-Altering Drugs

Drugs	Potential Adverse Effects
Anticholinergics	Confusion[a], constipation, increased intraocular pressure
Antidepressants Tricyclics	Hypotension[b], cardiac arrhythmias[b], syncope[c], anticholinergic effects, considerable potential for adverse drug interactions
MAO inhibitors	Hypotension, considerable potential for adverse interactions with drugs and tyramine-containing foods
Narcotics	Confusion at times accompanied by hallucinations[a], respiratory depression, constipation, acute urinary retention, dependence
Phenothiazines	Hypotension[b], syncope[b,c], lethargy[c], induced parkinsonism, cholestatic jaundice, photosensitivity reactions, hypothyroidism, hypothermia, constipation
Sedatives, hypnotics, and minor tranquilizers[d]	Confusion at times accompanied by hallucinations[a], syncope[c], increased nocturnal restlessness, agitation, urinary incontinence, dependence

[a] Prominent in persons with organic brain syndrome.
[b] Prominent in persons with coronary artery disease and conduction defects.
[c] Prominent in persons with cerebrovascular disease.
[d] Barbiturates associated with most prominent effects; benzodiazepines with least prominent.

Aspirin, Acetaminophen, and NSAIDs

The nonnarcotic analgesics are effective in the elderly, with the NSAIDs being particularly helpful for arthritic pains. However, the risk of gastric side effects such as ulceration and gastrointestinal bleeding is quite real. Renal toxicity from these drugs may also be increased and careful monitoring of renal function is needed when the NSAIDs are prescribed on a chronic basis. In addition, the low ceiling effect of the NSAIDs often results in increasing doses being unable to provide effective analgesia yet increasing toxicity.[16]

Hypnotics, Sedatives, Minor Tranquilizers, and Barbiturates

Altered pharmacokinetics associated with the aging process are most pronounced with those drugs classified as hypnotics, sedatives, or minor tranquilizers. Changes in drug effects associated with aging have been commonly observed with the barbiturates and minor tranquilizers. This increasing sensitivity may be related to several factors, including diminished metabolism or renal clearance or increased cerebral sensitivity secondary to an age-related neuronal loss.

Clinically, the use of barbiturates can be associated with confusion and paradoxical reactions such as agitation, restlessness, and even hallucinations.[17] The morning following barbiturate ingestion is often characterized by a "hangover" effect that may result in confusion and unsteady gait. The use of barbiturates in the elderly may, therefore, be associated with a number of adverse effects. Fortunately, the presence of milder sedatives and tranquilizers allows many of the complications associated with barbiturate use to be avoided.

Benzodiazepines

Benzodiazepines have also been shown to have a more pronounced effect when used in the elderly, although the severity of the response is less than with the barbiturates. In normal individuals, the terminal plasma half-life of diazepam (Valium) exhibits a linear increase with age ranging from a half-life at age 20 of 20 hours, to a half-life of 90 hours at age 80.[18] Diazepam clearance from plasma and plasma binding, however, are not age-dependent. In elderly patients, therefore, diazepam should not be prescribed on a specific fixed-dose regimen in order to avoid the progressive sedative effects of the drug. Metabolic clearance of chlordiazepoxide (Librium) is similarly impaired in the healthy elderly. The use of high-dose flurazepam or nitrazepam in the elderly is also associated with a threefold increase in untoward reactions.[19]

Adverse reactions, however, can occur at any dose, and conflicting findings have been reported in the literature.[20,21,22] Observed changes may be due to an age-related impairment in hepatic enzyme activity or to differences in volume of distribution. Although the newer benzodiazepines may be associated with a lesser incidence of adverse effects, it is still most prudent to use caution when administering any of these drugs to the elderly and to carefully monitor the effects of these drugs over time.

Opioids

Opioids can provide effective analgesia in the elderly. However, susceptibility to their central depressant effects is considerably increased. The volume of distribution of morphine has been shown to decrease with age, resulting in increased plasma morphine levels and prolonged serum half-life. Plasma levels of morphine two minutes after intravenous injection rise twofold in persons over 50 years of age as compared to those under 50.[23] The diminished respiratory reserve seen in the elderly will also affect the response to opioids. This is especially true in individuals with chronic elevations of plasma carbon dioxide. The presence of liver disease can diminish the rate of biotransformation of an opioid accompanied by elevated plasma levels and respiratory depression.

The use of opioids in the elderly should occur only when nonopioid analgesics cannot provide satisfactory relief. Careful monitoring during their use is important as a longer duration of pain relief and an increase in serum levels will be seen. This is especially true with the use of long-acting opioids, such as methadone and transdermal fentanyl. Frequently, the dose initially used must be diminished after 48 hours. Any alteration in alertness or increasing duration of sleep should alert one to the need to lower the dose of narcotic.

The development of tolerance with continued opioid use in chronic pain, however, may be beneficial as tolerance to the respiratory depressant and sedative effect of narcotics occur early. Constipation may result in continuous administration and should be addressed proactively prior to actually prescribing opioids through the use of stool softeners and bulk laxatives.

It has been suggested that meperidine (Demerol) might be preferable to morphine or other more potent opioids due to a lesser effect on respiratory depression as well as diminished side effects of constipation and urinary retention. This potential benefit is outweighed by the potential risks of meperidine, due to the accumulation of normeperidine, especially in persons with renal impairment or in those taking monoamine oxidose inhibitor antidepressants. An age-related decrease in the proportion of meperidine bound to plasma protein may be as much as twofold. Yet its analgesic effect is of shorter duration than its half-life, often resulting in increasing the frequency of administration with toxic effects.[24] In patients tolerant to meperidine, increasing doses may be associated with hyperactivity and convulsions.

Similarly, long-acting opioids with an affinity for K receptors, such as levorphanol or methadone, should be used cautiously, as the elimination half-life is in excess of the duration of analgesia. Chronic use can result in tissue accumulation with resultant sedation and even respiratory depression.

The cholinergic action of many narcotic drugs may result in acute urinary retention when administered to men with enlarged prostates. Constipation, a frequent symptom in the elderly, will also be accentuated. At times an exacerbation of Parkinson's symptoms may occur. Although not life-threatening, these side effects can result in considerable discomfort. Opioid agonists-antagonists such as pentazocine should be avoided due to the high risk of agitation and delirium.

Phenothiazines

The phenothiazines have been used extensively in elderly patients, most often in the nursing home setting for those with senile brain syndromes. Although these drugs are effective, hypotension, which is a common side effect, is much more prominent in the elderly. The elderly are also more susceptible to phenothiazine-induced Parkinsonism, as well as accidental hypothermia.

Electrocardiographic changes, well known to be a phenothiazine dose-related phenomenon, may be of particular concern in the elderly with cardiovascular disease. These changes may vary from mild repolarization abnormalities such as prolongation of QT intervals, flattening of T waves, and appearance of U waves to ventricular premature beats and even ventricular tachycardia and fibrillation.[25-30] Sudden death in patients receiving phenothiazines has been reported for more than a decade.

Although the phenothiazines are effective major tranquilizers, their use in the elderly, especially for those with cardiovascular disease, should be carefully considered. This is especially important as phenergan is often used with narcotics to enhance analgesia. If major tranquilizers are needed in this population, the use of the butyrophenones such as haloperidol (Haldol) is accompanied by a lesser incidence of adverse effects.[31]

Antidepressants

The administration of tricyclic antidepressants to geriatric patients, especially those with preexisting cardiovascular disease, can be associated with clinically important orthostatic hypotension.[32] Other adverse effects include cardiac arrhythmias, congestive heart failure, and symptoms such as urinary retention, which are due to their anticholinergic actions.

Age-related changes in the pharmacokinetics of the tricyclics have been demonstrated. Older individuals have been shown to exhibit high plasma levels and prolonged plasma half-lives of amitriptyline and imipramine.[33] Although all of the tricyclics are prescribed with equanimity, certain pharmacologic properties of the different drugs suggest some may be more advantageous. The orthostatic changes produced by imipramine and amitriptyline at relatively low doses warrant cautious use of these agents. Anticholinergic side effects are also of concern, and agents such as doxepin and amitriptyline should be carefully administered. Nonetheless, amitriptyline, imipramine, and desipramine have been shown to be quite help-ful in relieving neuropathic pain. Use of these agents should, however, begin with low doses to observe the presence of any untoward effects.

A number of new antidepressants have appeared on the market that are chemically unrelated to either the tricyclic or tetracyclic antidepressant and are believed to have minimal adverse effects on the cardiovascular system. These drugs include sertraline (Zoloft), bupropion (Wellbutrin) and fluoxetine (Prozac). Still, when used in the elderly, careful monitoring is needed.

Principles of Prescribing to the Elderly

Several of the principles advocated in prescribing analgesics need to be emphasized. As a group, the elderly are usually on multiple medications prior to the need for any analgesic, and at times may be confused as to the appropriate way to take their drugs (Table 16.6). In addition, failing eye-sight may prevent appropriate identification of medications or directions concerning their use.

Studies have indicated that for various reasons (Chapter 3), as many as half of the elderly do not take their medications as prescribed, with up to 35 percent misusing drugs to such a degree to have serious adverse effects.[34,35] Compliance has been reported to be the lowest for those drugs acting on the central nervous system, with misuse predominantly being underuse.[36,37]

Analgesic prescription to the elderly should be directed toward relieving pain as simply and as directly as possible. A thorough knowledge of the patient's existing medications is essential to avoid untoward drug interactions. The least potent analgesic capable of providing satisfactory analgesia should be prescribed with the directions for use clearly written. Most important, time

TABLE 16.6. Factors Promoting Poor Drug Compliance in the Elderly

Presence of senile cerebral changes
Diminishing eyesight
Need to take multiple medications
Feeling that pain cannot be relieved
Minimal symptoms
Isolated environment without sufficient support
Development of symptoms due to adverse drug interactions
Complicated, nonwritten directions

must be taken to carefully explain the reasons for prescribing the analgesic, the way it is to be taken, and the interactions it might have with other medications. These instructions should be clearly written and the person should be asked to review the information with the physician or other health care provider. If the person is part of a family unit or appears to be slightly confused, then instructions should be given to another family member or member of the staff concerned with that person's care.

SUMMARY

In summary, the aging process can modify the elderly's perception and response to pain as well as the dosage and type of analgesic drugs to be prescribed. The possibility of drug interactions are also increased, as this population is much more likely to be taking multiple medications for coexisting ailments. Finally, the appearance of multiple complaints may give the physician the feeling that the discomfort is less than that actually experienced. However, if the basic principles outlined above are kept in mind, there is no reason why pain in the elderly cannot be adequately diagnosed and effectively treated.

REFERENCES

1. Anand KJ, Hickey PR. Pain and its effects in the human neonate and fetus. *N Engl J Med,* 1987, 317:1321–1329.

2. Bhatt-Mehta V, Rosen DA. Management of acute pain in children. *Clin Pharmacol,* 1991, 10:667–685.

3. Walco GA, Cassidy RC, Schechter NL. Pain, hurt, and harm: The ethics of pain control in infants and children. *N Engl J Med,* 1994, 331:541–544.

4. U.S. Agency for Health Care Policy and Research. *Acute pain management: Operative or medical procedures and trauma.* Rockville, MD: U.S. Department of Health and Human Services, 1992.

5. Owens ME. Pain in infancy: Conceptual and methodological issues. *Pain,* 1988, 20:213–230.

6. Purcell-Jones G, Dormon F, Sumner E. The use of opioids in neonates. A retrospective study of 933 cases. *Anaesthesia,* 1987, 42:1316–1320.

7. Andrew W. *The anatomy of aging in man and animals.* New York: Grune & Stratton, 1971.

8. Gloth FM. Concerns with chronic analgesic therapy in elderly patients. *Am J Med,* 1996, 101 (Suppl. 1A): 19S–23S.

9. Melding PS. Is there such a thing as geriatric pain? *Pain,* 1991, 46:119–212.

10. Medina JL, Diamond S, Rubino FA. Headaches in patients with transient ischemic attacks. *Headache,* 1975, 15:194–197.

11. Zoob M. Differentiating the causes of chest pain. *Geriatrics,* 1978, 33: 95–101.

12. Stevenson IH, Salem SAM, Shepherd AMM. Studies on drug absorption and metabolism in the elderly. In: Crooks J, Stevenson IH (eds.). *Drugs and the elderly, perspectives in geriatric clinical pharmacology.* Baltimore: University Park Press, 1979:51–63.

13. Mitchard M. Drug distribution in the elderly. In: Crocks J, Stevenson IH (eds.). *Drugs and the elderly, perspectives in geriatric clinical pharmacology.* Baltimore: University Park Press, 1979:65–76.

14. Adelman RC. Age dependent effects in enzyme induction: A biochemical expression of aging. *Exp Gerontol,* 1971, 6:75–87.

15. Crooks J, O'Malley K, Stevenson IH. Pharmacokinetics in the elderly. *Clin Pharmacokinet,* 1976, 1:280–296.

16. Ferrell BA. Pain evaluation and management in the nursing home. *Ann Intern Med,* 1995, 123:681–687.

17. Dawson-Butterworth K. The chemopsychotherapeutics of geriatric sedation. *J Am Geriatr Soc,* 1970, 18:97–114.

18. Klotz U, Avant GR, Hoyumpa A, Schenker S, Wilkinson GR. The effect of age and liver disease on the disposition and elimination of diazepam in adult man. *J Clin Invest,* 1975, 55:347–359.

19. Greenblatt DJ, Allen MD, Shader RI. Toxicity of flurazepam in the elderly. *Clin Pharmacol Ther,* 1977, 21:355–361.

20. Kraus JW, Desmond PV, Marshall JP, Johnson RF, Schenker S, Wilkinson GR. Effects of aging and liver disease on disposition of lorazepam. *Clin Pharmacol Ther,* 1978, 24:411–419.

21. Greenblatt DJ, Allen MD, Locniskar A, Shader RI. Age, sex, and diazepam kinetics. *Clin Pharmacol Ther,* 1979, 25:227.

22. Shull HJ, Jr, Wilkinson GR, Johnson R, Schenker S. Normal disposition of oxazepam in acute viral hepatitis and cirrhosis. *Ann Intern Med,* 1976, 84:420–425.

23. Berkowitz BA, Ngai SH, Yang JC, Hempstead J, Spector S. The disposition of morphine in surgical patients. *Clin Pharmacol Ther,* 1975, 17:629–635.

24. Foley KM, Inturrisi CE. Analgesic drug therapy in cancer pain: Principles and practice. *Med Clin North Am,* 1987, 71:207–232.

25. Backman H, Elosuo R. The effect of neuroleptics on electrocardiograms. *Acta Med Scand,* 1968, 183:543 – 547.

26. Dillenkoffer RL, Gallant DM, Phillips JH. Electrocardiographic evaluation of mesoridazine (Serentil). *Curr Ther Res,* 1972, 14:71–72.

27. Fletcher GF, Kazamias TM. Cardiotoxic effects of mellaril: Conduction disturbances and supraventricular arrhythmias. *Am Heart J,* 1969, 78:135–138.

28. Levine DF, Marshall AJ. Cardiac arrhythmia induced by phenothiazine. *Lancet,* 1975, 3:990.

29. Leestma JE, Koenig KL. Sudden death and phenothiazines: A current controversy. *Arch Gen Psychiatry,* 1968, 18:137–148.

30. Peele R, Von Loetzen IS. Phenothiazine deaths: A critical review. *Am J Psychiatry,* 1973, 130:306–309.

31. Aman MG, Werry JS. The effect of methylphenidate and haloperidol on the heart rate and blood pressure of hyperactive children with special reference to time of action. *Psychopharmacologica,* 1975, 43:163–168.

32. Muller OF, Goodman N, Bellet S. The hypotensive effect of imipramine hydrochloride in patients with cardiovascular disease. *Clin Pharmacol Ther,* 1961, 2:300–307.

33. Nies A, Robinson DS, Friedman MJ, Green R, Cooper TB, Ravaris CL, Ives JO. Relationship between age and tricyclic antidepressant plasma levels. *Am J Psychiatry,* 1977, 134:790–793.

34. Wandless I, Davie JW. Can drug compliance in the elderly be improved? *Br Med J,* 1977, 1:359–361.

35. Smith DL. Patient compliance with medication regimens. *Drug Intel Clin Pharm,* 1976, 10:386–393.

36. Wade OL. Compliance problems. In J Crooks, IH Stevenson (eds.). *Drugs and the elderly: Perspectives in geriatric clinical pharmacology.* Baltimore: University Park Press, 1979:287–291.

37. National Institute on Drug Abuse. *Services research notes: Drug misuse by the elderly.* Rockville, MD: U.S. Department of Health and Human Services, Public Health Service, Alcohol, Drug Abuse, and Mental Health Administration, 1980.

Chapter 17

Relieving Pain in Malignant Disorders: The Acquired Immunodeficiency Syndrome and Cancer

THE ACQUIRED IMMUNODEFICIENCY SYNDROME

It has been more than a decade since the first case of the acquired immunodeficiency syndrome (AIDS) was identified in the United States. Infection with the human immunodeficiency virus (HIV), the cause of this disease, is felt to be present in more than 1 million people, with over 500,000 cases of AIDS having been reported to the Center for Disease Control and Prevention through October 1995.[1] In part, this number reflects the decision of the Center for Diseases Control and Prevention in 1993 to expand the criteria to allow the diagnosis of AIDS to be made. Between January 1, 1993 and March 31, 1993 a 20 percent increase in the number of AIDS cases occurred, compared to the same time frame in 1992.[2] The magnitude of this problem is evident when one realizes that worldwide it is estimated that 18 million adults and 1.5 million children have been infected with the human immunodeficiency virus, with 4.5 million having developed AIDS.

Epidemiology

Although initially described in this country as prevailing in the homosexual community, the demographics of HIV infection have, in fact, changed considerably, with heterosexual intravenous drug users representing 27 percent of AIDS cases now reported. In addition, the proportion of cases among non-IVDU (intravenous drug-using) heterosexual persons, women, African-Americans, and Hispanics has continued to escalate.[3] In the United States, AIDS is almost three times more common among African-Americans and Hispanics than in whites, representing 38 percent of all cases reported between 1993 and 1995. This racial disproportion is most prevalent in woman: in 1992, rates per 100,000 population in non-Hispanic blacks were 31.3, in Hispanics 14.6, and in whites 1.8. The largest proportional increase in AIDS reporting is in cases of heterosexual contact, which have increased from 3 percent of all AIDS cases between 1981 and 1987 to 10 percent between 1993 and 1995. Women are especially vulnerable, increasing from 8 percent of those affected between 1981 and 1987 to 17.5 percent between 1993 and 1995. In fact, in 1992, for the first time, the number of women infected through heterosexual contact exceeded the number infected through intravenous drug use.[4] Infection rates through heterosexual contact have been found to roughly parallel infectivity rates of sexually transmitted diseases; as the presence of STD increases, the chance of infection with HIV increases 10- to 100-fold.

The clinical manifestations of this disease are related to: (1) the actual effect of HIV on the immune system; (2) the effect of infections not ordinarily seen developing in the immunocompromised person (opportunistic infections); (3) the appearance of Kaposi's sarcoma; and (4) the effect of the virus on other organs. Mortality due to AIDS and its complications remains quite high; of the approximately 500,000 cases reported through October 1995, 62 percent have died. HIV infection was the third leading cause of death for persons aged 25 to 44 years in the United States, and the second leading cause of death in men in this group, representing 15 percent of all deaths.[5] Similar to HIV infection, mortality rates for black and Hispanic men were threefold and twofold respectively that of white men. This disproportion was even greater in women where mortality rates were 15-fold higher in black women and 5-fold higher in Hispanic women, as compared to white women.

However with consistent advances in treatment of the medical complications of AIDS, people are living longer. Between 1981 and 1987, of the cases of AIDS reported, 95 percent had died. This percentage decreased to 84 percent of cases reported between 1988 and 1992 and to 37 percent of cases reported between 1993 and 1995. While the magnitude of this improvement is skewed by temporal reporting factors, nonetheless, persons with AIDS have increasing chances of survival and the quality of their lives has become increasingly important.

Pain in Persons with AIDS

There are many reasons for a person with AIDS to be in pain (Table 17.1), with the intensity varying greatly depending on the underlying cause. When the pain is associated with an infectious agent, then aggressive treatment with appropriate antibiotics, antiviral, or antifungal agents

TABLE 17.1. Painful Symptoms in HIV Infection

SYMPTOM	CAUSE
Headache	Aseptic meningitis Cervical spine disease Cerebral diseases Cryptococcal encephalitis Toxoplasmosis Lymphoma Muscle tension headaches
Cutaneous Pain	Herpes zoster/simplex Kaposi's sarcoma
Extremity Pain	Guillain-Barré syndrome Mono- or polyneuropathy Herpes zoster Multifocal leukoencephalopathy
Orofacial Pain	Candidiasis Ulcers Peridontal disease Herpes zoster/simplex Parotid gland infection

hopefully will eliminate the infection and relieve the pain. In many circumstances, however, even with adequate treatment of an infection, pain will persist — especially in the terminal stages.

The most common reasons for chronic pain are the Guillain-Barré syndrome, herpes zoster infection with postherpetic neuropathy, and the predominantly sensory neuropathies. Whereas herpes infections can often be treated effectively with a variety of antiviral agents such a Idoxuridine, Vidarabine, and Acyclovir, the pain resulting from postherpetic neuropathy, Guillain-Barré syndrome, and the sensory neuropathics must be treated with the common available analgesics.[6,7] These include intrathecal and epidermal infusion of anesthetics, nerve blocks, and oral analgesics.[8] One survey of 100 persons with AIDS admitted to a hospice found more than half to be able to be treated only with oral analgesics. One-third of all recurring painful episodes was due to the presence of a peripheral neuropathy. For this reason combinations of narcotic analgesics with tricyclic antidepressants, such as amitriptyline or imipramine, often can provide considerable relief. Since AIDS is frequently accompanied by considerable depression, the use of antidepressants also has a value independent of the ability to enhance analgesia.

The use of marijuana in AIDS treatment as an antiemetic and appetite stimulant, especially when muscle wasting is prominent, remains controversial. Many with AIDS report great benefits. Unfortunately, despite attempts of physicians who care for AIDS patients to establish clinical trials to document its effectiveness, opposition by a variety of public agencies have prevented the initiation of such sorely needed studies.

Equally important to providing appropriate medication and surgical intervention when necessary to relieve pain is the need to be supportive and reassuring. The anxiety surrounding AIDS is probably equal to or greater than that seen in any other disease, including cancer. This is largely due to the stigma placed by society on those with AIDS. Presently, AIDS is a terminal disease and, unlike several forms of cancer, there is no known cure. It is therefore incumbent for those in the health professions to recognize this and to approach each person with AIDS in a compassionate, caring, and nonjudgmental manner. As with other painful conditions, the relief of pain and suffering are the primary objectives.

MALIGNANT DISEASES

Unfortunately, cancer remains an extremely common disease in our society, affecting over 8 million Americans and being responsible for approximately one out of every five deaths. Nowhere is concern over relief of pain more prominent than in individuals with cancer. Yet despite the fact that pain can be easily controlled, in over 90 percent of persons, the analgesia provided is less than optimal, resulting either in persistent pain or pain relief at the expense of obscuring mentation, thereby preventing a desirable level of function.[9,10,11,12,13,14] Inadequate pain relief is not only a perception of those with cancer. In a survey of almost 900 physicians who care for cancer patients, 86 percent believed that adequate pain medication was not provided for their patients. It is estimated that as many as one out of four patients with terminal cancer may die without adequate pain relief.[11] Yet even when surveys are performed among persons with metastatic cancer being treated at cancer centers, up to 42 percent of persons in pain are not provided with adequate analgesia. Such instances were found to be three times more likely in persons who were attending centers that treated predominately minorities. The risk of inadequate treatment was also increased if the patient was a woman, over 70 years of age, or actually functioning better than expected.[12]

There are many reasons for inadequate management of pain for cancer patients (Table 17.2). All can and must be effectively addressed and remedied by those providing medical care.

Prevalence

Not all persons with cancer experience pain. Surveys of hospitalized cancer patients found between 29 and 38 percent requiring analgesics.[10] It

TABLE 17.2. Reasons for Inadequate Pain Relief in Persons with Cancer

Inadequate knowledge resulting in:

  Considering development of dependence as an important issue

  Inadequate dose, schedule, and route of administration of narcotic

  Failure to administer a dose in accordance with individual needs

  Failure to use drugs other than analgesics to enhance analgesia

  Failure to appropriately assess coexisting psychological and social factors that might intensify pain

  Failure to utilize available nonpharmacologic techniques to relieve pain or enhance analgesia

Prevailing attitudes of health care providers, resulting in:

  Fear of creating addicts

  Concern with prescribing controlled substances

  Underestimating intensity of pain when a person has previously been on analgesics due to the belief person is exaggerating pain or manipulating health care providers to obtain narcotics

  Belief that psychosocial factors are not of primary importance in relieving pain

  Lack of understanding of beliefs and attitudes of different cultures or ethnic groups

Prevailing attitudes of persons with cancer pain:

  Reluctance to report pain

  Fear of becoming addicted to pain medications

  Fear of not being considered a "good" patient by expressing need for analgesia

Source: Adapted from Reference 9.

should be noted that these figures are probably greater than those seen among all patients with cancer, as these surveys were conducted in the hospital setting. Persons with advanced disease, however, experience pain much more frequently. Pain is seen in 60 to 80 percent of individuals at terminal care facilities.[11-13]

Diagnosis of Pain

There are three major categories of pain commonly seen in patients with cancer (Table 17.3): (1) pain due to direct tumor infiltration, (2) pain associated with cancer chemotherapy, and (3) pain unrelated to either the cancer or the therapy. The incidence of pain as a specific symptom of tumor involvement may vary greatly, depending on the type of tumor or the location of its spread. Primary bone tumors have the highest incidence of pain (85 percent), with leukemia being associated with a relatively low incidence (5 percent).[10,11,12,13,14]

Accurate diagnosis of the etiology of the pain is quite important because in many instances, the pain may be able to be controlled by nonpharmacologic modalities (Table 17.4) or, if drug therapy is warranted, by medications other than analgesic drugs. Failure to adequately assess the cause as well as the severity of the pain will almost invariably lead to its undertreatment.

MANAGEMENT OF PAIN

The approach to relieving pain in persons with cancer should focus on relief without impairment in function without regard to whether dependence will develop (Table 17.5). Inherent in the successful relief of pain is an involvement not only of patients but their families as well encouraging active participation in their care. Persons should be able to speak freely of their pain without feeling self-conscious or "weak." The physician should be aware of the nature of the pain, the location, its intensity, and aggravating or mitigating factors. Specific goals should be developed in accordance with the person's needs.

Discomfort Due to Chemotherapy

Pain or abdominal discomfort associated with nausea and vomiting are frequent concomitant syndromes of chemotherapy. The use of standard antiemetic agents provide variable relief (Table 17.6). Recently attention has been

TABLE 17.3. Classification of Pain in Cancer Patients

Associated with direct tumor infiltration
  Bone invasion
  Nerve or spinal cord compression
  Distension of the organs
  Blood vessel invasion or occlusion
Associated with cancer therapy
  Postsurgical
    Postmastectomy
    Postradical neck dissection
    Postnephrectomy
    Postthoracotomy pain
    Postlimb amputation
  Post chemotherapy
    Peripheral neuropathy
    Aseptic necrosis
    Steroid pseudorheumatism
    Postherpetic neuralgia
    Mucositis
  Postradiation syndromes
    Fibrosis of the brachial and lumbar plexus
    Myelopathy
    Radiation-induced second primary tumors
    Postherpetic neuralgia
Unassociated with cancer or cancer therapy
  Degenerative bone disorders
  Diabetic neuropathy
  Vascular disease
  Coronary artery disease

focused on the use of tetrahydrocannabinol (THC) as both an analgesic and an antiemetic in patients undergoing chemotherapy (Chapter 12). Some double-blind studies have found the analgesic activity of THC to be comparable to codeine, but associated with adverse side effects including drowsiness, hypotension, bradycardia, and dysphasia.[15,16] Studies concerning the effectiveness of THC as an antiemetic are more encouraging.[17,18] Although further investigation is warranted, THC does appear to be an effective antiemetic in patients undergoing chemotherapy with refractory vomiting.

Although synthetic THC is available by prescription (dronabiuol-Mauriuol), unfortunately many persons report an antiemetic effect can be

TABLE 17.4. Nonpharmacologic Therapies for Cancer

ABLATIVE	STIMULATORY	MISCELLANEOUS
Radiation	Cutaneous stimulation with heat or cold	Hypnosis
Nerve blocks	Acupuncture	Relaxation Techniques
Chemical	Transcutaneous electrical stimulation (TENS)	Distraction and refraining
Surgical	Exercise	
Neurosurgery and Surgery		
Excision		
Debulking		

TABLE 17.5. Objectives of Analgesia in Persons with Cancer

Develop therapeutic plan based on an individual assessment.
Prevent appearance of pain rather than symptomatic relief when it occurs.
Prescribe an analgesic regimen that leaves person alert and able to function.
Strive for oral or transdermal administration whenever possible.
Do not be concerned with development of dependence.
Address tolerance appropriately by increasing dose needed to provide relief.

obtained only by smoking marijuana. For reasons that are less than clear, federal and state authorities still do not permit the use of marijuana for these people even under well-regulated settings. Fortunately, the newer synthetic agents such as ondansetron (Zofran) have been shown to be highly effective in preventive chemotherapy-induced nausea and vomiting. These drugs, however, are exceptionally expensive and if not covered by insurance policies cause a considerable drain on one's financial resources.

Use of Nonsteroidal Anti-Inflammatory Drugs (NSAIDs)

NSAIDs have been found useful in providing analgesia in mild to moderate pain in persons with cancer. At times, combining an NSAID with

TABLE 17.6. Drugs Used to Treat Chemotherapy-Induced Nausea and Vomiting

Generic	Trade	Route
Chlorpromazine	Various	IM, PO, R
Dronabinol	Marinol	PO
Diphenidol	Vontrol	PO
Ondansetron	Zofran	IV
Metoclopramide	Reglan, Clopra, Maxolon, Octamide Reclomide	IM, IV, PO
Perphenazine	Trilafon	IM, IV, PO, R
Prochlorperazine	Compazine	IM, IV, PO, R
Promethazine	Phenergan, Prorex 50, Pentazine, Anergan 50 K-Phen-50, V Gan	IM, PO, R
Triflupromazine	Vesprin	IM, IV
Trimethobenzamide	Tigan, Trimazide, Triban, T-Gen, Arrestin, Ticon, Tiject-20	IM, PO, R

an opioid can provide additional relief. Several studies have suggested a special role for NSAIDs in relieving metastatic bone pain; however, better clinical trials are needed.

Use of Opioids

Althouth the presence of mild pain in patients with cancer can often be handled effectively with aspirin or acetaminophen, pain not responsive to the nonnarcotic analgesics is best managed with opioids. The specific opioid agents and the principles governing their use have previously been discussed (Chapter 6, 7, 13, and 14). When used appropriately, satisfactory analgesia without excessive sedation should be able to be achieved in over 90 percent of persons with cancer pain. Unfortunately, narcotics are often inadequately prescribed in these patients due to fear of addiction. It cannot be overemphasized that dependence should not be a major concern in persons with cancer. The overwhelming majority of patients with cancer neither experience euphoria while taking narcotics nor become compulsive drug takers. If the cause of pain is eliminated, there is little difficulty in withdrawing the narcotic.

Whenever possible, long-acting noninjectable narcotics should be used. These include sustained-relief morphine preparations (MS Contin, Orasmorph SR) methadone, or transdermal fentanyl. When using long-acting morphine it should be remembered that its duration of action is a result of its coating. The drug cannot be crushed or chewed. Although each of these drugs in equivalent doses is equally effective, their cost is not. The monthly cost of a 10 mg dose of methadone taken three times a day approximates $7.50 as compared to $81.90 for a 30 mg dose of MS Contin taken every 12 hours.*

The use of heroin, a subject that engendered much controversy a number of years ago is really a nonissue. Within minutes after heroin enters the body, it is converted to monoacetyl morphine and then morphine. Existing available narcotics provide analgesia that are effective orally and able to be administered relatively infrequently.

The development of tolerance to a specific narcotic dose can become a real problem. Clinically, tolerance is manifested by a request on the part of the patient for an increasing frequency of medication. This, in turn, is all too often interpreted by physicians, and even family members, as a sign of impending "addiction." Rather than assessing the existing pharmacologic regimen, the patient's pain is minimized, the frequency of medication is actually decreased, or a sedative or tranquilizer is added. It cannot be emphasized too strongly that in treating cancer pain, the development of tolerance or physical dependence are not signs of addiction.

Although tolerance to the analgesic effect will occur, the rate at which tolerance develops exhibits considerable individual variability. For reasons that remain unclear, some patients can obtain satisfactory analgesia using their initial regime for many weeks whereas others may need to increase their dose more often. At times, increasing pain due to progression of the cancer may also be a factor. Each person must therefore be individually evaluated.

The primary method in prescribing narcotics remains the use of sufficient amounts at intervals frequent enough to provide satisfactory analgesia with minimal side effects regardless of the amount of narcotic needed. "Customary optimal" doses of narcotics may be insufficient in a person with cancer pain. Administration of the narcotic at regular intervals will

---

*1995 Drug Topics Red Book: Pharmacy's Fundamental Reference. Montvale, New Jersey Medical Economics 1995: 335.

not only have few or no adverse effects, but may also even diminish the development of tolerance. At a time when narcotics can no longer provide relief, injectable narcotics may be given.

Patient-controlled analgesia on an outpatient basis has been shown to be both safe and reliable.[19] Although many physicians become anxious about patient-controlled analgesia (PCA), in fact there is no reason why this cannot be accomplished in as satisfactory a manner as self-injection of insulin by a diabetic patient. Allowing the patient to self-medicate helps to restore the loss of control often experienced by patients with advanced cancer. Administration of narcotics by epidural or intrathecal routes has also been reported to be effective.[20-22] More recently, implantable constant-flow pumps have been developed; these are capable of providing a steady dose of narcotic sufficient to relieve pain without the side effects related to varying dose levels.

Unfortunately many physicians fearful of using opioids appropriately to relieve pain will often turn to drugs perceived as less potent whose effectiveness is often overshadowed by their side effects. The frequent use of meperidine (Demerol) in increasingly high doses rather than more potent long-acting agents can result in central nervous system toxicity due to accumulation of its toxic metabolite, normeperidine. The use of agonist-antagonists such as pentazocine, butorphanol, nalbuphine, or buprenorphine can precipitate withdrawal in persons currently taking opiates, cause undesirable mood-altering effects in high doses, and may be associated with an "analgesic ceiling." Tranquilizers such as the benzodiazepines, often prescribed rather than utilizing an appropriate dose of opioid, have no analgesic properties and are associated with excessive sedation. Cocaine used in "Brompton's Cocktail" has not been shown to have a specific analgesic effect and is now usually deleted from the Brompton's mixture.

Adjuvant Drug Therapy

There are a number of drugs that have been found to be helpful in relieving pain in persons with cancer, especially when neuropathic pain is present (Table 17.7). Anticonvulsants have been most effective in lancinating or burning nerve pain when chemotherapy or radiotherapy are not being administered. Antidepressants have been able to provide additional analgesia in nerve pain and may result in lowering the dose of narcotic needed. Local anesthesia may also be of value in relieving neuropathic pain. Corticosteroids have been of most value in diminishing inflammation in the absence of infection, and in reducing elevated pressure in the central nervous system. Anxiety may often be relieved by concomitant use of neuroleptics such as methotrimeprazine and hydroxyzine.

TABLE 17.7. Additional Nonpharmacologic Therapies for Cancer

Site	Ablative	Stimulatory	Miscellaneous
Peripheral nerve	Nerve blocks	Transcutaneous electrical stimulation	
Nerve root spinal cord	Rhizotomy, cordotomy commissurotomy, extralemniscal myelotomy	Dorsal column stimulation	
Brainstem	Tractotomy: mesencephalon, pons, medulla	Periventricular stimulation	
Thalamus	Thalamotomy	Thalamic stimulation	
Cortex	Cingulotomy, frontal lobotomy		
Endocrine	Hypophysectomy, adrenalectomy, oophorectomy, testicular removal		Acupuncture, hypnosis

Source: Adapted from Foley (Reference 10).

Invasive Ablative and Stimulatory Procedures

Nonpharmacologic modalities for relieving pain have been reviewed by Foley.[10] Surgical procedures, stimulatory techniques, and ablation of tissue by chemicals (Table 17.8) have been shown to be helpful in specific settings. Most recently the use of radionuclide therapy with strontium 89 and other "bone-seeking" radio nucleotides have been found to be quite effective, accompanied by acceptable levels of toxicity treatment of intractable bone pain.[23]

Psychologic Support

Behavioral techniques such as relaxation and imagery exercises may be quite helpful. Focusing attention on stimuli as a distraction from pain perception (cognition distraction and refraining) and replacing negative thoughts with positive ones may be of value. Support groups and individual

TABLE 17.8. Nonanalgesic Pharmacologic Therapies Used for Cancer

DRUG	INDICATIONS	DISADVANTAGES
Anticonvulsants Carbamazepine Phenytoin	Neuropathic pain	May cause sedation, drug toxicity, bone marrow suppression
Antidepressants Amitriptyline Imipramine, Trazodone	Neuropathic pain	May cause sedation, some with anticoholinergic side effects
Antihistamine Hydroxyzine	Enhance opioid analgesia	May cause sedation in high dose respiratory depression
Corticosteroids Dexamethasone Prednisone	Brain metastasis, spinal cord compression	Prolonged use associated with gastritis, fluid and electrolyte disturbance, adrenal suppression, susceptibility to infections, altered immunity

Modified from Clinical Practice Guidelines Management of Cancer Pain, U.S. Department of Health and Human Services, 1994, pp. 44, 66.

psychotherapy can often help the person with cancer openly express fears and concerns rather than dealing with them in isolation. All of these approaches must be explored.[24,25]

Depression is the most common psychological symptom associated with cancer. Surveys attempting to estimate the prevalence of depression in cancer patients have varied considerably, depending on the characteristics of the population studied, the type of cancer, the stage of disease, and the criteria utilized to diagnose depression. Unfortunately, the physician's response is often one of complacency. Concern expressed by the family is met with retorts such as "Wouldn't you be depressed if you had this disease?" This attitude is obviously less than helpful.

In addressing the depression accompanying cancer, it is important to be certain first that there is no underlying problem that can be readily alleviated. Frequently, alterations in the metabolic milieu, such as electrolyte disturbances, or hormonal imbalances associated with neoplastic syndromes, can appear as psychological disturbances. Cerebral metastases will obviously also affect noncognitive, as well as cognitive, functions. Side effects of chemotherapy may precipitate changes in mental status. For example, treatment with steroids has long been associated with psychological changes. All of these factors must be evaluated in assessing the psychological function of a person with cancer.

Relationships may deteriorate with family members often floundering as to the most appropriate way to act. Condescension or solicitousness on the part of family or friends serve only to increase a person's frustration, anger, and alienation. Physicians, due to unconscious personal discomfort regarding death and dying, all too frequently spend little time with the patient, preferring to order medications from a distance. As the pain becomes more severe, there is a tendency to "recognize" the inevitability of death and to "snow" the patient with large amounts of narcotics rather than to try to titrate the narcotic drug dose according to the patient's needs.

Most patients with cancer want to talk about their disease and can accept the thought of death providing they can be assured that they will not be in severe pain or discomfort. The presence of unrelieved pain exacerbates deepening depression and anger. Elimination of the pain is often, by itself, associated with a marked improvement in personality as well as in self-esteem and the ability to deal with the illness.

Hospice Care

In patients with terminal disease, the use of a hospice has been demonstrated to be exceedingly effective in providing not only emotional support but also in surrounding the patient with a milieu conducive to tranquility and relief from anxiety.[26,27,28] The hospice, originally a way station for pilgrims coming from their journey to the Holy Land, in contemporary times has been shown to be capable of providing excellent terminal care. In 1985 only 150,000 patients received hospice care. The numbers of persons taking advantage of these facilities have increased dramatically. In 1992 this number increased to 246,000, and in 1994 to 300,000.[27]

The primary goal of the hospice is to return to the patient a sense of community, of belonging, and of personal worth (Table 17.9). Most frequently, those entering the hospice are in considerable pain due to inadequate analgesia. In such cases, appropriate use of analgesics might have obviated the need for a hospice. Even with adequate pain relief, however, a point is reached when symptoms cannot be adequately controlled and family and physician are unable to cope. The hospice can then provide a comfortable and secure setting, allowing the patient's final days to be as peaceful as possible. In addition to providing for a person's material needs, family members are available to assist them in adjusting to the final moment when death occurs.

The hospice is most appropriate for those patients who have accepted the incurability of their disease. Care is directed to supportive treatment. Extensive laboratory testing and specific chemotherapy is usually not administered. Although the establishment of vigorous life-support measures is discouraged, medical services appropriate to palliative therapy are well utilized.

Home Care

Although ultimately the hospice may be the best way for many to manage terminal pain, there are many barriers that may prevent a person from accepting this program (Table 17.10). Since the hospice often repre-

TABLE 17.9. Goals of Hospice Care

Comfort in terminal disease
Interdisciplinary approach
Meticulous medical and nursing care
Psychological support for patient and family
Participation of patient in decision-making process
Excellent analgesia
Coordination of medical care provided at home to allow for smooth transition to hospice entry
Availability regardless of ability to pay
Appropriate counseling of family members

TABLE 17.10. Barriers to Hospice Care

Reluctance of physician to relinquish management of patient
Accepting failure of therapy for care or remission
Psychological setting of limits that person may survive
Ineligibility for insurance to pay costs
Desire to die at home

sents the last resort in the management of neoplastic disease and implies defeat on the part of the physician as well as the patient in controlling the disease process, an intermediate stage is often psychologically desirable. For many patients, home care can provide a viable alternative.[29] In order to effect the transition from hospital to the home, the physician must relieve the anxieties of the patient as well as the family concerning the nature of the disease process, the outcome, and the specific measures that can be undertaken to provide analgesia. If analgesia cannot be obtained with oral medication, instructions can be given to allow for effective parenteral administration by either the patient or a family member. Dying at home rather than in a hospice or hospital setting may also be desirable for many persons. This objective should be able to be accomplished compassionately without the experience of pain.

SUMMARY

The management of a person with cancer who is in pain can be accomplished without impairing either autonomy or dignity. The approach that is most effective may ultimately be interdisciplinary, addressing psychological, social, and cultural issues with the same attention as given to the medical requirements. Comfort by those who direct the comprehensive care will be accompanied by an equal degree of comfort and confidence in the patient. In the end, this is the ultimate objective.

REFERENCES

1. Centers for Disease Control and Prevention, Atlanta, GA. First 500,000 AIDS cases — United States 1995. *Morbidity and Mortality Weekly Report,* 1995, 44(45): 849–852.

2. Centers for Disease Control and Prevention, Atlanta, GA. Impact of the expanded AIDS surveillance case definition on AIDS case reporting — United States, First Quarter, 1993. *Morbidity and Mortality Weekly Report,* 1993, 42:308–310.

3. Rubin R. Acquired immune deficiency syndrome: Epidemiology. *Scientific America,* February, 1993, 269:1–24.

4. Update: Acquired immunodeficiency syndrome — United States, 1992. *Morbidity and Mortality Weekly Report,* 1993, 42:547–551.

5. Update: Mortality attributable to HIV infection among persons aged 25-44 United States, 1990 and 1991. *Morbidity and Mortality Weekly Report,* 1993, 42:869–872.

6. Anderson DW, Bedder MD. Orofacial pain in AIDS patients: In: Janisse T (ed.). *Pain management of AIDS patients.* Boston: Kluwer Academic Press, 1991:73–90.

7. Rauck RL. Chronic pain syndrome in AIDS patients. In: Janisse T (ed.). *Pain management of AIDS patients.* Boston: Kluwer Academic Publishers. 1991:91–113.

8. Schofferman J. Pain: Diagnosis and management in the palliative care of AIDS. *J Palliat Car,* 1988, 4: 46–49.

9. *Cancer pain: Report of the Expert Advisory Committee on the management of pain in cancer patients.* Canada: Minister of Supply and Services, 1984, 1992.

10. Foley KM. The management of pain of malignant origin. *Curr Neurol,* 1979, 2:279–302.

11. Lipman AG. Drug therapy in terminally ill patients. *Am J Hosp Pharm,* 1975, 32:270–276.

12. Cleeland CS, Gonin R, Hatfield AK, Edmonson JH, Blum RH, Stewart JA, Pandya KJ. Pain and its treatment in outpatients with metastatic cancer. *N Engl J Med,* 1994, 330:592–596.

13. Twycross RG. Clinical experience with diamorphine in advanced malignant disease. *Int J Clin Pharmacol,* 1974, 7:184–198.

14. Ackerman LV, del Regato JA (eds). *Cancer: Diagnosis, treatment, and prognosis.* 4th ed. St. Louis: Mosby, 1970.

15. Noyes R, Jr, Brunk SF, Avery DH, Canter A. The analgesic properties of delta-9-tetrahydrocannabinol and codeine. *Clin Pharmaco Ther,* 1975, 18:84–89.

16. Noyes R, Jr, Brunk SF, Avery DH, Canter A. Psychologic effects of oral delta-9-tetrahydrocannabinol in advanced cancer patients. *Compr Psychiatry,* 1976, 17:641–646.

17. Moertel CG, Reitemeier RJ. Controlled clinical studies of orally administered antiemetic drugs. *Gastroenterol,* 1969, 57:262–268.

18. Sallan SE, Zinberg NE, Frei E III. Antiemetic effect of delta-9-tetrahydrocannabinol in patients receiving cancer chemotherapy. *N Engl J Med,* 1975, 293:795–797.

19. Kerr IG, Sone M, Deangelis C, Iscoe N, MacKenzie R, Schueller T. Continuous narcotic infusion with patient controlled analgesia for chronic cancer pain in outpatients. *Ann Intern Med,* 1988, 108:554–557.

20. Driessen JJ, de Mulder PH, Claessen JJ, Van Diejen D, Wobbes T. Epidural administration of morphine for control of cancer pain long term efficacy and complications. *Clin J Pain,* 1989, 5:217–222.

21. Follett KA, Hitchon PW, Piper J, Kumar V, Clamon G, Jones MP. Response of intractable pain to continuous intrathecal morphine: A retrospective study. *Pain,* 1992, 49:21–25.

22. Shir Y, Shapira SS, Shenkman Z, Kaufman B, Magora F. Continuous epidural methadone treatment for cancer pain. *Clin J Pain,* 1991, 7:339–341.

23. Robinson RG, Preston DF, Spicer JA, Baxter KG. Radionuclide therapy of intractable bone pain: Emphasis on strontium-89. *Seminars in Nuclear Medicine,* 1992, 22:28–32.

24. Chapman CR. Psychologic and behavioral aspects of pain. In: Bonica JJ, Ventafridda, V. (eds.). *Advances in pain research and therapy,* Vol. 2. New York: Raven Press, 1979, 45–58.

25. Pither CE, Nicholas MK. Psychological approaches in chronic pain management. *Brit Med Bull,* 1991, 47:743–761.

26. Potter JF. A challenge for the hospice movement. *N Engl J Med,* 1980, 302:53–55.

27. Skelly F. Hospice. *American Medical News,* March 28, 1994, 37:7–12.

28. Bulkin W, Lukashok H. Rx. for dying: The case for hospice. *New Engl J Med,* 1988, 318:376–378.

29. Rosenbaum EH, Rosenbaum IR. Principles of home care for the patient with advanced cancer. *JAMA,* 1980, 244:1484–1487.

Chapter 18

Persons Tolerant to
or Dependent upon Opioids
and Pain of Undocumented Etiology

INTRODUCTION

Although management of pain may often present a problem to the physician not thoroughly familiar with analgesic agents, the problem is most severe in persons who already have a tolerance to narcotics or who are truly dependent. This large heterogenous population can be classified into four major categories: (1) persons currently dependent on physician-prescribed narcotics secondary to an underlying medical disorder; (2) persons dependent on street narcotics without any underlying medical disorder preceding narcotic use, (3) persons currently dependent on methadone prescribed through a methadone maintenance program, and (4) persons with pain of undefined origin.

NARCOTIC DEPENDENCY ASSOCIATED
WITH UNDERLYING MEDICAL DISORDERS

Satisfactory analgesia in narcotic-dependent persons with underlying medical disorders, although not difficult to achieve, rarely occurs. Indeed, the existing narcotic dependency is frequently the result of a failure to achieve pain relief associated with a continuous administration of escalating doses of various narcotic drugs, as well as sedatives and tranquilizers. The painful medical conditions most frequently associated with narcotic dependency are: (1) blood dyscrasias such as hemophilia and sickle cell or sickle cell C disease, (2) chronic bowel diseases such as regional enteritis, (3) lower back or disc syndromes refractory to surgical manipulation, and (4) severe unremitting headaches regardless of etiology.

In many instances, when a physician sees such a patient for the first time, it is difficult if not impossible to determine if an organic basis for the pain is present, although the basic underlying disorder is not questioned. Some of these people may be taking narcotics for their mood-altering effects yet are sincere in their protestations of persistent pain. They are extremely knowledgeable about analgesic agents and quite definite about their ability to tolerate or obtain relief from specific drugs. They usually prefer and request the more potent oral short-acting narcotics or parenteral agents for relief. Frequently, there is a considerable concomitant use of hypnotics, sedatives, or tranquilizers.

General Therapeutic Approach

The first principle of management is to develop a positive physician-patient relationship. This is not easy as these people have seen many physicians and are often extremely suspicious of and hostile to suggestions to change their existing therapeutic regimen. Often their past encounters with physicians and the health care system have been far from optimal. It is, therefore, extremely important for the physician to be nonjudgmental and to seriously consider whether any further medical studies are needed to obtain an accurate diagnosis. If an acute reason for the pain is present, relief should be promptly provided. Unfortunately, rarely is a diagnosis readily available.

Second, a determination should be made as to whether the patient is receiving adequate psychological support. This is quite important in allowing one to openly express concerns over the underlying disease process and may result in a decreased need for analgesics (Chapters 4, 13, and 14).

Third, an assessment should be made to determine whether everything possible is being done to prevent an exacerbation of the pain or to provide relief with available appropriate nonpharmacologic modalities. Attention to these details can be of great value in treatment of extremely common disorders that may progress to chronic disability if untreated. Even when a person presents with a considerable degree of dependence, institution of appropriate pharmacologic therapy may effectively relieve existing pain and allow a reduction in analgesic requirements.

In many instances of prolonged narcotic use, relief of the pain has become secondary to the reinforcing mood-altering effects of the drugs. In such cases, it is important for the physician to explain the risks of continued narcotic use and to explain the appropriateness of either switching from parenteral to oral use, or changing from a short-acting to a long-acting analgesic.

Hematologic Disorders

Sickle Cell Disease

Sickle cell disease is not a rare occurrence among the African-American community, as the gene for this disorder is carried by 8 percent. Painful crises are seen not only in sickle cell anemia but also occur in patients with combined traits such as sickle beta thalassemia and hemoglobin SC disease. Approximately 20 percent of persons with sickle cell disease experience severe pain with only 30 percent rarely having pain.[1] Unfortunately, when a painful crisis occurs, interactions with physicians or other health care providers are often far from satisfactory. There are several reasons for this. First, although the pain in sickle cell crisis can be quite intense, few — if any — objective findings may be seen. This unfortunately can result in the belief that the patient's expression of pain is out of proportion to that experienced, resulting in a hesitancy to prescribe adequate doses of analgesics. In fact, the frequency of painful crises in sickle cell disease is a measure of clinical severity and correlates well with early death. Complaints of pain should always be taken seriously, regardless of the physical findings.[2]

Second, very often the physician does not realize that a person with sickle cell disease, in an attempt to control the minor pains that are experienced, may have a tolerance threshold to narcotic analgesics and therefore will need a greater analgesic dose than ordinarily prescribed.

Third, since the analgesic prescription is often written PRN with the frequency of administration often beyond that appropriate for the drug's pharmacokinetics, excessive time occurs between injections. This results in a recurrence of pain, increasing anxiety and ultimately, a need to prescribe a larger dose of narcotic in order to achieve the same effect. All of this is quite unnecessary. Providing pain relief to persons with sickle cell crisis is not at all difficult if one follows several basic rules.

Despite the lack of objective findings, a person in sickle cell crisis has severe pain that should be addressed as promptly as possible. Since the pain will persist for at least 48 to 72 hours, writing analgesic orders on an "as needed" basis (PRN), serves no purpose other than to increase anxiety, discomfort, and ill feeling toward the physician and staff. Analgesics should be administered "around the clock" at a frequency consistent with their duration of action. Finally, one must determine if the person has been taking narcotic analgesics at home in an attempt to relieve the pain. If so, tolerance exists, and an increased dose of narcotic must be prescribed. Adjunctive measures such as hydration and treatment of any existing infection are also mandatory.

Any of the available narcotics may be used to treat sickle cell crisis. However, for reasons less than clear, most physicians select meperidine (Demerol), usually at a dose that is too low and administered too infrequently to provide effective analgesia. Meperidine can relieve pain provided it is given in appropriate dosage at no longer than three-hour intervals. However, in persons with a high tolerance threshold to narcotics, increased doses must be given. In the presence of compromised renal function, which frequently occurs in sickle cell disease, one must be quite cognizant of the possibility of normeperidine accumulating with resultant seizure activity (Table 18.1).[3] Morphine should remain the drug of choice although other narcotic analgesics, including the mixed agonist-antagonists, have also been effective.

Recently, several studies have evaluated the use of patient-controlled analgesia (PCA) with morphine in persons with sickle cell crisis. By using PCA, a person is able to obtain relief whenever the pain starts to increase. Studies have demonstrated that PCA is not only a safe and effective means of providing analgesia in adults, but also is quite helpful in treating children.[4] In addition, when compared to the standard use of narcotics on a PRN basis, PCA provides a much more rapid relief of pain.

When the pain has been resolved, the narcotic analgesic should be slowly tapered at a rate of 20 percent every 12 hours if only several days of

TABLE 18.1. Reasons for Meperidine Toxicity Appearing in Persons with Sickle Cell Disease

Increased amounts of meperidine needed due to tolerance to narcotics
Presence of renal dysfunction can result in decreasing excretion and accumulation of normeperidine
Alkaline urine may exist diminishing normeperidine excretion
Concomitant injection of phenobarbital or hepatic enzyme-inducing drugs that enhance meperidine metabolism
Coadministering phenothiazine (Phenergan) to enhance analgesia may also lower seizure threshold
Existence of previous seizure history

Adapted from Reference 3.

treatment were required. However, if longer periods of analgesia existed, then the taper should be more gradual, based on individual needs.

In prescribing analgesics for home use, when patients with sickle cell disease start to have pain, a long-acting rather than a short-acting narcotic is much more effective. Oral controlled-release morphine in one study decreased admissions for sickle cell pain by 44 percent and emergency room visits by 67 percent.[5] Recognition that sickle cell patients may have an intermittent chronic pain syndrome can allow for more effective analgesia, as well as a strengthening of the doctor-patient relationship.

Finally, the psychosocial aspects of the disease should be addressed. Children should be taught ways to cope with their pain, as well as control it through methods other than taking analgesics. However, when these methods do not control the pain, analgesia should be used promptly rather than letting the intensity of the pain increase until it can be managed only by hospital admission.

Hemophilia

Hemophilia is the second hematologic condition often associated with painful crisis. Unlike sickle cell disease, the acute pain experienced in hemophilia is virtually always secondary to an episode of unexpected bleeding. Although the spontaneous bleeding may occur anywhere, most often pain is associated with bleeding in the body joints. Initially the bleeding may not be visible; however, the pain may be severe. Since the immediate goal of treatment is to provide the appropriate missing coagulation factor as quickly as possible, physical evidence of a large bleed may not be present. In other instances, signs of joint bleeding, such as swelling and increased skin temperature, may be obvious. In either instance, a person with hemophilia complaining of pain should be believed and treated with analgesics. However, the route of administration should never be intramuscular.

Chronic pain most often localized to the joints as a result of deformities due to multiple episodes of bleeding are also not uncommon in hemophilia. In such instances, the person may be on a maintenance regimen of analgesics and may have a considerable tolerance level. When a recurrent or an acute exacerbation of pain is experienced, this tolerance must be taken into account when assessing the dose of narcotics to be used. A narcotic agonist-antagonist should not be prescribed if maintenance therapy had consisted of a narcotic analgesic until several days have passed since the last narcotic dose.

Finally, as a result of multiple transfusions of blood or coagulation factors, a number of persons with hemophilia have become HIV-positive and have developed clinical AIDS. Pain management in these individuals should be no different than in others with AIDS. The primary goal is compassionate relief of pain and discomfort.

Gastrointestinal Disorders

There are a variety of gastrointestinal disturbances that may be associated with acute or chronic painful episodes (Table 18.2). As with other medical conditions, treatment with diet and medications that address the underlying medical condition is primary. The pain may be often relieved without the need of analgesics.

Regional Ileitis and Ulcerative Colitis

Persons with chronic bowel disease, however, often have recurrent abdominal pain despite appropriate medical or surgical therapy. In fact, often surgical therapy, even when indicated can, at times, result in complications causing additional pain and discomfort. Individuals who have

TABLE 18.2. Gastrointestinal Disorder Associated with Chronic or Intermittent Pain

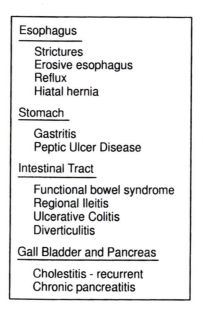

Esophagus

    Strictures
    Erosive esophagus
    Reflux
    Hiatal hernia

Stomach

    Gastritis
    Peptic Ulcer Disease

Intestinal Tract

    Functional bowel syndrome
    Regional Ileitis
    Ulcerative Colitis
    Diverticulitis

Gall Bladder and Pancreas

    Cholestitis - recurrent
    Chronic pancreatitis

experienced severe ileitis and its attendant complications are often in chronic pain and have tried, usually unsuccessfully, a variety of narcotic analgesics. In order to enhance analgesia and diminish anxiety, which is often is seen by the physician as the primary problem, frequently one of the benzodiazepines or other sedatives may be taken concomitantly.

Although most mild abdominal pain can be treated satisfactorily with codeine preparations, panegyric, lomotil, or tincture of opium, those with severe disease present a therapeutic challenge. Consistent with the principles that should be followed in management of all persons with chronic pain, the physician should listen carefully to the therapeutic regimen found to be most effective. In some instances, especially when extensive surgery has been performed, absorption of oral analgesias is impaired; thus, many oral medications do not appear to provide effective relief. The existing level of tolerance may also be such that what appears to be excessive doses of narcotics are requested to relieve the pain. Once again, the approach should be nonjudgmental and consistent with the person's history and needs.

Long-acting oral narcotics for persistent severe pain are preferable if intestinal absorption is adequate. If not, then transdermal fentanyl may be helpful for severe unremitting pain. Postoperatively, patient-controlled analgesia can be most effective not only in relieving pain, but also in decreasing the inevitable anxiety associated with analgesics prescribed on an "as needed" basis. In persons who have had multiple surgical procedures, pain is rarely adequately controlled. PCA allows the opportunity to achieve a degree of autonomy which psychologically will also be extremely helpful. Finally, the debilitation that accompanies severe bowel disease is such that psychological support is often of considerable value. There is no reason why persons with chronic bowel disease cannot lead a comfortable productive life without the anxiety associated with chronic pain.

HEROIN ADDICTS

There are few who engender as much anger and hostility among physicians and other health care providers as alcoholics and heroin addicts. The diagnosis of either condition immediately serves to make the person's complaints and past medical history suspect. This is most unfortunate as not only do these feelings often interfere with appropriate care, but in addition, they are quickly detected by the patient, resulting in a vicious circle of mutual antagonism and hostility.

The three medical issues a physician confronts in treating a heroin addict are: (1) the current state of the addiction, (2) the etiology, and (3) the severity of the pain. Due to a feeling of distrust of the medical establishment, rarely, if ever, will an addict willingly give an accurate history of his or her narcotic habit. Fear of physician disbelief, accompanied by the frequent refusal by physicians to prescribe appropriate amounts of narcotics, result in a considerable upward distortion of narcotic needs. Even when the person is honest and the physician appropriately concerned, it is extremely difficult to quantitate the daily dose of narcotic required to prevent withdrawal due to the extreme variability in potency of street heroin.[6]

Preventing Withdrawal

In assessing the appropriate narcotic dose to be prescribed, it is best, therefore, to forget about the person's stated need and to begin therapy immediately with an oral narcotic agent. Methadone, with its long duration of action, is the drug of choice. Once the presence of active heroin addiction has been confirmed, 15 to 20 mg of oral methadone can be administered. The person should be observed over the next 4 to 12 hours to determine if objective symptoms of early withdrawal occur. If such symptoms appear, an additional 5 to 10 mg of methadone can be given orally every six hours as needed. Usually most heroin users will not require more than 20 to 40 mg of methadone daily, regardless of existing habit. After an adequate daily methadone dose has been ascertained, this may be given in a single administration. Detoxification can subsequently be accomplished by decreasing this dose by 10 to 20 percent every three days.

Diagnosis

The presence of pain in the heroin user requires a careful history and physical examination. Although heroin users are frequently at risk for superficial infections secondary to the injection of contaminated material under unsterile settings, heroin also serves as an analgesic as well as an euphoric so that medical attention for mild painful conditions is rarely sought. However, progression of infections with the formation of deep-seated abscesses or osteomyelitis is associated with considerable pain that is unable to be relieved adequately by street heroin.

Other ominous causes of pain may also exist.[7] Chest pain may result from septic pulmonary emboli, endocarditis, papillary muscle rupture, or, more rarely, coronary artery ischemia due to occlusion of the coronary arteries by vegetations. Arterial emboli may cause severe localized pain or abdominal crises if associated with splenic infarcts or occlusion of the abdominal vessels. The presence of a coexistent alcohol abuse may be associated with recurrent attacks of pancreatitis. Finally, any cause of pain unrelated to drugs may also be seen and must be addressed.

Providing Pain Relief

It is a common belief that addicts demand more analgesic medication than others due to their desire to remain high rather than having an increased tolerance accompanying habitual narcotic use. Although such motivation may, on an individual basis, play a role, it is more likely that the need for greater doses of analgesics is related to an actual decrease in pain tolerance and pain threshold. Pain perception studies in methadone-maintained and drug-free ex-addicts with matched nonaddict subjects found former heroin users to have a lower pain threshold but not a lower pain tolerance than nonaddicted subjects.[8,9,10]

Whether these observations have practical importance with respect to clinical management of pain remains to be determined. It is clear, however, that heroin addicts do feel pain and will require a somewhat higher dose of a narcotic analgesic, depending on the extent of their tolerance. Analgesia should be able to be provided without difficulty if the physician is able to overcome his or her own biases and the development of an adversarial relationship. Severe pain should be treated with parenteral narcotics when indicated, in a stepwise fashion, until pain is relieved without producing excess sedation. Due to the synergistic effects of narcotics with hypnotics and tranquilizers, combinations of these agents should not be used.

Once the underlying cause of the pain has been removed, the narcotic dosage may be rapidly decreased to a "maintenance" level, with subsequent detoxification as previously described. It is important to emphasize that giving inadequate amounts of narcotics to relieve pain will result in considerable anxiety. This, in turn, will necessitate an escalation in dose needed for analgesia. This will not only seriously interfere with the physician-patient relationship, but will also result in intermittent administration of excessive doses of narcotics.

Prior to detoxification, however, it is essential to assess the need and/or the wish of the person for therapy for the primary addiction. If therapy is to be provided, it should begin while the person is in the hospital. Appropriate social service evaluation should be made available. If it is felt that maintenance therapy is warranted, this can be started during the hospital stay to diminish the chances of a person injecting heroin when discharged.

PERSONS IN METHADONE MAINTENANCE

A considerable number of former heroin addicts function productively in methadone maintenance programs. It is estimated that 114,000 persons are currently in treatment in methadone programs across the country with approximately 40,000 residing in New York State. It is therefore quite important for physicians and other health care providers to be knowledgeable about the management of pain in this population.

Persons on chronic methadone maintenance do not have an impaired perception to pain as compared to either drug-free ex-addicts or nonaddicts. Despite the daily ingestion of a medication that would certainly be analgesic in nontolerant subjects, several investigations have shown that persons on methadone maintenance, similar to drug-free ex-addicts, have a significantly lower pain threshold when compared to nonaddicted subjects.[7,10] Development of pain in the methadone-maintained patient will, therefore, occur in a manner similar to that seen in those not on narcotics and must be managed accordingly.

Providing Pain Relief

Methadone is a potent analgesic in the nontolerant individual. When a person on chronic maintenance therapy is in pain, certain principles should be followed when pain appears. First, the use of a nonnarcotic analgesic such as acetaminophen, aspirin, or NSAID may be quite helpful, especially in the presence of inflammation. The use of a narcotic analgesic with agonist-antagonist properties, such as pentazocine (Talwin) or any of the more recently developed analgesic antagonists (Chapter 7), will result in immediate withdrawal symptoms and is therefore contraindicated. The use of an oral mild narcotic analgesic will probably be ineffective due to the high degree of tolerance already present. This degree of tolerance is directly dependent on the maintenance dose of methadone. Considerably less tolerance exists with a daily maintenance dose of 20 mg compared to one of 40 or 100 mg.

If the pain is modest to severe, then parenteral narcotics may be used. It should be emphasized that although a patient on methadone maintenance will have a considerable tolerance threshold to narcotics, this tolerance is based on a single oral dose of methadone given every 24 hours. Parenteral administration of short-acting narcotic agents in doses equal to slightly greater than that usually prescribed is effective. However, if the pain persists, this dose should be increased. Adjunctive agents such as tranquilizers should be used cautiously, if at all, to avoid excessive sedation. As discussed earlier, both the tricyclic antidepressants and the benzodiazepines have been shown to potentiate the sedative and depressant effects of methadone.

If a person on methadone maintenance is admitted with pain and is unable to take anything by mouth, there are several ways of obtaining analgesia and preventing withdrawal.[11] The total daily dose of methadone may be divided in either half or in thirds and administered intramuscularly every 8 to 12 hours. Additional analgesia can be provided parenterally with a short-acting narcotic. When the pain has subsided, the short-acting narcotic is discontinued and the person is kept on the usual methadone maintenance dose.

A second method is to administer only a short-acting narcotic in dosage sufficient to both relieve pain and prevent withdrawal. This may require a greater narcotic dose than usually needed for analgesia. Since this technique will usually disturb the prior steady methadone level, it is infrequently used.

Theoretically it is also possible to administer only methadone parenterally in doses sufficient to overcome tolerance and to provide analgesia. Practically, this is usually not well tolerated, resulting in oversedation without adequate analgesia. It essential to remember that persons on methadone maintenance are dependent but not addicted. This distinction is not trivial. Failure to distinguish between those two conditions is often responsible for the inadequate care given, resulting in needless pain and anxiety (Chapter 3).

PAIN OF UNDOCUMENTED ETIOLOGY

The use of these regimens discussed above, with the provision of appropriate psychologic support, may allow a number of persons to considerably diminish their narcotics requirement without a recurrence of pain. This is an extremely time-consuming process and one that puts increasing demands on health care personnel. It must be said, however, that even under the best of circumstances, there are persons with underlying medical disorders without demonstrable cause of pain unable to accept either psychological intervention or dose reduction.

In this setting, the physician is confronted with a moral dilemma. There is no question that the patient has a medical condition that can be associated with pain, is currently complaining of pain in the absence of what is considered to be sufficient objective findings, and is clearly dependent on narcotic analgesics, using these drugs at a much greater than desirable frequency. The difficult decision that physicians address is whether they should (1) continue to prescribe the narcotic as requested, (2) refuse to prescribe any drug whatsoever, or (3) establish reasonable limits beyond which additional medication will not be prescribed.

Unfortunately, the usual approach to this problem is to make an immediate referral to a consultant in the hope of obtaining additional evaluative studies to document a cause of the pain or, more likely, to place the burden of making such a decision on another's shoulder. Although this feeling is understandable, it is rarely helpful. Frequently, referral initiates a chain reaction, whereby the patient is directed from physician to physician in a never-ending attempt to find the specific cause of the pain or new, untried therapeutic maneuvers. This, in turn, creates anger and frustration on the part of the patient, interfering with the development of any physician-patient relationship. It is also accompanied by an increase in narcotic consumption in order to relieve anxiety. In the end, the person learns how to manipulate the system, receiving prescriptions for smaller quantities of narcotics from several physicians, who may feel that the problem is being adequately managed and are only too happy to provide these prescriptions rather than be confronted by the patient's anger and anxiety.

At times, a referral may be made to a pain clinic. These clinics can be extremely helpful in providing an overall assessment of the problem, as well as exploring the possibility of nonpharmacologic intervention in providing pain relief. Unfortunately, not only is there often a great deal of resistance on the part of the patient to enter this setting, but additionally, there are insufficient numbers of these clinics to accommodate those who might benefit from their services.

Most often the person will ultimately return to the referring physician with a feeling of being manipulated, a great degree of hostility, and, unfortunately, the presence of unremitting pain. It is at this point that a final decision must be made as to the best way of addressing the problem. It has been my personal experience that in such situations, the most reasonable approach is for the physician to set boundaries with respect to the development of a reasonable analgesic regime, discussing the matter fully in a nonconfronting manner. A clear message is given that while everything possible will be done to provide relief from pain and additional support, the physician cannot merely function as a supplier of drugs.

REFERENCES

1. Shapiro BS. The management of pain in sickle cell disease. *Pediatric Clin of North Am,* 1989, 36:1029–1045.

2. Platt OS, Thorington BD, DJ, Milner PF, Rosse WF, Vichinsky E, Kinney TR. Pain in sickle cell disease: Rates and risk factors. *New Engl J Med,* 1991, 325:11–16.

3. Payne R. Pain management in sickle cell disease. Rationale and techniques. *Annals of the NY Acad of Sci,* 1989, 565:189–206.

4. Holbrook CT. Patient-controlled analgesia pain management for children with sickle cell disease. *J Assoc Acad Minor Phys,* 1990, 1:93–96.

5. Gonzalez ER, Bahal N, Hansen LA, Ware D, Bull DS, Ornato JP, Lehman ME. Intermittent infection vs. patient controlled analgesia for sickle cell crisis pain: Comparison of pain in the emergency department. *Arch Intern Med,* 1991, 151:1373–1378.

6. Halpern M. Analysis of drug samples seized by New York police shows much adulteration. *National Association for Prevention of Addiction to Narcotics, Newsletter,* 1964, 2:2.

7. Stimmel B. Medical complications. In: Stimmel B (ed.). *Heroin dependency: Medical, economic, and social aspects.* New York: Stratton Intercontinental Medical Book Corporation, 1975: 138–186.

8. Einstein S (ed.). Methadone maintenance. New York: Marcel Dekker, 1971.

9. Martin JE, Inglis J. Pain tolerance and narcotic addiction. *Br J Soc Clin Psychol,* 1965, 4:224–229.

10. Ho A, Dole VP. Pain perception in drug-free and in methadone-maintained human ex-addicts. *Proc Soc Exp Biol Med,* 1979, 162:392–395.

11. Regarding methadone treatment: A review. *COMPA,* 1995, New York, NY.

Index

Page numbers followed by the letter "t" indicate tables; those followed by the letter "i" indicate illustrations (figures).